a medicine of the future...
beyond mechanics to the domain of mind and spirit

"Dr. Richard Gerber has brought together an extensive compilation of information on human energy systems that serves to make clear the significant bioenergetic principles emerging in our time for the development of a new 'Einsteinian Medicine.' I would recommend it equally for the researcher's reference, the layperson in search for the meaningful, or for the student looking for hints to the changing paradigms of the near future."

Dolores Krieger, R.N., Ph.D.
professor of nursing, New York University; author of Therapeutic Touch

"Anyone who is aware of the recent trends in medicine will realize that modern physicians—like the physicists before them—have begun to deal with finer and finer forms of energy both in the diagnosis and treatment of human illness. This trend can only continue. It is sure to bring with it the recognition of increasingly subtle expressions of our minds and bodies, which will require correspondingly subtler approaches in therapy. One does not kill flies with shotguns nor manipulate electrons with hammers; and neither will many human maladies be 'fixable' with our current shotguns and hammers, our drugs and surgical procedures. Dr. Richard Gerber has provided a valuable step in thinking about the higher reaches of human beings—that rarefied domain where consciousness and body come together, where mind and matter meld. He points to a medicine of the future and describes a rationale for its existence. But he does not ask us to wallow in wild mysticism and forsake the therapies which have served us well. Rather, he asks us to complete the picture of mankind, whose luminous expressions are hardly hinted at in the mechanical ways in which we have for too long described ourselves. He wisely describes the inner game of healing, in which no healer can be effective who has not attained to higher knowledge. He takes us beyond mechanics to the domain of mind and spirit, and shows how these issues will become crucial factors in the medicine of the future."

Larry Dossey, M.D.
author, Space, Time and Medicine

"[Dr. Gerber has] been quite bold in writing about a broad range of healing arts and sciences—and equally bold in the esoteric depth in which [he has] discussed them. This is the only book which seeks to explain all major forms of energy (vibrational) healing and their relationships in such detail. I am delighted that [he has] chosen to write comprehensively on topics which deserve this lucid and thorough discussion. I know [he is] risking the scorn of the establishment when [he] emphasizes the esoteric, the subtle, and the nontraditional, but a book like this is long overdue. Bravo! [Dr. Gerber has] written a book which should be read by all people in the healing professions."

Robert Leichtman, M.D.
author, Returns *series*

"What a masterpiece! For the first time we have a scientific review of energy healing with a powerful overview of the whole subject. This book also presents a reasonable theory backed by voluminous references and personal experiments. I predict it will be the standard reference for all researchers and teachers. My hat's off to you, Richard."

Dael Walker
director, Crystal Awareness Institute

"For thirty years now there has been a slow shift in paradigm of healing from the monotheism of scientific medicine toward a concept of holistic medicine and more recently one which has been called sometimes energy medicine. Dr. Gerber's use of the word vibrational falls into this category. This is a book for those at the interface. It covers extremely well the transition from science to metaphysics and will serve as a useful guide to those ready to begin the path toward energy consciousness. Unfortunately, the deeper search needed to establish 'the etheric world of energies' remains to be done and until it is completed satisfactorily, scientists and physicians steeped in the 'Newtonian model of reality' are unlikely to be ready to begin thinking along these lines. This is a good example for those individuals who are beginning to open their consciousness."

C. Norman Shealy, M.D., Ph.D.
founding president, American Holistic Medical Association

VIBRATIONAL MEDICINE

"The human body is made up of *electronic vibrations*, with each atom and element of the body, each organ and organism, having its electronic unit of vibration necessary for the sustenance of, and equilibrium in, that particular organism. Each unit, then, being a cell or a unit of life in itself has the capacity of reproducing itself by the first law as is known of reproduction-division. *When a force in any organ or element of the body becomes deficient in its ability to reproduce that equilibrium necessary for the sustenance of physical existence and its reproduction, that portion becomes deficient in electronic energy.* This may come by injury or by disease, received by external forces. It may come from internal forces through lack of eliminations produced in the system or by other agencies to meet its requirements in the body."

—Edgar Cayce (1928)
from *There Is A River* by Thomas Sugrue
(italics added)

VIBRATIONAL MEDICINE

Richard Gerber, M.D.

NEW CHOICES
FOR HEALING OURSELVES

BEAR & COMPANY
SANTA FE, NEW MEXICO

Library of Congress Cataloging-in-Publication Data

Gerber, Richard, 1955-

    Vibrational medicine: new choices for healing ourselves/by
Richard Gerber; introduction by Gabriel Cousens; foreword by
William A. Tiller.

        p.   cm.
    Bibliography: p.
    Includes index.
    ISBN 0-939680-48-3   ISBN 0-939680-46-7 (pbk.)

    1. Mental healing.   2. Vital force—Therapeutic use.
3. Alternative medicine. I. Title.
RZ401.G35   1988
615.5—dc19   88-3515
                                            CIP

Available in both paperback (ISBN 0-939680-46-7) and hardcover
(ISBN 0-939680-48-3) editions.

Bear & Company
Santa Fe, NM 87504-2860

Cover photo by Richard Gerber is an electrophotograph of a small
serapegia leaf.

Cover & interior design by Angela C. Werneke

Typography by Copygraphics, Santa Fe

Printed in the United States of America by R.R. Donnelley

9 8 7 6 5 4 3 2 1

*This book is dedicated
to the vast spiritual Hierarchy
which silently works to uplift
the human condition.*

SPECIAL NOTICE TO
THE READER

Although this book was written by a physician and discusses various methods of healing, it is not meant to give specific recommendations of advice for the treatment of particular illnesses. This book is an examination of the mechanisms of a variety of alternative therapies that may hold promise as adjunctive treatments to conventional medical approaches. The book is not intended to be a replacement for good medical diagnosis and treatment. Therefore, before attempting to use any of the mentioned therapies within this book, it is suggested that the reader seek the expertise of a trained physician or enlightened health-care practitioner for diagnosis, treatment, and guidance in the selection of particular therapeutic modalities.

Richard Gerber, M.D.

PERMISSIONS

Special thanks to Gurudas for permission to quote extensively from *Flower Essences and Vibrational Healing,* copyright © 1983 by Gurudas, published by Brotherhood of Life, Inc., Albuquerque, New Mexico. Thanks also to Dr. Robert Leichtman for permission to quote material from *Nikola Tesla Returns,* copyright © 1980 by Ariel Press, and *Einstein Returns,* copyright © 1982 by Light, published by Ariel Press, Columbus, Ohio. Sections from *The Keys of Enoch,* copyright © 1977 by J. J. Hurtak, reprinted by permission of the author, James J. Hurtak, published by The Academy for Future Science, Los Gatos, California. Quotes from *Esoteric Healing* by Alice A. Bailey, copyright © 1953 by Lucis Trust, published by Lucis Press, Ltd., appear by permission of Perry Coles and the Lucis Trust. Special thanks to John Ramsell and The Dr. Edward Bach Healing Centre for permission to quote material by Dr. Edward Bach, appearing in *Heal Thyself,* copyright © 1931 by The Dr. Edward Bach Healing Centre, reprinted by Keats Publishing Co, New Canaan, Connecticut. Thanks also to Mirtala Bentov for permission to use material from her late husband Itzhak Bentov's book, *Stalking the Wild Pendulum,* copyright © 1977 by Itzhak Bentov, published by E. P. Dutton, New York. A special thank-you to Wally Richardson for permission to quote extensively from *The Spiritual Value of Gem Stones,* copyright © 1980 by Wallace G. Richardson, published by DeVorss and Company, California. Thanks also to DeVorss and Company for permission to quote from *Through the Curtain* by Shafica Karagulla and Viola Petit Neal, copyright © 1983 by Shafica Karagulla, M.D. The Illness/Wellness Continuum from *Wellness Workbook* by John W. Travis and Sarah Ryan, copyright © 1972, 1981 by John W. Travis, M.D., published by Ten Speed Press, 1981, was adapted by permission of the authors. Special thanks also to Dr. William Tiller for permission to reprint graphs and materials quoted.

CONTENTS

LIST OF DIAGRAMS

ACKNOWLEDGMENTS

This book is a culmination of more than twelve years of reading, study, research, and inner search. Although there are many scientists, psychics, and scholars who are mentioned throughout the book, there have been a few who have had a profound influence on my thinking. From these special individuals and their writings I have drawn much inspiration and insight, which has served to stimulate my own creative thinking and model building. They stretched my thinking to such a degree that they irreversably changed my perception of myself, of humanity as a whole, and of the universe. The vast physical realm is but a small part of an even greater and more wondrous multidimensional reality, of which we, as human beings, have infinitely more control than is immediately apparent. By helping myself and others to begin to appreciate the limitless boundaries of human potential (especially with regard to the realms of healing), these special individuals have helped to pave the way before me.

For their pioneering efforts and inspiring words, I wish to thank the following individuals: Marilyn Ferguson, Robert Monroe, Carl Simonton, Anne and Herbert Puryear, Judith Skutch-Whitson and William Whitson, Abram Ber, Robert Leichtman, Dolores Krieger, Brugh Joy, Bernard Grad, Alice Bailey, Jane Roberts and Seth, Hilarion, Itzhak Bentov, Russell Targ and Harold Puthoff, Stanley Krippner, Shafica Karagulla, Viola Petit Neal, Ken Pelletier, Meredith Lady Young, Albert Einstein, William Tiller, Nikola Tesla, Edgar Cayce, Edward Bach, Kevin Ryerson, Gurudas, Gabriel Cousens, Geoffrey Hodson, Charles Leadbeater, Rudolph Steiner, Thelma Moss, David Bohm, Dael Walker, Charles Tart, David Tansley, Harry Oldfield, Elmer and Alyce Green, Marcel Vogel, James Hurtak, Semyon and Valentina Kirlian, Ion Dumitrescu, Victor Inyushin, Lou Golden, and John Fetzer. Through their writings, actions, or creative assistance, these people are, in part, responsible for the writing of this book.

In a metaphorical sense, the writing and production of this book has been somewhat like a birth. My publishers at Bear and Company, Barbara and Gerry Clow, and their excellent editorial and artistic staff—managing editor Gail Vivino and designer Angela Werneke, have been like spiritual midwives in helping to deliver this child through its long gestation and birth process. I would like to thank them for their assistance, creative insight, and their willingness to work with my own inner vision of how this book should be. I would especially like to thank my wife, Lyn, for her many hours of editing and rewriting many portions of the book with me, without whose assistance and patience this book would not have manifested in such a readable and flowing format.

I would like to express special thanks to Dr. William Tiller and Dr. Gabriel Cousens for taking time out of their busy schedules to write the foreword and introduction to this book. Their input in the final stages of writing was especially helpful.

I also wish to acknowledge Steven P. Jobs and his original Mac development team at Apple Computer, Inc. for their creative vision in producing the Macintosh computer. Without my Macintosh (with which this entire book was created) and its ability to synthesize ideas, pictures, and graphics so intuitively and easily, I would probably have never taken the time to put into writing a project of this scope and size.

FOREWORD
by William A. Tiller, Ph.D.

Until recently, science and traditional Western medicine have considered that living organisms operate largely by means of the following sequence of reactions:

Equation 1.

FUNCTION $\longleftrightarrow$ STRUCTURE $\longleftrightarrow$ CHEMISTRY

When an organism was not functioning properly, the cause has been ascribed to structural defects in the system arising out of chemical imbalances. It was recognized that chemical level homeostasis may have been dependent upon a connection with a deeper level energy structure in the organism, but no clear discrimination of this connection was made. More recently, a growing awareness has developed of the interactions between chemical states and electromagnetic fields. Studies in neuropsychiatry show us that small electric currents between specific brain points give rise to the same behavioral changes that are observed with certain specific brain-stimulating chemicals. Small direct current (D.C.) electric currents $(10^{-12}$ amp/mm^2 to 10^{-9} amp/mm^2) applied to leukocytes in vitro have been shown to produce cell regeneration, while larger current densities were shown to produce cell degeneration. Such studies have been extended to enhance fracture healing in animals and humans. Thus, although we do not yet understand the detailed pathways whereby electric and magnetic fields couple into the cellular metabolism, it is clear that Equation 1 should be replaced by:

Equation 2.

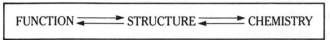

FUNCTION $\rightleftarrows$ STRUCTURE $\rightleftarrows$ CHEMISTRY $\rightleftarrows$ ELECTROMAGNETIC ENERGY FIELDS

An illustration of Equation 2 is Wolf's law of bone structure changes, which states that if one bone receives a non-uniform stress for an extended period of time, that bone will grow new trabeculae in the exact locations needed to maximally support this new stress distribution. The physical

strain field is manifested in fibers and collagen which are both piezoelectric, so that an electrostatic field is produced with specific orientation and
polarity. This electrostatic field, with its associated microcurrents, causes
ion and colloid redistribution in the local body fluids to specific locations
where agglomeration and gelation set in. These new semisolid structures
age and calcify, eventually forming the microstructures making up trabeculae. One can readily imagine the more subtle stresses of an emotional or
mental nature setting the foregoing chain of sequences in motion.

Equation 2 has an obvious defect in that it overlooks mental effects.
Under hypnosis, the human body has exhibited truly remarkable feats of
strength and endurance attesting to an unconscious mind/structure link.
In aikido, Zen, and yoga disciplines, we see a conscious link between the
mind and both structure and function. Recent studies in the area of biofeedback techniques show that directed mind cannot only control various
autonomic body functions such as skin temperature and pain, but can also
repair the body. Finally, on another front, modern psychotherapy has
shown that certain chemical treatments influence mental states, and that
certain mental treatments influence chemical states. The point is that
"mental fields" are additional contributions that should be placed on the
right side of the reaction chain given in Equation 2. Other fields, not yet
clearly discriminated, also appear to play a part in this reaction chain. Let
us label them all under the heading "subtle energy fields" and rewrite
Equation 2 as:

Equation 3.

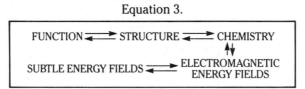

Equation 3 is a reasonable representation for a living organism, a cell,
or a membrane. Each item in the reaction chain maintains its conditions
of homeostasis via immediate support from the item on its right. The development of serious imbalance in any particular item in the chain leads,
in time, to obvious disruption of homeostasis for the item to the left. Thus,
to develop an early warning system concerning the chemical homeostasis
of a biological system, a device must be created that monitors the electrical
nature of the biological system. In order to gain information concerning
future disruptions of of the bioelectric system, the subtle energy fields of

the entire biological entity must be monitored. At the moment, there is very little knowledge concerning the nature and character of those subtle energy fields, therefore electrical system monitoring must be used as a basis for early warning. This is a happy circumstance because our technical competence has grown significantly in this area over the past few decades.

A number of electrical devices are presently available for rapid diagnosis of the body's state of health and for the treatment of imbalances in that condition. Many holistic-health practitioners are beginning to utilize these devices, and it has become important to understand how they function on an electrical level and what they actually measure in the human body. Using basic information on the electrical properties and response behavior of both macroscopic and microscopic (acupuncture points) areas of skin, it has been possible to account for all the key characteristics of the three major diagnostic instruments on the market. One of these instruments, the Voll Dermatron, is also utilized in the selection of homeopathic remedies for the patient. It thus forms a narrow bridge across the chasm between the domains of electromagnetic energy and subtle energy shown in Equation 3. In order to strengthen that bridge and to eventually give it quantitative underpinnings, we need to gain a clearer understanding of the basic nature of homeopathy and how it relates to traditional Western medicine.

One might say that it was the emphasis on disease rather than on health that split apart allopathic and homeopathic practice. The physical body reveals the obvious materialization of disease; the relationship to the more subtle aspects that relate to health is not so easily measured. Conventional allopathic medicine deals directly with the chemical and structural components of the physical body. It can be classed as a truly objective medicine because it deals with nature on a purely four-dimensional space/time level, and thus has developed much direct laboratory evidence to support its physiochemical hypotheses. This has occurred because the reliable sensing ability of both humans and instrumentation presently operates on that level.

Homeopathic medicine, on the other hand, deals indirectly with the chemistry and structure of the physical body by dealing directly with substance and energies at the next, and more subtle, level. It must be classed as a subjective medicine at this time for the following reasons: 1) It deals with energy that can be strongly perturbed by the mental and emotional activity of individuals, and 2) there has not been any diagnostic equipment available to support the homeopathic physician's hypothesis.

Both theoretical structure and an experimental laboratory for studying subtle energies are essential ingredients for the generation of a correct scientific foundation for homeopathy. A postulation concerning the former allows a testing via the latter, so that a bootstrap process can be invoked to inch our way towards the desired goal. Because of this, Equation 3 must be altered to the following form:

Equation 4.

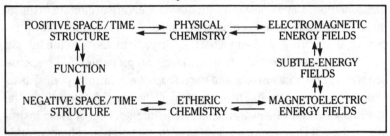

Allopathic medicine follows the upper path between the subtle energy fields and the functioning state of the human, while homeopathic medicine follows the lower path between these two domains. In essence, discriminating between the subtle energies of Equation 3 leads to the series-parallel circuit of Equation 4, wherein two different levels of chemistry and energy operate in two different space/time frames.

This book by Richard Gerber, M.D., is an attempt to present a conceptual bridge between current allopathic medicine and future subtle-energy medicine. It is a broad-ranging book that tries to set a qualitative and somewhat speculative perspective. One does not need to agree with all the details given in this book to appreciate its overall synthesis. It is this overall synthesis of information, and this grand perspective, that Dr. Gerber hopes readers will take away with them.

I liked the book, have enjoyed reading it and think that it is a timely contribution. I do not agree with all of it but, in the main, it is consistent with my personal view of the bottom line, which is:

We are all elements of spirit, indestructible and eternal, and multiplexed in the divine. We contain a unique mechanism of perception which is mind. In my theoretical modeling, mind consists of three levels—the instinctive, the intellectual, and the spiritual—and mind is postulated to function in a six-dimensional space lattice.

This mind creates a vehicle for experience (a universe, a world, a body) and each person, as a spiritual being plus perception mechanism, invests in that vehicle which runs a continuously programmed course. The being is connected to the vehicle via the emotional circuitry. The stuff used for the construction of this vehicle or *simulator* is of dual or conjugate nature. One part, which is electrical in nature and travels at velocities less than that of electromagnetic light, is of positive energy and positive mass. It forms the *physical* part of the simulator. The other part, which is magnetic in nature and travels at velocities greater than that of electromagnetic light, is of negative mass and negative energy. It forms the *etheric* part of the simulator. The total sum of these two energies is zero, as is the sum of their entropies. Thus, the total simulator or vehicle is created out of what we call "empty space," the space of mind, via a fluctuation type of process. This vehicle world (simulator) is just the "world of appearances and form," the world of relative reality that we shape with our minds. Outside of that is the absolute! It is necessary to learn to penetrate the foibles of the "relative" in order to appreciate the "absolute." However, all who read this book are presently in the simulator and, when we talk about holistic health and a new medicine, it must be the medicine of that material, the simulator material. We know a great deal about one aspect of the simulator material (the physical) but very little about its conjugate part (the etheric). Now is the time to begin serious investigation of the etheric, and to develop an etheric material science to balance our present, physical, material science. This book is a significant contribution to the new awareness needed to support such a task.

PROFESSOR WILLIAM A. TILLER, PH.D.
DEPARTMENT OF MATERIAL SCIENCES AND ENGINEERING
STANFORD UNIVERSITY
JUNE 1987

INTRODUCTION
by Gabriel Cousens, M.D

Sir Arthur Edington once said, "Verily it is easier for a camel to pass through the eye of a needle than for a scientific man to pass through a door. And whether the door be barn door or church door, it might be wiser that he should consent to be an ordinary man and walk in rather than wait till all the difficulties involved in a really scientific ingress are resolved." In *Vibrational Medicine*, Dr. Richard Gerber not only helps us walk through the door to an understanding and acceptance of vibrational medicine, but he examines the doorway as well. This book is an encyclopedic and comprehensive coverage of vibrational medicine. The author creates a clear model of the human organism from the physical to the etheric. He then goes on to include the subtle energetic harmonics of the spiritual planes as well. In this book we begin to understand the human organism as a series of interacting multidimensional energy fields. By developing this model in scientific terms and backing it up with some of the recent exciting clinical and laboratory research, this book allows the reader to more fully appreciate the body/mind/spirit language that is developing in holistic health today. The reader should remember, however, that models are not necessarily real, but serve as conceptual tools to enhance a functional understanding. Even the idea of energy is a concept. If those within the mass consciousness of medicine were able to remember that the Newtonian mechanistic approach is also only a model based on two-hundred-year-old concepts, the transition to the Einsteinian quantum model would be taking place with much less resistance. It is unfortunate that mainstream medicine still acts as if it believes the Newtonian concepts—that have been proven to be an inaccurate model for the last 50 years—are real.

Dr. Gerber does a particularly excellent job of creating a working model of the physical-etheric interface. He nicely clarifies the relationship of acupuncture meridians, as detected by Dr. Motoyama's AMI device, and uses sophisticated Kirlian photography diagnosis to show how the etheric body forms a type of holographic magnetic grid which communicates with the electrically based matter and cells of the physical body. The meridian system is the key interfacing system between the etheric and the physical.

It is nicely pointed out that the interface is diagnostically important because disease states can be detected at the etheric level before they manifest on the physical plane. It therefore follows that if diseases can be detected at this etheric level, they can be prevented. Because Dr. Gerber explains in detail the scientific instumentation which is being developed and used to diagnose at the physical-etheric interface, it gives credibility to this physical-etheric interface that most skeptics would find hard to ignore.

The Tiller-Einstein model outlined in the book, which describes the etheric energies as negative space/time, faster-than-light magnetoelectric energies, gives an additional deeper and fresh insight into the physical-etheric interface, and into matter-energy relationships in general. It also helps us to understand the difficulty in measuring these etheric/magneto-electric energies, because they are not detected by the standard electromagnetic positive space/time instrumention. It is nice to read about the current research in these areas, in which these etheric/magnetoelectric energies are currently being measured by biological systems such as enzyme function, crystallization effects on water, and the shifting of the water hydrogen-oxygen bonding angles.

The book thoroughly, clearly, and gently opens the reader's mind to the conclusion that we, as human organisms, are a series of interacting multidimensional subtle-energy systems, and that if these energy systems become imbalanced there may be resulting pathological symptoms which manifest on the physical/emotional/mental/spiritual planes. It describes how these imbalances can be healed by rebalancing the subtle energy templates with the right frequency of vibrational medicine. This is the essence of the foundation of vibrational medicine. Dr. Gerber further correctly points out that when the human organism is weakened or not in balance, it oscillates at a different or less-harmonic frequency. This abnormal frequency reflects the general state of the cellular energetic balance. If a person is not able to rebalance or increase his or her energetic mode to a normal frequency, then either a general or a specifically tuned frequency input is needed. This is the role that vibrational medicine plays.

This book gives an excellent overview of the different vibrational medicine approaches. What is particularly enjoyable is the way Dr. Gerber relates them to his general model. It is a very helpful synopsis of vibrational medicine that can be understood both by the lay public and by health professionals who are interested in learning about vibrational medicine.

As we shift from the materialist, mechanistic, Newtonian worldview to the Einsteinian, quantum, mechanical holism, medicine and the people who practice it will also change. We will newly embrace the holistic view that has been with us for thousands of years. It is an understanding that not only does the healer see health from a holistic perspective as part of an overall relationship with the universe, but the healer lives as an example of such a whole and harmonious way. I saw this being actively practiced by some Ayurvedic physicians in India, and heard about it in Taoist healers, American Indian medicine men/women, and Hunza healers. In our Western culture it has been practiced for over two thousand years by the Essenes, who produced such healers as John the Baptist, John the Divine, and, of course, Jesus. This tradition reemerged around the 1400s from Constantine the African, who studied Essene texts in the Monte Cassino monastery and then taught them at the Salerno school of medicine in Italy. Today, as there have always been, there exist evolved healers who continue to carry on these harmonistic holistic healing traditions that Dr. Gerber romanticizes and hopes for. Their commitment to love and health can never be stopped by whatever medical system has political power. This book paves the way for greater support for these healers.

It is important to understand that the type of healing which these healers share comes from their own harmony and love. It is a holism that is not based on the latest far-out diagnostic tool, or on one or two progressive healing approaches, but from the perspective of being involved in every aspect of the healing. It is a simple and whole person multi-leveled energetic approach, rather than a series of fragmented alternative therapies to which the client is referred.

This book is part of a new and growing medical consensus that says, as Dr. Gerber writes, "A system of medicine which denies or ignores its existence (spirit) will be incomplete because it leaves out the most fundamental quality of human existence, the spiritual dimension." He points out, which is clarified in detail in my book, *Spiritual Nutrition and the Rainbow Diet*, that "the tissues which compose our physical form are fed not only by oxygen, glucose, and chemical nutrients, but also by higher vibrational energies which endow the physical form with the properties of life and creative expression." Health is a total balance of our subtle energetic systems with the forces of our physical vehicle and also with the forces of Mother Nature. Many healers feel that in a state of harmony in which we are absorbing many levels of energy, even the use of megavitamins, as suggested in this book, may act as stimulants which may actually bring the system into a state of imbalance.

Although vibrational medicine is a boon to the future of health for this country and the world, health ultimately does not depend on vibrational medicine or the physician/healer/priests, but on people learning to live in a whole, harmonic, and loving way in every aspect of their lives. As we learn to live whole lives in which there is a balance of love and harmony with all levels of self, creative work, family, society, and the ecology of the planet, there will be a constant rebalancing, healing, and regeneration of ourselves. We will have learned, as Dr. Gerber humorously puts it, about the "Owner's Consciousness Maintenance Manual." One of the most important aspects of this book is that it gives a new scientific paradigm which strongly supports what healers and educated people have known about health for thousands of years. It delivers the understanding in a scientific manner that allows us to make a graceful transition from the atomistic fragmented Newtonian understanding of health to the unbroken wholeness of the Einsteinian quantum mechanical worldview. For anyone who is interested in vibrational medicine and needs to examine the door before walking through, this book is an absolute must.

May we all know health, love, and harmony on every level of our being.

GABRIEL COUSENS, M.D.
OCTOBER 1987

Dr. Cousens is a holistic physician and author of
Spiritual Nutrition and the Rainbow Diet.

PREFACE

This book is an exploration into the various mechanisms of healing. It is an introduction to a new system of thinking about health and illness in general. This system of thought examines human functioning from the perspective of multiple interactive energy systems. It is an attempt to go beyond the current medical paradigm of illness in order to understand at a deeper level why our thoughts and emotions affect our physiology, and also to comprehend how therapies as simple as herbs, flowers, and water can be such powerful healers.

My approach to understanding this growing field known as "vibrational medicine" stems from eleven years of personal research in alternative methods of healing during my years of medical training and practice as an internist. I have attempted to build upon the foundations of accepted medical knowledge in order to bridge the gap between science and metaphysics.

From my earliest years in medical school I sensed that there were simpler, less invasive methods of healing illness than prescribing potent drugs with toxic side effects and performing surgery with its accompanying risks. Admittedly, drugs and surgery have brought help and healing to many thousands in need, and have succeeded in wiping out numerous epidemic diseases. Unfortunately, there are still many chronic illnesses for which current medical therapy offers only palliative treatment. My own practice in internal medicine is still dependent upon these therapeutic modalities. I would very much like to be able to do without surgical and medical tools but, at this time, they are still very important. For many years I have sought to discover diagnostic methods and therapeutic tools that would be less invasive, less costly, less toxic, and of greater healing benefit to patients. That was one of the underlying reasons behind my search to understand the true nature of healing. It is my conclusion that vibrational healing systems hold the key to extending our current medical knowledge toward an improved understanding, diagnosis, and treatment of human ailments.

Medical science has done much to investigate the mechanisms behind disease, but it has only recently begun to study the reasons that people stay healthy. Scientists have tended to focus upon the microscopic/micromolecular mechanisms behind disease causation, but have often lost sight of the bigger picture. Also, mainstream medicine suffers from an extreme narrow-mindedness in thinking because of its steadfast focus upon the Newtonian worldview of people as sophisticated biological machines. Vibrational healing philosophies have the unique perspective that human beings are more than flesh and blood, proteins, fats, and nucleic acids. The body would be but a pile of disordered chemicals were it not for the animating life-force that maintains and organizes our molecular substituents into living, breathing, thinking individuals. This life-force is part of the spirit that animates all living creatures. It is the so-called "ghost in the machine." It is a unique form of subtle energy that has yet to be fully grasped by the scientists of the twentieth century. This spiritual dimension is an aspect of human nature that is not taught in medical school nor well understood by most physicians. But the spiritual element is a part of human existence that must be taken into account if we are to truly understand the basic nature of health, illness, and personal growth.

One of the primary reasons that physicians have such a hard time in accepting the validity of alternative healing methods is that they see the physical body as the only dimension of human existence. Given that one must somehow influence physical/cellular systems with gross molecular methods such as drugs or surgery, it is little wonder that the therapeutic effectiveness of weak dilutions of substances, like those used in homeopathy, have been misunderstood and discredited by the orthodox medical structure. Homeopathy works at an energetic level which is not yet understood by most medical thinkers.

It is only recently that scientists have acknowledged that the mind can influence the biomolecular mechanisms that regulate the body. For many years doctors thought that consciousness was something the brain produced, similar to the gall bladder producing bile. Consciousness was considered merely a by-product of the central nervous system machinations. Neurophysiologists have long sought the area of the brain that is the center of free will and decision making. Although they may identify regions of grey matter that participate in the process of executing commands, researchers will look long and hard before they ever discover the real seat of consciousness in the brain.

The brain, albeit a complex biocomputer, still needs a programmer to instruct the nervous system how to perform and what acts to accomplish. That conscious entity which uses this biomechanism of the brain and body is the human spirit or soul. That which we refer to as the spiritual domain is part of a series of higher dimensional energy systems which feed directly into the computer hardware we call the brain and body. It is these higher dimensional systems, our so-called subtle energetic anatomy, that science has yet to recognize. Alternative systems of healing are often effective because they can correct abnormal patterns of function in the higher dimensional systems which control cellular physiology and behavioral patterns of expression.

The acupuncture meridians, the chakras and nadis, the etheric body, and other higher systems are parts of human multidimensional anatomy that have been described by ancient schools of healing throughout the world. Western science has long ignored descriptions of ethereal components of physiology because their existence could never be documented by anatomical dissection. After all, who had ever seen a so-called meridian under the microscope? Only now has Western technology evolved to the point that we are beginning to get the earliest of confirmations that subtle-energy systems do exist and that they influence the physiologic behavior of cellular systems.

Throughout my years of research, I have tried to piece together scientific evidence to substantiate the existence of an extended subtle-energy human anatomy. It is only through the acceptance of this multidimensional framework of functioning that scientists can begin to comprehend the true nature of human physiology and the reasons for illness and wellness. The evidence that I have assembled comes from a variety of disciplines and researchers. Many of the studies which I have put together are known to those within the parapsychological and holistic medical communities. However, I have added new insights to the existing studies.

Many alternative-medicine studies are unfamiliar to the mainstream medical practitioners, who vehemently claim there is no good evidence to substantiate the effectiveness of practices like psychic healing. One of the reasons why most doctors have never read about alternative healing studies in their medical journals is because there is a Catch-22 associated with vibrational healing research. The Catch-22 is that an established medical journal would never publish anything of a controversial nature without references from another established journal. Since no one in this controversial field can get anything into the orthodox medical journals to begin with, there are obviously no established sources of credible references to quote. Therefore the medical journals are safe in their ivory towers of scientific dogmatism.

It is the purpose of this book to demonstrate that healing via systems that affect the elements of human subtle-energy anatomy is just an extension of existing medical science. The Newtonian paradigm of physics was extended by the Einsteinian viewpoint. Likewise, this book will show how the principles of what I call Einsteinian medicine go beyond the limited Newtonian clockwork universe to comprehend human beings from the perspective of interpenetrating, interactive energy fields.

The studies which I have assembled as evidence for our extended subtle anatomy are a collection of clinical observations and experimental findings from a variety of interdisciplinary researchers. Some studies have been replicated by other researchers in other laboratories, while others have not. Viewed by themselves, these studies might be considered weak evidence for the phenomena and energy systems whose existence I am attempting to substantiate. But if viewed collectively, like many small colored tiles assembled into a larger mosaic, one can observe the greater picture. That greater picture is the extended viewpoint of humans as multidimensional beings of energy. Quantum physics and experiments in high-energy particle physics have shown us that, at the particle level, all matter is really energy. Einsteinian medicine is a viewpoint that tries to put the Newtonian picture of biomachinery into the perspective of dynamic interactive energy systems.

If we are beings of energy, then it follows that we can be affected by energy. Even orthodox medicine has begun its evolutionary progression toward the development of energy methods of treatment. Therapeutic radiation to treat cancer, electricity to halt pain, and electromagnetic fields to stimulate healing of fractures are but the first developments of a newly evolving perspective within the medical community. The energies employed by those who use vibrational methods of healing also deliver measured quanta of energy to patients. However, the energy delivered by these therapies exists in frequencies far beyond those measured with conventional detection equipment. As unbelievable as it might seem, this higher dimensional energy is predicted by Einstein's famous equation, $E = mc^2$.

This book was also written to communicate to others the insights that I have derived from my research over the last eleven years. I feel that I have achieved a new synthesis of understanding in a field that badly needs some

type of theoretical foundation upon which to build a new science of healing and understanding human illness. This book will perhaps stimulate
further thinking about human health and illness in new ways. I consider
it a kind of explorers' guidebook to a newly emerging region of scientific
endeavor.

It is my sincerest hope that there will be those within the general public, as well as within the diverse medical communities, who will read this
book with an open mind. There are many radical ideas within this book
and not all will find a home in every reader's mind. As with any book, I
hope the reader will examine my book with an open yet critical attitude,
accepting that information or knowledge which rings true for him or herself. There is no one book which has all the answers. Certainly this is but
a transitional model, waiting to be expanded upon, changed, and reshaped
by newly acquired experimental evidence.

The key issue here is experimental validation. What is truly needed
is a multidisciplinary healing research center which can study the elements
of the model that I have elaborated upon within this book. I have long envisioned a kind of Mayo Clinic of healing research which could study the
many dimensions of healing phenomena within an academic research setting. Such a center would be staffed by medical personnel from all fields
of study, i.e. by doctors, nurses, and medical researchers, but also by acupuncturists, healers, herbalists, clairvoyant diagnosticians, engineers, chemists, physicists, and a host of others. There would be an interdisciplinary
team which could design experiments to measure the subtle energies of
human function and observe how they are affected by different modalities
of healing. Within the center there would be all manner of existing diagnostic technologies, from brainwave mapping and magnetic resonance imaging to more unconventional techniques such as electroacupuncture
monitoring. A wide variety of resources would be brought to bear in trying to understand the basic nature of healing and the potential effectiveness of the healing modalities presented within this book and elsewhere
within this developing field.

The center would be a place where physicians and healers of all back-
grounds and disciplines would come to not only offer their advice in de-
signing experiments, but also to teach each other their various healing
skills. It would be a place where the healers themselves would come to
learn and to be healed. As various modalities of healing were shown to be
effective in limited studies, clinical trials would begin in a larger outreach

through various affiliated clinical-treatment centers. All research would be collated and organized through a computer network, which would make interorganizational networking much easier. For affiliated centers, an ongoing research file access to healing studies would be available through computer linkups. Such a center would publish its own journal of research which would hopefully come to be recognized as a quotable reference source and hence eliminate the Catch-22 of healing research.

Interestingly, many of the healing modalities discussed in this book are often less expensive and considerably less toxic or risky than conventional medical and surgical methods. There is great potential for reducing the runaway costs of medicine if doctors begin to incorporate alternative therapies on an everyday basis. I do not advocate doing away with all drugs and surgery. However, the effectiveness of existing medical technologies can be greatly augmented by *adjunctive* alternative therapies. When vibrational healing methods have progressed to the point that they can repeatedly and consistently offer therapeutic options that drugs and surgery cannot provide, then we will begin to see that greater shift away from standard methods of practice. In the future, homeopathic remedies and flower essences may be recognized as useful for treating various chronic ailments, but I will still rely on a good vascular surgeon to treat a ruptured aortic aneurysm.

The point is that we must begin to investigate alternative healing methods for what they can teach us about ourselves as evolving spiritual beings, as well as for their treatments of ailments for which orthodox medicine can do very little. My hope is that people will examine the contents of this book in a critical yet open manner, and hopefully come away with a better understanding of themselves as multidimensional beings of unlimited healing and growth potential.

RICHARD GERBER, M.D.
JULY 7, 1987

Vibrational Medicine
NEW CHOICES
FOR HEALING OURSELVES

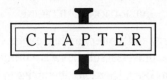

CHAPTER I

Of Holograms, Energy & Vibrational Medicine:
AN EINSTEINIAN VIEW OF LIVING SYSTEMS

The current practice of medicine is based upon the Newtonian model of reality. This model is primarily a viewpoint which sees the world as an intricate mechanism. Doctors conceptualize the body as a type of grand machine which is controlled by the brain and peripheral nervous system: the ultimate biological computer. But are human beings really glorified machines? Or are they complex biological mechanisms which are in dynamic interplay with a series of interpenetrating vital energy fields. . . the so-called "ghost in the machine"? This book is an introduction to a new viewpoint of healing that encompasses an evolving picture of matter as an expression of energy. This new field of healing, based upon the Einsteinian paradigm, is called vibrational medicine.

The Einsteinian paradigm as applied to vibrational medicine sees human beings as networks of complex energy fields that interface with physical/cellular systems. Vibrational medicine uses specialized forms of energy to positively affect those energetic systems that may be out of balance due to disease states. By rebalancing the energy fields that help to regulate cellular physiology, vibrational healers attempt to restore order from a higher level of human functioning.

The recognition that all matter is energy forms the foundation for understanding how human beings can be considered dynamic energetic systems. Through his famous equation, $E = mc^2$, Albert Einstein proved to scientists that energy and matter are dual expressions of the same universal substance. That universal substance is a primal energy or vibration of which we are all composed. Therefore, attempting to heal the body through the manipulation of this basic vibrational or energetic level of substance can be thought of as vibrational medicine. Although the Einsteinian viewpoint has slowly found acceptance and application in the minds of physicists, Einstein's profound insights have yet to be incorporated into the way doctors look at human beings and illness.

Present-day Newtonian models of medical thinking see human physiological and psychological behavior as dependent upon the structural hardware of the brain and body. The heart is a mechanical pump which delivers oxygen and nutrient-rich blood to the organ systems of the body and the brain. Doctors think they understand the heart so well that they have invented mechanical replacements to take over the function of the failing natural heart. Many physicians see the primary role of the kidney as an automatic filtration and exchange mechanism. Doctors have mechanically duplicated the kidney's ability to filter out impurities and toxins by creating hemodialysis machines. Although advancements in biomedical technology have given doctors a wider variety of spare parts to replace diseased organs and blood vessels, the greater knowledge of how to reverse or prevent many diseases is still (sadly) lacking.

Mechanical analogies have offered great utility in explaining the behavior of the physical world since the time of Isaac Newton. The Newtonian thinkers saw the universe as an orderly, predictable, yet divine mechanism. It would follow that human beings, like their Creator, would also be constructed in a similar fashion. During Newton's era, it was easier to think of human anatomy in terms of intricate biological machinery. So prevalent was this mechanistic viewpoint that thinkers of Newton's day saw the entire universe as a grand clockwork. Doctors' perspectives on the inner workings of human beings have changed very little in the evolution of scientific thought over the ages. Present-day physicians still see the human body as a complex machine. They have merely become more sophisticated in studying biological clockwork mechanisms at the molecular level.

The first Newtonian medical approaches were surgical. Early surgeons worked under the basic premise of the human body as a complex plumbing system. The present-day surgeon may be seen as a specialized "bio-plumber" who knows how to isolate and remove a "diseased" component and how to reconnect a system so that it may again function properly. More recent developments in drug treatments have provided newer ways to "fix" the failing body. Although different in philosophy, drug therapy is still Newtonian in that it operates from the perspective of the body as a complex biomechanism. Instead of using knives, as in surgery, doctors use drugs to deliver magic bullets to the appropriately targeted tissue of the body. Different drugs are employed to strengthen or destroy the aberrantly functioning cells, depending upon the medical need. Advances in molecular biology have allowed magic bullets to be targeted with improved specificity, in hopes of creating drugs with greater efficacy and less overall toxicity to the body. Although both pharmacologic and surgical approaches have provided significant strides in the diagnosis and treatment of human illness, both subscribe to the Newtonian view of the human body as an intricate clockwork mechanism of physical organs, chemicals, enzymes, and membrane receptors.

The Newtonian mechanistic viewpoint of life is only an approximation of reality. Pharmacologic and surgical approaches are incomplete because they ignore the vital forces which animate and breathe life into the biomachinery of living systems. In a machine, the underlying principle is that the function of the whole can be predicted by the sum of its parts. However humans, unlike machines, are more than the summation of a pile of combined chemicals. All organisms are dependent upon a subtle vital force which creates synergism via a unique structural organization of molecular components. Because of this synergism, the living whole is greater than the sum of its parts. The vital force creates order in living systems and constantly rebuilds and renews its cellular vehicle of expression. When the life-force leaves the body at death, the physical mechanism is slowly degraded into a disorganized collection of chemicals. This is one of the unique principles which distinguishes living from nonliving systems, and people from machines.

This animating life-force is an energy which is currently unaddressed by today's Newtonian mechanistic thinkers, whose opinions predominate orthodox medicine. These subtle forces are not dealt with nor discussed by physicians because there are no currently acceptable scientific models which explain their existence and function. Science's current inability to deal with the vital forces animating the human frame is partly due to the conflict between Eastern and Western belief systems that occurred many ages ago. This difference in worldviews is actually a deeper sign of the schism between religion and science that took place thousands of years ago. The application of the Newtonian model to explain the workings of the human body was a reflection of scientists' attempts to take human function out of the realm of the divine and into the mechanistic world that they could understand and manipulate. The mechanization of the human body represented a further movement away from religious explanations of the mystical forces that moved humans through life and, just as mysteriously, into sickness and death.

Present-day medical views are deeply entrenched within a Newtonian worldview which is hundreds of years old. The Newtonian model had been important in assisting mechanical and theoretical advancements in the era of the Industrial Revolution. However, this model was eventually found to be plagued with many shortcomings as physicists gained more experience with the phenomena of electricity and magnetism. The Newtonian world-view similarly lacks an adequate explanation for the role of the vital forces in living systems. Although vitalism was popular at one time in medicine's past, overconfidence with technology and science has tossed aside such philosophies in favor of mechanistic models of organic life.

The Newtonian view is based upon early models of mechanistic be-havior that were derived from observation of nature. Acceleration and gravity were analyzed by Newton from his observations of a falling apple. He applied mathematics to his observations and deduced various laws of motion which described what he had seen. These early Newtonian laws enabled scientists to make predictions on the way mechanical systems would behave. For its time, the Newtonian model was quite advanced. Through his development of calculus, Newton gave scientists a tool for probing the observable universe. This led to new directions in scientific discovery and enabled the creation of many inventions which have since benefited humanity. But Newton's laws dealt primarily with the force of gravity as it acted upon moving bodies in the Earth's gravitational field. His models were unable to explain the behavior of electricity and magnetism in later years. Eventually, new models of the universe had to be invented to accomodate these curious energetic phenomena.

Scientists are again beginning to discover forces that do not fit into the conventional Newtonian model of reality. Although not acknowledged as such by orthodox scientists, the energies of the life-force are being studied by various researchers who recognize their vital importance to living sys-tems. Unfortunately, the majority of biological researchers and physicians are still working from a Newtonian model of living systems in which the human body is seen as a cellular mechanism. Researchers do not yet recognize the primary role of vital life-energies that animate the body. Although medicine has increased its sophistication by focusing on cellular interactions at the molecular level, physiologic models are based strictly upon the behavior of dense physical matter. These models exclude the contributions of bioenergetic fields which influence cellular patterns of growth and physical expression.

There is a new breed of physician/healer that is evolving today who seeks to understand the functioning of human beings from the revolutionary view of *matter as energy*. These spiritual scientists look to the human body as an instructional model by which we can begin to understand, not only ourselves, but also the inner workings of nature and the secrets of the universe. By realizing that *humans are beings of energy*, one can begin to comprehend new ways of viewing health and illness. This new Einsteinian viewpoint will not only give future doctors a unique perspective on the causes of disease, but also more effective ways by which human beings can be healed of their suffering.

Instead of conventional drug and surgical approaches, *vibrational medicine attempts to treat people with pure energy*. This theoretical perspective is based upon the understanding that the molecular arrangement of the physical body is actually a complex network of interwoven energy fields. The energetic network, which represents the physical/cellular framework, is organized and nourished by "subtle" energetic systems which coordinate the life-force with the body. There is a hierarchy of subtle energetic systems that coordinate electrophysiologic and hormonal function as well as cellular structure within the physical body. It is primarily from these subtle levels that health and illness originate. These unique energy systems are powerfully affected by our emotions and level of spiritual balance as well as by nutritional and environmental factors. These subtle energies influence cellular patterns of growth in both positive and negative directions.

Conventional medical wisdom is misguided by the notion that one can cure all illness by physically repairing or eliminating abnormal cellular systems. Through drugs and surgery, doctors try to reroute dysfunctional components, such as atheromatous arteries, much as a high-tech plumber might try to fix a clogged drain. They use chemicals to increase blood flow past cholesterol blockages, and when that fails, they use a balloon plunger or even a laser beam to blast away the dysfunctional debris. More commonly, a new pipe is carefully stitched in place to bypass the old clogged artery. The key to treating such recurring conditions of disease may not lie in simple, "quick-fix" physical solutions, but in the realm of repatterning the organizing energy fields which direct the cellular expression of dysfunction.

There is an aspect of human physiology that physicians have not yet understood and only reluctantly acknowledge. This dimension of human physiology is the domain of Spirit as it relates to the physical body. The spiritual dimension is the energetic basis of all life, because it is the energy of spirit which animates the physical framework. *The unseen connection between the physical body and the subtle forces of spirit holds the key to understanding the inner relationship between matter and energy.* When scientists begin to comprehend the true relationship between matter and energy, they will come closer to understanding the relationship between humanity and God.

The evolving field of science which will bring humankind to this new level of understanding is vibrational medicine. Vibrational medicine attempts to heal illness and transform human consciousness by working with the energetic patterns that guide the physical expression of life. We will eventually discover that *consciousness itself is a kind of energy that is integrally related to the cellular expression of the physical body.* As such, *consciousness participates in the continuous creation of either health or illness.* Vibrational medicine, as the science of the future, may contain clues which will help doctors solve the mystery of why some people remain healthy while others are continually in a state of dis-ease.

When physicians come to better understand the deeper interrelationship between body, mind, and spirit, and the natural laws guiding their manifestation upon our planet, then there will be a truly holistic medicine. We are indeed a microcosm within a macrocosm, as oriental philosophers have long understood. The principles seen within the microcosm often reflect larger principles governing the behavior of the macrocosm. Patterns of order within nature repeat themselves on many hierarchical levels. If one can make sense of universal laws as they are expressed in matter at the micro level, then it becomes easier to make sense of the cosmic whole. When humans truly understand the physical and energetic structures of their minds and bodies, they will be that much closer to comprehending the nature of the universe and the forces of creation which link them with God.

The Marvels of Laser Light:
Holography as a New Model of Reality

To understand Einsteinian medicine, we can use a working knowledge of light or, more specifically, laser light. Laser light, as applied in laser beams and holography, is a very special type of light known as coherent light. Coherent light is extremely orderly, with all of its waves moving in step like soldiers marching in a parade. Laser light has had numerous applications in science, medicine, and industry. Video discs, fiberoptic telecommunication, and laser eye surgery are now common applications of coherent laser light. The study of pictures produced by using laser light to illuminate subject matter is called holography. The hologram is a special three-dimensional picture created by energy interference patterns. Holograms also demonstrate a unique principle in nature which shows that every piece can contain the essence of the whole. The hologram provides us with a new and unique model which may help science to understand the energetic structure of the universe as well as the multidimensional nature of human beings.

A hologram is made by sending a single laser beam through an optical device known as a beam splitter in order to create two laser beams which originate from the same source. One of the beams, designated the "reference beam," passes through a diffusing lens that spreads it from orderly pencil-thin rays into a flashlight-like beacon.

This beam is directed by mirrors to fall upon an unexposed photographic plate. Meanwhile, the second beam, referred to as the "working beam," undergoes an initial fate similar to that of the reference beam by passing through a second diffusing lens. The difference between the two beams is that light from the working beam is used to illuminate the object being photographed. The light from the working beam bounces off the object, and then falls upon the photographic plate.

What happens at the photographic plate is the basis for both holography and a new way of understanding the universe. When the pure unaffected reference beam meets with the reflected light of the working beam, an interference pattern is created. This interference pattern is produced by the waves of one beam mixing and interacting with the waves of the other beam.

It is the interference pattern created by laser light and captured on the photographic film that produces the phenomenon which we call a holo-

Diagram 1.
CREATION OF A HOLOGRAM

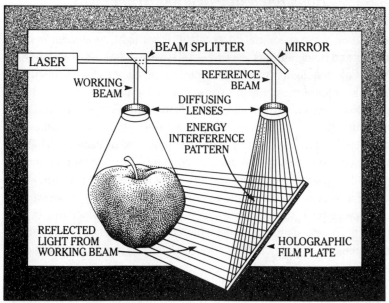

gram. It is quite unlike any photograph taken using ordinary or incoherent light.

An interference pattern is a phenomenon for which there are many simple examples in nature. One example is the interference pattern created by simultaneously dropping two stones into a quiet pool of water. Each stone creates a series of ever-expanding circular waves travelling outward from their respective centers. As the two groups of circular wave fronts meet, they interact and form an interference pattern.

This pattern is similar, in principle, to the interference pattern created by the mixing of the laser beams in front of the photographic plate. The photographic emulsion captures the interference pattern, and the hologram is born. What is remarkable about this piece of film is that by shining a pure beam of laser light similar to the reference beam through the hologram, one is able to view in three dimensions the object recorded by the working (reflected) beam. In effect, by supplying a reference beam, the hologram recreates the working beam as recorded within the interference pattern on the film. The working beam, which was the light which interacted with the object being photographed, holds within its altered waves a record of its interaction with the object.

Holograms are truly three-dimensional. Certain holograms permit one to walk all the way around the projected image and see it from above and below as if the image were real. The other remarkable property of holograms is that one can cut away a small piece of the holographic film, hold it up to laser light, and still see an entire, intact, three-dimensional image of the photographed object.

Diagram 1 illustrates the creation of a holographic picture of an apple. This hologram, when viewed under the illumination of incoherent light, such as the light from an incandescent light bulb, reveals no apple. The observer sees only a smoky haze, the result of the laser-produced interference pattern. If the holographic film is viewed with illumination from a source of coherent laser light, it reproduces the reference beam that helped to create the original interference pattern, and the apple is revealed with all its three-dimensional characteristics. If a small piece of that holographic apple film is now cut away and examined under the illumination of laser light, a smaller, yet intact, whole apple can be seen.

The reason for this is the fact that *the hologram is an energy interference pattern. Within this pattern, every piece contains the whole.* That is, one could take a hologram of an apple, cut the film into fifty pieces, and

Diagram 2.
INTERFERENCE PATTERN
CREATED BY DROPPING TWO STONES INTO WATER

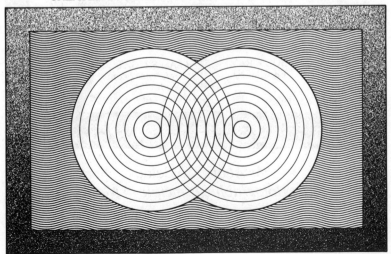

each piece when viewed through laser light would reveal its own miniature apple.

The holographic model sets a precedent for new ways of understanding Einsteinian medicine and provides a totally new way of looking at the universe. Utilizing the holographic model, it is possible to arrive at conclusions one might not come upon by utilizing simple deductive reasoning and logic.

Fifty tiny apples from fifty pieces of a single apple photograph is far from what one would predict utilizing assumptions of a Newtonian universe. How then does one apply holographic theory to understanding phenomena in nature? The simplest place to begin is with the human body itself.

Diagram 3.
THE HOLOGRAPHIC PRINCIPLE:
EACH PIECE CONTAINS THE WHOLE

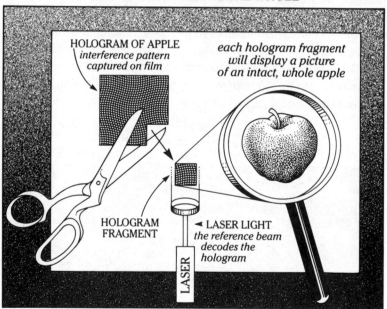

"As Above, So Below":
The Holographic Principle in Nature

At a highly symbolic level, the holographic principle that "every piece contains the whole" can be seen in the cellular structure of all living bodies. Scientific discoveries in the world of cellular biology have demonstrated that every cell contains a copy of the master DNA blueprint, with enough information to make an entire human body from scratch. This realization is the basis for experiments in cloning living cells. In creating a duplicate of a lower life-form, such as a frog, cloning techniques are employed in which the DNA material from a fertilized frog's egg is removed and exchanged for the DNA material from an adult frog's intestinal cell. Because the instructions within each body cell contain the same library of information found in every other cell, it is possible to produce a completely identical frog without utilizing sexual reproduction. This is a kind of technologic virgin birth. The potential of the genetic blueprint is expressed in an appropriately supportive environment such as a fertilized egg. The fact that *every cell within the human body contains the information to create an entire duplicate body mirrors the holographic principle whereby every piece contains the information of the whole.*

The holographic principle may also be of value in understanding the bioenergetic fields associated with the physico-chemical structure of the human body. Science has come far in its understanding of the natural growth, development, and repair of living systems. Much of this understanding is an outgrowth of our sophisticated deciphering of the genetic code within the nucleus of the living cell. The nucleus is clearly a control center for the complex processes and interactions taking place within and between cells. Our understanding of the DNA-containing chromosomes within the nucleus has furthered our knowledge of such phenomena as cellular replication, growth, and the differentiation of primitive embryonic cells into specialized cells that carry out specific functions within the body. However, our knowledge of DNA has been inadequate thus far to explain how differentiated cells in the developing human fetus find their way to the appropriate spatial locations where they will carry out their specialized functions.

Suppose we trace the steps in the growth and development of a human being from the stage of the newly fertilized egg. At the time of conception, a sperm unites with an egg, thereby providing a stimulus for the entire growth process to begin. In uniting a sperm and an egg, a cell is produced that carries half the chromosomal content from the mother and half from the father. This genetic material will provide the information for the final expression of this new human being. The single cell begins to undergo a process of self-replication and soon is transformed into a tight little ball of many formless, undifferentiated cells. Somehow these formless cells must take on the shape of nerve, bone, muscle, and connective-tissue cells and migrate to their appropriate positions to work together as a whole human body.

To help fill in the missing biological information, suppose we make an analogy between a Little League baseball team and the development of human cells. We wish to take a group of undifferentiated little children and form them into a cohesive functioning unit: a baseball team. Let us further suppose that these children are of school age, are able to read, and have limited attention spans. To teach these children how to play baseball, we first elect a captain of the team who will assign appropriate roles to each player. The captain hands out a booklet entitled "How to Play Baseball" to all the team members. Because the children have limited attention spans, they are each given a book in which dark construction paper covers all the pages concerning information not directly relevant to their assignment. The first baseman receives a booklet with dark paper covering all but the pages on "How to be a First Baseman," and so on for each of the players.

This analogy relates to the developing human in the early stage of development. As with the little-league team, human development begins with a group of tiny undifferentiated components—in this case, cells. Similar to the booklet on "How to Play Baseball" given to all the would-be baseball players, each cell is endowed with a master library of "How to Build and Maintain a Human Being." This library is contained within the DNA-assembled genetic code in the nucleus of each cell. The cell reads the genetic code by using a process known as transcription. During transcription, information from DNA is transcribed or copied onto an intermediary RNA molecule which is then used to carefully assemble the various functional and structural proteins of the cell. The DNA is coated with specialized proteins known as histones and non-histones that perform a function similar to the dark construction paper used in the baseball booklets. These unique proteins selectively block from transcription of the genetic code those portions that are not pertinent to the functioning of the particular cell in which that DNA text resides. For instance, a developing muscle cell has the construction-paper equivalents covering all of the pages of its DNA manual except those instructing "How to be a Muscle Cell." This process is known as differentiation of cells. It is similar to an undifferentiated player being assigned a "job" or position to play. That cell (or player) now has very specific functions.

Today's state-of-the-art knowledge of molecular biology and DNA fully explains how this process of differentiation occurs in the developing cells of the growing human embryo. DNA contains all of the information necessary to instruct each cell how to do its particular job, how to manufacture its proteins, etc. What DNA does not explain, however, is how these newly differentiated cells travel to their appropriate spatial locations in the developing baby's body. In order to understand how this process is likely to work, we must return to our baseball analogy.

When we last left our little-league players, they had just gone home to read about their unique functions in playing a coherent and organized game of baseball. They have now become well versed in their respective functions and the rules of the game; however, there is still one missing ingredient before they can play. The missing element is a playing field and baseball diamond. In order to play baseball, the team must orient themselves in space on the playing *field*. The term "field" has been carefully chosen in this analogy because it is more than metaphorically represented in the case of the developing human being. It is highly likely that the spatial organization of the cells is ordered by a complex three-dimensional map of what the finished body is supposed to look like. This map or mold is the function of a bioenergetic field which accompanies the physical body. *This field or "etheric body" is a holographic energy template that carries coded information for the spatial organization of the fetus as well as a roadmap for cellular repair in the event of damage to the developing organism*. There is mounting scientific evidence, albeit unknown to the vast majority of scientists, to support the hypothesis of such a holographic energy body.

The Scientific Evidence: A Search for the Etheric Body

The earliest evidence to support the existence of a holographic energy body is the work of neuroanatomist Harold S. Burr at Yale University[1] during the 1940s. Burr was studying the shape of energy fields around living plants and animals. Some of Burr's work involved the shape of electrical fields surrounding salamanders. He found that the salamanders possessed an energy field roughly shaped like the adult animal. He also discovered that this field contained an electrical axis which was aligned with the brain and spinal cord.

Burr wanted to find precisely when this electrical axis first originated in the animal's development. He began mapping the fields in progressively earlier stages of salamander embryogenesis. Burr discovered that *the elec-*

Diagram 4.
SURFACE ELECTRICAL POTENTIAL
OF A SALAMANDER

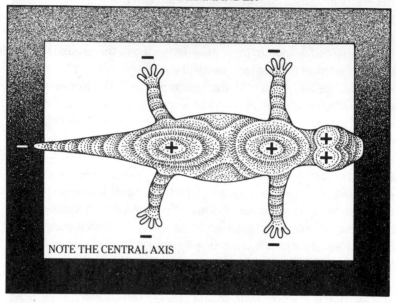

NOTE THE CENTRAL AXIS

trical axis originated in the unfertilized egg. This discovery contradicted the conventional biological and genetic theory of his day.

Burr theorized that the electrical axis aligned with the nervous system of the adult salamander was synonymous with the axis present in the unfertilized egg. His research to support this theory involving a "tagging" procedure. Since amphibians like the salamander produce very large eggs, it was possible to use direct visual observation through a biomicroscope to label the electrical axis of the unfertilized salamander egg. Burr injected tiny droplets of a dark indelible ink into the axial region of the egg utilizing a micropipette technique. He discovered that the dark ink always became incorporated into the brain and spinal cord of the developing salamander.

Burr also experimented with the electrical fields around tiny seedlings. According to his research, the electrical field around a sprout was not the shape of the original seed. Instead the surrounding electrical field resembled the adult plant. Burr's data suggested that any developing organism was destined to follow a prescribed growth template and that such a template was generated by the organism's individual electromagnetic field.

Contemporary research has lent further credence to Burr's theories of bioenergetic growth fields. There is also increasing evidence supporting the holographic nature of these bioenergy fields which comes from experimental work in the area of electrographic photography. Electrography, or Kirlian photography, is a technique whereby living objects are photographed in the presence of a high frequency, high voltage, low amperage electrical field. This technique was largely pioneered by the Russian researcher Semyon Kirlian[2] from whom the process has acquired its name. Kirlian's first research began in the early 1940s at about the same time Burr was measuring electromagnetic fields around living objects.

Both scientists developed experimental techniques that were capable of measuring changes in the energy fields of living systems. Burr's approach utilized conventional voltmeters and revealed data in the form of microvoltage levels. Kirlian studied the same electrical fields of the body, but his electrographic techniques translated Burr's electrical measurements into the visual characteristics of an electrical corona. Burr and Kirlian found that diseases like cancer caused significant changes in the electromagnetic fields of living organisms. Burr had made this revelation by studying superficial skin measurements taken with his voltmeter. Kirlian recorded corona discharge images of the body to confirm the disease-associated energy field changes. Since Kirlian first developed his novel approach to studying the bodies of plants and animals through the use of electrophotography, numerous other investigators, including the author of this book, have confirmed the diagnostic potential inherent in electrographic recording techniques.

Electrophotography (in its most basic form) is based upon observations of a phenomenon known as the corona discharge. Electrically grounded objects in high-frequency electrical fields characteristically demonstrate spark discharges between the object and the electrode generating the field. The term "corona discharge" arises from the observation of discharge patterns around circular objects, where the spark pattern along the edge of the object resembles the outer corona of the sun during an eclipse. When a piece of photographic film is interposed between the object and the electrode, the spark discharge is captured on the recording emulsion. The corona is the result of electron discharge trails that represent millions of electrons streaming from the object to the photographic plate upon which an object rests. Depending upon the type of film used and the energetic characteristics of the electrical field generator, beautiful colors and spark patterns are observed in the electrographic image in what has been described as the "Kirlian aura."

There are numerous biophysical factors such as temperature, moisture, local microenvironment, pressure, etc. which can physically affect the final discharge.[3] In spite of the many variables which can affect the picture, numerous investigators have succeeded in obtaining relevant biological information from the appearance of the electrical coronas photographed around human fingertips. Corona discharge patterns of human fingertips reveal significant diagnostic information pertaining to the presence of cancer,[4] cystic fibrosis,[5] and other diseases in the body of the individual whose finger is photographed.

Even more interesting than fingertips are the beautiful discharge patterns photographed around various types of leaves. A unique phenomenon recorded by electrophotography, which is especially relevant to our discussion of bioenergetic growth templates, is the "Phantom Leaf Effect." This effect can be observed when the upper third of a leaf is cut off and destroyed. The remaining leaf fragment is then photographed by the electrographic process. Examination of the amputated leaf electrophotograph reveals a picture of an intact, whole leaf. The amputated portion still appears in the photo of the leaf even though the missing leaf fragment has been physically destroyed.

Various physical explanations for the phantom have been invoked by skeptical scientists. Critics suggested that the phantom effect resulted from leaf moisture on the photographic plates. Keith Wagner, a researcher at California State University, seems to have refuted this skepticism.[6] Elegant electrographic studies by Wagner demonstrated that the phantom portion of the leaf could still be photographed through a clear lucite block which had been placed where the phantom was to appear. The ghost-like phantom appeared consistently, even though moisture could not pass through the plastic barrier.[7]

Clues from the Phantom Leaf: The Etheric Body as a Hologram

The implication of the Phantom Leaf Effect is that some type of organized energy field is interacting with the electrons of the corona discharge of the remaining leaf in the area of the phantom. This interaction registers as an orderly discharge pattern. The discharge pattern retains the spatial integrity and organization of the missing leaf portion. Allen Detrick[8] has performed phantom leaf experiments in which both sides of the phantom have been captured by photographing the amputated leaf on either side. This would be equivalent to slicing off the upper fingers of a hand and taking electrographs of the front and back of the hand. One electrograph would show phantom fingerprints whereas the other electrograph would demonstrate phantom fingernails. The three-dimensional spatial and organizational properties of such a biological energy field would seem to be holographic in nature. Even more convincing evidence to support this idea has come from recent developments in electrographic recording techniques.

Studies by I. Dumitrescu in Rumania, utilizing a scanning technique based on the electrographic process, added a new twist to the Phantom Leaf Effect. Dumitrescu cut a circular hole in a leaf and then photographed the leaf with his electrographic equipment. The image revealed was that of a

Diagram 5.
PHANTOM LEAF PHENOMENON
adapted from a photo by I. Dumitrescu

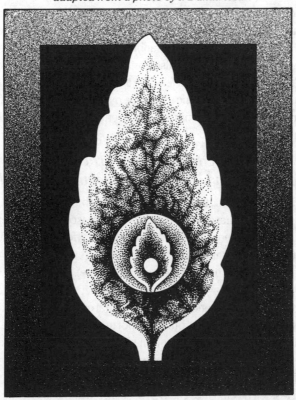

tiny intact leaf with a smaller hole in it (see Diagram 5).[9] The smaller leaf appeared inside the area where the circular portion of the leaf had been cut away. Dumitrescu's phenomenon resembles the holographic photo of the apple that was discussed earlier in the chapter. When a fragment of the apple hologram was removed and held up to laser light, a small intact apple was revealed. This is exactly what happened in Dumitrescu's experiment! A leaf appeared within a leaf! Dumitrescu's results with the Phantom Leaf Effect would seem to confirm the holographic nature of the organizing energy field that surrounds all living systems.

In metaphysical literature, this energy field that surrounds and penetrates living systems is referred to as the "etheric body." It is said that the etheric body is one of many bodies contributing to the final expression of the human form. The etheric body, in all likelihood, is an energy interference pattern similar to a hologram.

There is speculation that the application of the holographic model can be extended even further. Perhaps the universe itself is a gigantic "cosmic hologram." *That is to say, the universe is a tremendous energy interference pattern*. By virtue of its likely holographic characteristics, every piece of the universe not only contains but also contributes to the information of the whole. The cosmic hologram is less like a holographic still photo frozen in time than it is like a holographic videotape dynamically changing from moment to moment. Let us examine the theoretical evidence for such a holographic universe.

News from the World of Particle Physics: Matter as Frozen Light & Its Implications for Medicine

There is an esoteric statement that says "as above, so below." One level of meaning to this phrase is that things on a microscopic level seem to parallel or mirror events on a macroscopic level. A further interpretation is that as we come to understand ourselves more fully (below), we may come to better understand the universe around us (above).

Let us examine the world from the perspective of a single cell. The DNA within the nucleus encodes the structural-physical expression of the cell's activity. But the DNA is only an information manual containing instructions that still must be acted upon by some intermediate actors in the cellular scheme of things. Those actors in the cellular scenario are the enzymes, the protein-bodied workers that carry out the many, everyday biochemical tasks. The enzymes catalyze specific reactions of chemicals either to create structure through molecular assemblies or to provide the electro-chemical fire to run the cellular engines and ultimately keep the entire system working efficiently. Enzymes are actually composed of proteins, which are themselves collections of amino acids strung together in linear array like colored beads on a thread. The various positive and negative charges on the amino acids, by virtue of electrostatic attraction and repul-sion, cause the string of beads to "self-assemble" into a functional three-dimensional structure. At the center of this structure is found the "active site" (or business end) of this macromolecule where the chemical reactions are catalyzed. The DNA molecule encodes and assigns the sequential ar-rangement of the various "colored" amino acids for each type of protein in its genetic structural memory.

We now know that molecules are aggregations of yet tinier particles called atoms. Only within the last century has Western technology evolved to the point of being able to answer the question, "What are atoms?" It has now become common knowledge that atoms are further reducible to even smaller particles called electrons, neutrons, and protons. All matter is com-posed of infinitely different arrangements of atomic and subatomic par-ticles, such as electrons. But what exactly IS an electron?

This question has caused feverish debate within the scientific com-munity for nearly a century. Answering this fundamental question is a pivotal point in the understanding of the atom and, indeed, the structure of the universe. It is also a turning point in the evolution of our understand-ing of physics and the unique concept of "complementarity." Complemen-tarity is the concept which suggests that the world is no longer only black and white but is made up of various shades of grey. It is a concept which accepts the peaceful coexistence of two seemingly different, or even op-posite properties, existing simultaneously within the same object. Nowhere does complementarity find greater application and confusion than in the description of the properties of electrons.

In the early twentieth century, scientists noted that in certain exper-iments electrons appeared to behave as tiny billiard balls. They would ca-reen off each other in collisions, similar to balls colliding on a pool table. To the mechanistic thinking of the Newtonian physicists, this was a predic-table pattern of particle behavior. The confusion began to set in when other experiments demonstrated properties suggesting that electrons behaved more like waves of light. The famous example of the electron's odd, wave-like behavior is the "double-slit experiment." The results of this experiment demonstrated that a single electron appeared to pass through two holes simultaneously. This feat was quite unprecedented for the tiny billiard ball which the electron was supposed to represent. Yet other tests showed that if one aimed two beams of electrons at each other, they did indeed bounce off each other like tiny billiard balls. Waves, but not particles, can pass through two windows simultaneously. So what then are electrons, which can seemingly do both? It appears that electrons display the complementary behaviors of both waves and particles simultaneously. Two mutually exclusive properties of energy and matter coexist within a single electron. This is the true essence of the principle of complementarity. The electron is neither pure particle nor pure energy. It displays elements of both. Some physicists have resolved the dilemma by conceptualizing electrons to be "wave-packets."

The wave/particle duality of subatomic particles like electrons is a reflection of the energy-matter relationship first elaborated upon by Albert Einstein with his famous $E = mc^2$ in the early 1900's. Matter and energy are now known to be interchangeable and interconvertible. *This means that one cannot only convert matter into energy, but it should be possible to convert energy into matter.* Although physicists have not yet accomplished this feat artificially in their laboratories, this event has actually been observed and captured in the photographic records of cloud chambers in experimental nuclear facilities.

A cosmic ray—a highly energetic photon of light—when passing in the vicinity of a heavy atomic nucleus, leaves its imprint on film as it spontaneously becomes a particle/antiparticle pair. The photon changes form to become two mirror-image particles. Literally, energy becomes matter. This is the reverse of what happens when matter and antimatter meet and annihilate each other, releasing tremendous amounts of energy.

This interconversion of light into matter and vice-versa would seem curious behavior, rather like apples becoming oranges and then changing back to apples. But are we really seeing the interconversion of two wholly different substances? Is it possible that we are observing an event more analogous to the change of state of some primary universal substance (i.e., solid ice vaporized into steam, or liquid condensed steam [water] frozen back into ice)? This interpretation gives new "light" to the wave/particle nature of particles like electrons.

Consider the example of the high-energy photon becoming two particles. At the point of conversion from energy to matter, the photon (a quan-

Diagram 6.
BIRTH OF MATTER FROM ENERGY

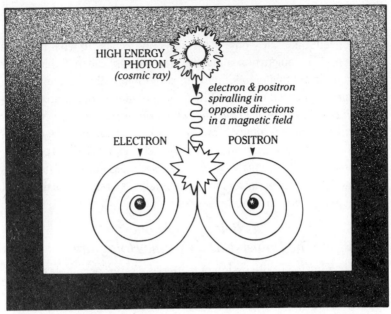

HIGH ENERGY PHOTON *(cosmic ray)*

electron & positron spiralling in opposite directions in a magnetic field

ELECTRON   POSITRON

tum of electromagnetic energy or light) slows down to become a particle. In doing so it attains some of the properties attributable to solids (i.e., mass) and yet still retains some of its wave-like properties. These wave-like properties are hidden except in certain experiments where beams of electrons are treated like beams of photons, as in an electron microscope. In a simplistic sense, a packet of light has been slowed down and frozen. This particle of frozen light might be viewed as a miniature energy interference pattern or a microcosmic energy field occupying an infinitessimal space. And so we see how the macroscopic illusion of solidity melts away when one delves into the subatomic world of particle physics. Add to this realization the fact that the atom is made up mostly of empty space. The minute particles that do fill this void are, in fact, frozen packets of light. When viewed from the microcosmic level, *all matter is frozen light!*

Matter is composed of highly complex, infinitely orchestrated energy fields. The combinations are governed by various "laws of nature" which physics has sought to discover. The term "fields within fields" has been appropriately applied to this theoretical model. If we apply this to living systems, the cellular matrix of the physical body can be seen as a complex

energetic interference pattern interpenetrated by the organizing bioenergetic field of the etheric body. This understanding of *matter as a specialized
energy "field"* is a revolution in thought and is the central theme and basis
for discussion throughout the rest of this book. It is also the departure point
from conventional "Newtonian" medical approaches" to what I call the
"Einsteinian" paradigm of healing: the practical application of this clearer
understanding of matter to human illness. Vibrational medicine is a systems approach based upon the Einsteinian paradigm of healing. *Vibrational medicine attempts to interface with primary subtle energetic fields
that underlie and contribute to the functional expression of the physical
body.* Whereas the Newtonian pharmacokinetic approach deals primarily
with molecular interactions such as enzymes and receptors, this new energetic model will allow doctors to conceptualize systems of healing that
work at a more primary, subtle energetic level.

"As Below, So Above":
The Universe as a Cosmic Hologram

Returning to our discussion of matter as a series of complex and integrated energy fields, it might be said that matter is a type of energy interference pattern. Consider our speculation that the "etheric body" is a
holographic energy template that guides the growth and development of
the physical body. The etheric body is felt by many to be a body of matter
—so-called "etheric matter." In this case, the matter is of a higher frequency
nature. That is, the particles vibrate at a higher frequency so that etheric
matter is perceived differently. Remember, *if matter has light-like properties, then it is probable that matter may have frequency characteristics.* Matter in the so-called "physical universe" is merely matter of a particular density or slower frequency.

Etheric matter is referred to in the Eastern esoteric literature as "subtle
matter," or matter which is less dense than physical, i.e., of a higher frequency nature. The etheric body appears to be a subtle counterpart of the
physical body, possibly somewhat like the phantom leaf. Our etheric body
is an energy interference pattern with the characteristics of a hologram. It
is likely that there are subtle counterparts to the physical universe made
up of matter of higher frequencies. If the energy interference pattern of a
single etheric body acts as a hologram, might not the entire universal energy interference pattern represent a vast cosmic hologram? If this is true,
then by virtue of the holographic principle whereby every piece contains

the whole, there are profound implications for information being stored within the seemingly empty space around us! The fact that limitless amounts of information might be enfolded into the structure of the universe is an idea gaining more and more attention from theorists such as Nobel prize-winning physicist David Bohm.[10] Bohm has presented convincing scientific arguments for what he calls the "implicate order" of the holographic universe. In such a universe, higher levels of order and information may be holographically enfolded in the fabric of space and matter/energy.

If indeed there exists such a cosmic hologram, then every piece of the universe contains information concerning the makeup of the entire cosmos. Unlike a static hologram, the cosmic hologram is a dynamically moving system that changes from micosecond to microsecond. *Because what happens in just a small fragment of the holographic energy interference pattern affects the entire structure simultaneously, there is a tremendous connectivity relationship between all parts of the holographic universe.* If one were to view God as "all there is," then, through the holographic interconnectivity of space, God could simultaneously be in contact with all creations. The ultimate question, of course, is how does one tap into this information about the cosmos which is enfolded into the structure of space within and around us? How do we decode the cosmic hologram? As we all occupy a small area of real estate within the universe, we all, in a sense, own a "piece of the rock." Can we tune into this information being broadcast? Do we even own the right kind of radio receiver for listening to the broadcast?

This type of holographic reasoning may provide an explanation for some of the successful research in "remote viewing" at Stanford Research Institute in Palo Alto, California.[11] Remote viewing is a term created by Russell Targ and Harold Puthoff, two laser and quantum physicists who have headed this interesting research effort in psi. Remote viewing subjects were sealed in rooms with observers and asked to identify remote geographical locations selected randomly during the time of the experiment. The test sites were visited by a second experimenter at the same time that the first test subject was asked to describe the remote location(s). Many individuals were found who could identify in great detail the remote locations chosen. In certain cases, "star performers" such as Ingo Swann were not only able to identify distant target sites that were not on conventional geographic maps, but were also able to accurately pinpoint weather conditions at the site during the time of the remote viewing attempt. Mr. Swann, a New York artist, has participated in research that has produced convincing data on remote viewing of Jupiter, Mars, and Mercury. Mr. Swann and another gifted subject, Harold Sherman, were able to supply accurate observations of planetary conditions on Jupiter and Mercury that could only later be confirmed by NASA satellite missions. Some of the planetary data supplied by the "psychic space probe" ran contrary to contemporary astrophysical predictions. But several years later, satellite telemetry data validated what Swann and Sherman had psychically observed.

Is it possible that individuals with this type of remote viewing perceptual ability are tapping into and decoding their own piece of the cosmic hologram? Remember, each piece of the hologram contains the information of the whole. Because the universal hologram is a dynamic energy interference pattern, it is continually changing from moment to moment. This would explain how Swann was not only able to identify an island in the Indian Ocean (where there was also a secret French-Soviet meteorological station) but also to view weather conditions on the island at the time.

The cosmic hologram is likely to be composed of overlapping energy interference patterns of many different frequencies. Each frequency-specific holographic pattern would carry information of a unique nature relative to the characteristics of that frequency domain. For example, there would be a subpattern of the universal hologram created from the interference pattern of frequencies in the realm of "physical" matter as opposed to "etheric" matter. Tapping into this frequency hologram would allow one to glean information about the physical structure and surface of the planets, such as in Swann's remote viewing experiment of the planets Jupiter and Mercury. Tapping into the "etheric" frequency band of the cosmic hologram would allow one to tap into information of an "etheric" or higher-dimensional nature beyond the physical plane.

The cosmic hologram might be viewed as a multiplexing of many overlapping frequency holograms, each of which would contain information of a slightly different nature about the universe. An interesting analogy might be made with our view of the cosmos through an optical telescope as compared to observation through an x-ray or radiotelescope. An optical telescope's photograph of a star may look dim and uninteresting when compared with the brilliant image seen when the same star is looked at in the x-ray spectrum of energy. *Different types of observing devices can be focused on the same area of space, and relay wholly different pictures to the eyes of an onlooking astronomer. The varying data will be caused by variations in the frequency band of the observational devices.* This would suggest that there are many levels of frequency-specific information that may be tapped into by reading and decoding one's piece of the cosmic hologram. The nature of decoded information will depend upon the frequency band of energy received, as well as the skill and sensitivity of the observer's perceptual mechanisms.

The fact that everyone (from housewives to Pentagon generals) tested at Stanford was able to do remote viewing, implies that all people have the potential to tap into this level of information storage inherent within the cosmic hologram. Remote viewing is a unique example of how the exploration of inner space may lead to new discoveries in outer space. These and other psychic abilities are part of the extended repertoire of human potential that scientists are only now beginning to discover. Higher states of consciousness, such as those demonstrated by remote viewers, may play an integral role in understanding and decoding the holographic universe.

The holographic model allows us to comprehend information structures from the level of the single cell all the way up to levels of cosmic order. It provides a unique way of viewing the hidden qualities of matter at both the microscopic and macroscopic levels. At the micro level, cells of living organisms display organizing principles which demonstrate that every piece contains the whole. Similar information storage patterns are seen in conventional holograms. At a higher organizational level, the growth of the entire organism is guided by an invisible etheric overlay or template which is also similar to a hologram in its three dimensionality. "Phantom leaf" electrographs confirm that, within this energetic field pattern, every piece contains the information of the whole.

Holograms are based upon the unique properties of energy interference patterns. Physicists have recently concluded that subatomic particles, such as electrons, are actually tiny energy-interference patterns. Since these building blocks of the physical universe are energy interference patterns, they may also display holographic properties. If holograms can be generated by interference patterns at the subatomic and organismic levels (as in the etheric body), then holographic principles might also govern interactions at the macrocosmic level of the entire universe. Thus, holographic principles which organize structure and information content within the human body may also be reflected in patterns of order throughout the cosmic whole.

The universe displays ascending hierarchies of structure based on

repeating patterns of organization at the micro and macro levels. For instance, electrons orbiting the atomic nucleus resemble a miniature solar
system. Other such patterns of order, such as holographic structuring, may
be similarly represented at the cosmic level. This is one interpretation of
the phrase, "as above, so below."

If holographic information encoding does exist at micro and macro
levels of universal organization, can one extract meaningful data? Remote
viewing studies suggest that human consciousness has the potential to
view and decode information inherent within holographic structures at
many levels. Coherent and focused consciousness of the type achieved in
successful remote viewing may have qualities similar to coherent, reference
laser beams used to display and decode more conventional holograms.

Ordinary light from incandescent light bulbs is known as incoherent
light. Incoherent light moves randomly, with light waves travelling chao-
tically in all directions. One might think of average human thought as random and incoherent. Conversely, laser or coherent light is highly focused,
with all light waves travelling in step, similar to soldiers marching in a
parade. If the energy produced by an incandescent bulb were to be made
coherent, the resulting focused laser beam could probably burn a hole
through a steel plate. One can extend the analogy to the production of
coherent thought activity (as reflected by increased brain wave coherence.)
In addition to being highly focused and ordered, coherent light can also
decode holograms. There is also some evidence to suggest that increased
coherence of brain wave activity may be associated with other psychic
events such as psychokinesis and remote viewing. Scientific studies of
transcendental meditators tend to confirm this "coherence" hypothesis.
Long-term meditators attempting certain psychic feats (also known as sid-
dhis) were found to have brain wave patterns of increased energetic coherence during psychic events.[12] Other researchers have also found a definite
shift in brain wave frequencies toward the delta/theta range (1-8 cycles/sec-
ond) along with increased hemispheric synchronization during human
psychic functioning.[13,14]

The key principle here is that coherent consciousness may display
properties which go beyond ordinary waking consciousness. Going from
incoherent random thought to coherent consciousness may be as powerful a transition as going from incandescent light to the brilliant energy of
a laser beam. By achieving this highly focused level of awareness we may
be able to tap into normally unconscious or latent human abilities. Medita-

tion and other mental disciplines may condition or "program" the physical and "subtle energetic" hardware of our sophisticated nervous system to gain access to higher levels of information. These techniques may allow one to selectively tune the brain/mind receiver to specific frequency bands of energetic input, similar to tuning the station dial on a radio.

Achieving such specialized states of consciousness may allow an individual to gain access to hierarchical levels of information enfolded within the structure of matter/energy fields and space itself. Expanded human awareness may be the most important tool for exploring the holographic universe and the multidimensional human being. Remote viewing studies, such as those conducted at Stanford, point toward the hidden and unexplored potentials that all human beings may possess. As human consciousness evolves toward developing these unique potentials, we shall begin to see a greater acceptance and understanding of the principles of vibrational medicine and the hidden wonders of the holographic universe.

Chapter Summary:
New Energetic Principles for a New Age

Medicine that is directed toward an understanding of energy and vibration, and how they interact with molecular structure and organismic balance, is a slowly evolving field known as vibrational medicine. In a real sense, vibrational medicine is Einsteinian medicine, since it is Einstein's equation which gives us the key insight toward understanding that energy and matter are one and the same thing. The current model of medicine is still Newtonian in character, for pharmacokinetic therapy is based upon a biomolecular/mechanistic approach. Surgery is an even cruder approach of Newtonian mechanistic roots. The healing arts must be updated with new insights from the world of physics and other allied sciences.

Medicine is at the threshold of discovering a hidden world of unseen energies that will help to diagnose and heal illness as well as allow researchers to gain new insights into the hidden potentials of consciousness. The etheric level of energy will be the first of these unseen worlds to be explored by enlightened scientists. Researchers will discover that the etheric body is an energetic growth template which guides the growth and development as well as the dysfunction and demise of all human beings. Based upon the evolved insights of these enlightened reseachers, medicine will begin to comprehend that it is at the etheric level that many diseases have their origins.

The understanding of our multidimensional nature and the application of subtle energetic medical approaches will allow medicine to evolve beyond its present-day needs for drugs and surgery to less traumatic and more natural systems of healing. In addition, the recognition of our relationship to these higher frequency energy systems will ultimately lead to a fusion of religion and science as scientists begin to recognize the spiritual dimension of human beings and the laws of expression of the life-force. The trend of "holism" in medicine will ultimately move physicians toward the recognition that, for human beings to experience health, they must enjoy an integrated relationship between body, mind, and spirit.

The patterns by which energy becomes crystallized in matter are dependent upon subtle forms of expression which already exist at the etheric and higher levels of the multidimensional universe. Energy and matter of the etheric levels of vibration play an important role in guiding the expression of the life-force through the varying forms of nature. This realization will be the creative fire behind the next greatest level of discovery in medicine: the discovery of how our etheric body participates in health and disease. And this important etheric energy/matter insight might also lead scientists to recognize the relationship between humankind and its Creator.

The holographic model and the energetic basis of matter gives new food for thought to those who live according to a Newtonian way of life. To many it will be hard to accept, but such is the nature of evolving science.[15] Exploring the ways in which information may be decoded from the cosmic hologram will ultimately give rise to new methods in science which will be dependent upon the state of consciousness of the scientist. We will see special methodologies and areas of research arise which have been referred to as "state-specific sciences."[16] This means that future scientists will have to be trained to enter specially receptive states of consciousness while they are also learning the academic foundations of their respective sciences. If astrophysicists could learn to decode the cosmic hologram and inwardly explore the planets as Ingo Swann has demonstrated, just think how our understanding of the universe could be expanded.

In the future, states of consciousness will be recognized as important tools for exploring the sciences. New areas in vibrational medicine will demand specialized mind training to probe the energetic structure of the human body. Medical developments in this direction will greatly amplify the powers of physical diagnosis and will eventually result in earlier disease detection than with conventional methods currently in use. The ability to sense the subtle energetic fields of people will be greatly enhanced by technologic achievements in the areas of electrographic imaging. However, it is likely that our inherent perceptual abilities will outperform such technologies for many years to come. The key to making this realization a practical reality is the discovery of methods which will teach us to utilize our extrasensory perceptual skills. When we learn to more fully use the hidden natural potentials of the human mind, we will move closer toward tapping into the subtle energetic elements of the multidimensional universe.

This book is an attempt to present a coherent model for understanding the subtle energetic structures of the human body. It provides a rational basis upon which to understand ancient systems of healing as well as future methods of energetic diagnosis and therapy. One of the central concepts behind this new way of thinking is the realization that we are multidimensional beings. We are more than just flesh and bones, cells and proteins. We are beings in dynamic equilibrium with a universe of energy and light of many different frequencies and forms. We are composed of the stuff of the universe which, as we have already discovered, is actually frozen light. Mystics throughout the ages have referred to us as beings of light. It is only now that science has begun to validate the basic premise behind this statement.

This chapter has attempted to present the energetic foundations which will allow the reader to understand the remainder of the book. Each succeeding chapter builds upon the foundations of the previous one. In a sense, this book is both a textbook of energetic medicine as well as an illustrated history of its evolution throughout the ages. These lessons in vibrational medicine ultimately demonstrate how healing with modalities such as flower essences, gem elixirs, and homeopathy is possible and is based upon an understanding of our subtle energetic anatomy. Many individuals are using essences, elixirs, and homeopathy, but few understand the premise behind their usage.

The first four chapters of this book attempt to lay a foundation for understanding the multidimensional human being. They form a synthesis of experiments and discoveries that have never been assembled nor looked at in such a manner as to create support for the argument that we are beings with both physical and subtle energetic components. There is an entire level of subtle energetic anatomy that is virtually unknown to physicians and health care professionals who propose to treat the whole human being. It is by influencing these subtle energetic pathways, which the life-force follows, that many alternative medical practices are successful in affecting human illness.

In chapters 5 through 11, ancient and modern systems of subtle energetic diagnosis and treatment will be discussed, including acupuncture, radionics, and healing with crystals. Each of these alternative medical approaches is effective via its ability to influence various components of our subtle energetic anatomy, such as the etheric body. Our physical form is intimately related to etheric and other subtle energetic interference patterns which determine the flow of the life-force. When the relationship between the higher vibrational energies and physical matter is understood, we will be better able to comprehend the patterns governing the flow of the life-force through the physical body. Vibrational medical approaches will ultimately be proven effective because they are able to positively influence the human body's subtle energetic pathways. These pathways include the acupuncture meridian system, the chakras, and the etheric body. These little-known energetic systems contribute to the final physical expression of the human form in both health and illness. Only when we are able to understand the role these systems play in maintaining physiological balance will we realize the true relationship between "wholeness" and "dis-ease."

The final two chapters of the book integrate and speculate on the direction towards which medicine will shift in the New Age. It is an introduction to the way medicine will be practiced in the future. In the New Age, our inner understanding of Einsteinian physics will allow the development and application of techniques for diagnosis and healing which will transcend present-day Newtonian limitations.

Key Points to Remember

1. Most orthodox approaches to healing, including drugs and surgery, are based upon the Newtonian viewpoint that the human body is a complex machine.

2. The Einsteinian viewpoint of vibrational medicine sees the human being as a multidimensional organism made up of physical/cellular systems in dynamic interplay with complex regulatory energetic fields. Vibrational medicine attempts to heal illness by manipulating these subtle-energy fields via directing energy into the

body instead of manipulating the cells and organs through drugs or surgery.

3. The holographic principle says that every piece contains the information of the whole. This principle is mirrored in the fact that every cell in the human body contains the master DNA library on how to create an entire human being.

4. The etheric body is a holographic energy field or template that carries information for the growth, development, and repair of the physical body. While the genes within the DNA direct the molecular mechanisms which govern the development of individual cells, the etheric body guides the spatial unfoldment of the genetic process.

5. At the quantum level of subatomic particles, all matter is literally frozen, particularized energy fields (i.e. frozen light). Complex aggregates of matter (i.e. molecules) are really specialized energy fields.

6. Just as light has a particular frequency or frequencies, so does matter have frequency characteristics as well. The higher the frequency of matter, the less dense, or more subtle the matter. The etheric body is composed of matter of a higher frequency than physical matter and so is referred to as subtle matter.

7. The universe itself may be a tremendous energy interference pattern with the same characteristics of a hologram. By decoding a small piece of the universal hologram, one may unfold information about the whole universe stored within the matrix. The selective focusing of consciousness via psychic attunement may hold the potential for such decoding of the universal hologram.

8. The movement of the life-force into the physiological/cellular systems is guided by the subtle patterns within the etheric body as well as by higher frequency inputs into the human energetic system. Various vibrational healing modalities, such as homeopathy, flower essences, and crystals, can influence these subtle patterns to improve human functioning and heal illness.

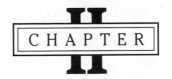

CHAPTER II

Newtonian vs. Einsteinian Medicine:
HISTORICAL PERSPECTIVES ON THE ART & SCIENCE OF HEALING

The state of the art in hospital medicine is synthetic drug therapy. This sophisticated approach to disease intervention is based on knowledge of Newtonian billiard-ball mechanics, molecular biology, drug receptor interactions, and pharmacokinetics. Presently, manmade agents are manufactured in test tubes and administered to patients in precisely calculated dosages. To evaluate a drug's effectiveness, doctors will look for precise relations between drug dosage and therapeutic patient responses. Scientific advances in pharmacological medicine have all but antiquated the use of once-common natural or herbal remedies.

The Newtonian model of synthetic drug therapy does allow physicians to make reliable predictions of drug behaviors and to eliminate certain side effects of natural remedies—but at what expense? Perhaps there are important energetic healing factors which have been left out in the scientific transformation of herbal medicine to drug therapy. Perhaps it is time to integrate the Einsteinian concept of matter as energy into our system of disease intervention. The Einsteinian view of matter as energy may present new reasons for re-examining the healing properties of the natural plants from which today's synthetic drugs were derived. To understand why medicine has remained focused on its present Newtonian level of modeling, it may be useful to examine the history and evolution of drug therapy from its earliest roots.

Herbal Medicine:
Drug Therapy's Earliest Beginnings

Contemporary physicians tend to view herbal medicine as a somewhat primitive approach to healing. The image of the herbalist envisioned by most scientific doctors is that of the traditional healer or "witch doctor." The true "jungle medicine" as practiced in tribal societies consists of administering various herbs and roots indigenous to the geographical region, as prescribed for specific maladies, by a traditional healer. Although this might be the nature of the healing arts in various primitive African tribes today, it also describes the way medicine was practiced by doctors in Europe and Asia for centuries.

Among the earliest known records describing the practice of herbal medicine is the *Pen Ts'ao*. This document, left by an ancient Chinese herbalist, dates back to the year 2800 B.C. and lists 366 plant drugs used to heal various ailments. Perhaps the most famous of the early herbal medical textbooks was the original *Materia Medica*. It was created in the first century A.D. by Pedanius Dioscorides, an army surgeon from Asia Minor.[1] In his book known as *De Materia Medica* (or "About Medicinal Trees"), Dioscorides attempted to organize all the current medical information on plant drugs into one informative text. Each entry concerning a particular plant gave a detailed account of the plant's medicinal properties, a small drawing of the plant, the ways the plant was to be prepared for administration, dosage suggestions, and possible toxicities.

From a historical perspective, herbal medicine lies at the very roots of modern drug therapeutics. Herbs contain various active chemicals that have particular physiologic effects relative to the amounts given. Many of the drugs in use today have their origins in well-known herbs used for treating illness by early healer/physicians. Scientific research in pharmacology has validated many of the beneficial therapeutic effects which have been attributed to commonly used herbs. Few people realize that common aspirin had its origins in herbal medicine. It is only recently that modern physicians have begun to comprehend the varied molecular mechanisms by which aspirin has its beneficial effects.

The prototype example of today's drugs borrowing from yesterday's herbal medicines is the foxglove leaf and its primary active agent, digitalis. Herbalists in the late 1700s knew that the foxglove plant was efficacious in the treatment of fluid retention due to heart disease. Later, twentieth-century scientists discovered that digitalis was the active ingredient in foxglove which endowed the plant with beneficial cardiac effects. By utilizing modern research techniques, doctors have come to understand the cellular and molecular effects that enable digitalis to assist the failing heart. Because of great strides in technology and organic chemistry, digitalis (or rather its its synthetic counterpart, digoxin) is now manufactured in test tubes and beakers. Modern doctors have dispensed with the plant source of digitalis in favor of the pure synthetic drug. Utilizing synthetic digoxin, exact dosages based on a patient's body weight and age may be given. Blood levels of the drug can be easily monitored for maximum therapeutic vs. toxic effects. In a sense, drug therapy is a cleaner form of herbal medicine. By isolating the active substances within known healing plants, the herbs themselves are replaced by pills and "potions" which contain synthetic versions of the active plant ingredients.

One criticism of the newer drug approach as compared to herbal medicine is that there are so many different substances present within the natural plant that it is sometimes hard to distinguish and isolate all of the physiologically therapeutic chemicals. When a patient takes a pill containing a single active drug, he or she might be missing out on further therapeutic benefits had he/she ingested the original healing plant. These extra ingredients contained within the herb may offer additional aid toward resolving the patient's illness. Unfortunately, there are few available research studies which compare herbal treatment of diseases with synthetic drugs derived from the same plants.

The drug proponents counter with an argument stating that there is considerable variability of active drug concentration within different samples of harvested plants. By giving a measured amount of pure drug, it is much easier to scientifically calculate and administer appropriate dosages for patients based upon various parameters, including age, weight, body surface area, etc. It is also easier to establish the predictability of drug effects as well as minimize toxicities when calculated amounts are given. Both schools of thought might have valid arguments if, in fact, they were only studying dosage-related drug effects. Homeopathy, an offshoot of herbal medicine, may suggest additional reasons why the primary plant can be more valuable than the chemically synthesized drug.

Homeopathic Medicine: A Radical Step Beyond Herbs

The discovery and development of homeopathic medicine is credited to Samuel Hahnemann (1755-1843), a brilliant German physician.[2] Because of his disillusionment and dissatisfaction with the medical approaches of his day, he developed a system of treatment based on the unique principle of "like cures like." This principle was found in early Greek medical writings and existed in the German folk medicine of Hahnemann's day. His new system of healing was based upon a discovery made concerning the effects of cinchona bark on malaria.

At the time that Hahnemann practiced, cinchona was the treatment of choice for malaria. One of the prime symptoms of malaria is intermittent fevers. Hahnemann experimented upon himself by taking multiple doses of cinchona for several days. To his surprise, the cinchona caused him to have all the symptoms of malarial intermittent fever. In other words, the treatment for malaria reproduced the symptoms of malaria in a healthy individual. It was this discovery that caused him to search through the various texts of medical literature of his day for information on the principle of "like cures like." This he later formalized into a concept known as the *Law of Similars*.

Hahnemann reasoned that cinchona worked to cure malaria because it created an artificial illness within the body, similar to malaria, which stimulated the body's own defense mechanisms into action. Such bodily defenses were activated by a principle known in the Hippocratic school of medicine as *Vis Medicatrix Naturae*. In translation, it might be referred to as "the healing powers of nature." If cinchona cured by the principle of "like cures like" (treating diseases with medicines known to reproduce the symptoms of the illness), then other drugs might be used in the same way once their actions upon a healthy person had been determined.

In current homeopathic vernacular, Hahnemann had conducted a drug "proving" of the plant substance, cinchona. Symptoms which appeared most frequently after ingesting cinchona were intermittent fevers. Therefore, intermittent fevers and other physical complaints induced by the drug established the proving of cinchona. Another term which has been used to describe this grouping of common symptoms is the homeopathic "drug picture." The drug picture is a portrait of an idealized person who has ingested the drug in question. It describes the total symptom complex of the individual including physical, emotional, and mental disturbances. Usually, the drug picture is the result of compiling the most frequent symptoms which have occurred among many individuals taking the drug. It is almost humorous to note that orthodox physicians would consider this a compiling of side effects as opposed to therapeutic associations! According to the Law of Similars, Hahnemann deduced that it was possible to cure a patient's illness by matching his symptom complex to the drug picture of a particular remedy. In order to treat a wide variety of illnesses which were present in the world, he would need to know the drug pictures of many different remedies. Hahnemann set out to establish reliable provings for other therapeutic substances in hopes of expanding his new system of treatment to other diseases.

While a professor at Leipzig University, Hahnemann instituted a series of provings whereby a group of healthy students (science's perennial guinea pigs) were given small doses of a particular plant or other substance, and their common reactions were recorded. Each student kept elaborate notes of their reactions: physical, emotional, and mental. The symptoms that appeared most frequently among many individuals taking the substance constituted a proving of the drug in question. Based upon the drug provings (common reactions found to each drug), a new *Materia Medica* began to evolve. *Indications for the healing use of a particular plant remedy was determined by the symptoms the plant induced in a healthy person.*

According to this new principle of "like cures like", cinchona was ideal for treating malaria because it reproduced malaria's symptoms in someone healthy. A homeopathic remedy was chosen to treat an illness based upon its ability to reproduce the patient's "total symptom complex" in an otherwise healthy person. This was not the same as adding together medicines that cumulatively reproduced all of the patient's symptoms. (This, we shall later see, is one of the primary differences between contemporary, or allopathic medicine, and homeopathic medicine).

One interesting note about the symptom complex pieced together by the prescribing homeopath is that mental and emotional symptoms were given equal or greater weight than physical symptoms. Modern physicians tend to do quite the opposite, attributing greater significance to physical than to emotional and mental symptoms. From this perspective, homeopathy was one of the first holistic medical disciplines that gave attention to alterations of both mind and body in a search for the appropriate cure.

On the basis of the Law of Similars, Hahnemann began to empirically treat patients. In each case, he selected a medicine based on the principle of giving the sick individuals a substance which would reproduce their symptoms in healthy persons. Often the individuals would experience an initial worsening of their symptoms (the so-called "healing crisis"), after which the illness resolved completely. This observation led Hahnemann to believe that his remedies produced an illness in the patient similar to the one already present, which stimulated the body's natural defenses.

Hahnemann treated many illnesses with great therapeutic success utilizing the principle of "like cures like". In the course of his medical research he made yet another discovery. After experimenting with diluting the remedies given to patients, he was surpised to find that *the greater the dilution, the more effective the medication!!* The process of repeated dilution seemed to make the remedies more potent. Hahnemann referred to this technique as "potentization." Very dilute solutions of homeopathic substance were used to coat tablets of milk sugar, which could then be ingested by patients. So dilute were his homeopathic remedies that in many of the medicines given, *there was not a single molecule of the original herb present!* Hahnemann's observation of greater efficacy from increasingly weaker concentrations would certainly contradict many of the accepted principles of dose-related effects in pharmacokinetics!

The ability of homeopathic drugs to have effectiveness without containing amounts of their substance necessary for measureable physiologic effects would seem to be impossible at first glance. Many allopathic doctors, in scoffing at the lack of theoretical efficacy in treating patients with such small drug doses, use the term "homeopathic dosage" in jest when referring to conventional medicines given in inadequately small doses for the "necessary" effects. Physicians' lack of belief in medicines that are of infinitesimal concentrations is based upon an even stronger belief in conventional principles of drug therapy and pharmacokinetics. Hahnemann's observations do not fit in with the Newtonian principles of action and reaction which underly current medical thinking. According to pharmacokinetic reasoning, one must have significant dosages of drugs to produce measureable, reproducible, physiologic effects. Conventional physicians have learned that for administered drugs to have therapeutic effects upon the body's cellular receptors, they must be given in dosages adequate to produce measureable blood levels.

It is possible for a substance of undetectable concentration to have effects upon the physical body. Homeopaths believe that microdoses interact with the human subtle energetic system which is so integrally related to the physical cellular structure. How this is possible is not well understood at this time even by the homeopathic physicians themselves. A possible rationale for how homeopathic medicines may work will be presented here, but first a bit of research on some seemingly unrelated subjects must be discussed. This material will give a background and foundation for the explanation of homeopathic energetic principles that will follow. By understanding the energetic mechanisms behind homeopathy, it will also be easier to comprehend how other "subtle energy" or "vibrational" medicines work. Surprisingly, we first need to delve into the subtle energetic properties of ordinary water, the most abundant substance on our planet.

The Wonders of Water: What Makes It All Possible

Water is a very special substance. It covers two-thirds of the surface of planet Earth. It also constitutes 99 percent of the molecules making up the human body. There is much known about the basic physical properties of water, but very little was known, until recently, about the subtle-energy properties of water. Much of the preliminary evidence for these special properties comes from studies on the effects of "laying on of hands healing" conducted in the 1960s. Of all the healing research carried out during that period, the most significant groundbreaking work was done at McGill University in Montreal by Dr. Bernard Grad.[3]

Grad was interested in finding out if psychic healers had real energetic effects upon patients, above and beyond what might be due to belief and "charisma." He wished to separate the physiologic effects of emotion (the so-called placebo effect) from true subtle energetic effects on living systems. To study this phenomenon, he created a series of experiments which substituted plant and animal subjects for human patients in order to eliminate the known effects of belief. Of greatest relevance here is Grad's work with barley seeds. To create a "sick plant patient," Grad soaked barley seeds in salty water, which is a known growth retardant. Rather than work directly with the seeds, Grad had a healer do a laying-on-of-hands treatment on a sealed container of salt water which was to be used for germinating the seeds. The barley seeds were placed by lab assistants in salt water taken from untreated or healer-treated water containers arbitrarily labelled "One" or "Two". Only Grad knew the correct identity of the salt-water bottles.

The seeds were separated into two groups, differing only in the salt water with which each group was initially treated. Following saline treatment, the seeds were placed in an incubator and studied for signs of germination and growth. Percent germination of seedlings was calculated and statistically compared between the two groups. Grad found that seeds ex-

posed to healer-treated water sprouted more often than those in the regular
saline group. Following germination, the seedlings were then potted and
placed in similar conditions of growth. At the end of several weeks, the
plants were statistically compared for height, leaf size, weight, and chlorophyll content. Grad discovered that plants watered with the healer-treated
water were of greater height and chlorophyll content. His experiment was
repeated a number of times in the same laboratory with similar positive
results. Following publication of Grad's work, other labs in the United
States had success in reproducing his results utilizing different healers.

Because of his success, Grad utilized the same experimental protocol
to test other subtle energetic effects upon seedling growth rate. Of particular
interest was Grad's success in stimulating the growth rate of plants utilizing water treated with common magnets! Although skeptical scientists
hypothesized that Grad's healer was cheating by palming magnets, sensitive magnetometers were unable to detect such fields around the healer's
hands. More recent studies by Dr. John Zimmerman, utilizing ultrasensitive SQUIDs (Superconducting Quantum Interference Devices) as magnetic measuring tools, have detected weak but significant increases in the
magnetic field emanations of healers' hands during the healing process.[4]
Although the signals emitted by healers' hands during healing were several
hundred times that of background noise, these levels of magnetism were
still significantly weaker than those produced by the magnets which Grad
was using in his experiments. (This finding will have great significance
when we later discuss the nature of healing energy.)

Another unusual variation thought up by Grad consisted of giving
water to psychiatric patients to hold. This same water was then used to treat
barley seeds. Interestingly enough, water energized by patients who were
severely depressed had the reverse effect of healer-treated water in that *it
suppressed the growth rate of seedlings!*

Because of the positive growth effects attributed to the healer-treated
water, Grad carried out chemical analysis on this water to see if energizing
had caused any measureable physical changes. There were significant
changes in infrared spectroscopy analyses of healer-treated water. This test
revealed that the atomic bond angle of the water had shifted slightly from
normal. Minor shifts in the molecular structure of healer-treated water also
produced decreased hydrogen bonding between water molecules. Testing
confirmed a significant decrease in the surface tension of healer-treated
water, a result of the altered hydrogen-bonding between the energized

water molecules. Curiously, magnet-treated water showed similar decreases in surface tension as well as positive effects in stimulating plant growth.[5] Studies by Douglas Dean and Edward Brame,[6] and more recently, Stephan Schwartz with Edward Brame and others,[7] have replicated Grad's findings of alterations in infrared spectroscopy and bond-angle changes in healer-treated water.

This material has been presented not so much for its relevance to psychic healing but because of the significance of these findings in illustrating the subtle energetic properties of water. This is a critical point which has been missed by most researchers familiar with these experiments on healing. It would appear that water can be "charged" with and then "store" various types of subtle energies. Subtle energy of both a beneficial and detrimental nature can be stored, as evidenced by Grad's studies utilizing healers and depressed patients. Treated water was able to induce measureable changes in plant physiology and growth, although there were no physical substances added to nor detected in the water. During the process of energizing, the healers had no physical contact with the water within the sealed flasks. Their hands were separated from the water by the glass walls of the containers.

These experiments on the subtle energetic properties of water have relevance in examining the known principles of drug therapy vs. the unknown mechanisms of homeopathy. According to modern pharmacokinetic theory, it is important to give patients a high-enough drug dosage to obtain therapeutic blood levels. Most drugs cause what are known as dose dependent effects. The higher the amount of drug given, the more potent the physiological effects. Conversely, in homeopathy, the more dilute the drug dosage the more powerful its effects. Drug solutions used to make homeopathic remedies are so dilute they are unlikely to contain even single molecules of the original substance, yet they appear to have powerful healing effects. This would seem to be paradoxical in view of the physical need for adequate numbers of drug molecules to achieve the desired therapeutic effect.

Although cases of successful treatments of illness using homeopathic remedies have not been presented here, many physicians have documented homeopathic cures of physical diseases.[8] Assuming that homeopathy does work, we are confronted with evidence that is unexplainable by the current cause-and-effect analysis of Newtonian dynamics as applied to pharmacology. The failure of the Newtonian theories to account for such observable, repeatable effects suggests that these theories are inadequate or incomplete. Returning to healer-treated water, we are presented with a case, similar to homeopathy, whereby a medicine containing no physical molecule of drug is able to have curative powers. Is it possible that there is something besides drug molecules in homeopathic and healer-treated solutions that offers therapeutic benefits? The Einsteinian or subtle energetic model may suggest reasons for the possible healing properties of such dilute molecular solutions.

A Subtle Energy Model for Healing with Homeopathy

In order to understand how homeopathy works, we must first analyze certain aspects of homeopathic theory and practice. It will also be necessary to reassess our current model(s) of illness and wellness. The best place to start is with the preparation of homeopathic remedies (as they are called by practitioners of this art).

The remedies are usually prepared by taking the primary plant (or other substance) and soaking it in alcohol. A drop of this tincture is removed and added to either 10 or 100 parts of water. (Dilutions using a 1:10 ratio are referred to in potencies of "X". Those using the ratio of 1:100 are called "C." This will become more clear momentarily.) The container of water and tincture is shaken forcefully in a process known as "succussion."

Diagram 7.
PREPARATION OF HOMEOPATHIC REMEDIES

		1/100	1/100	1/100	1/100	1/100
HERB + ALCOHOL		(H_2O)	(H_2O)	(H_2O)	(H_2O)	(H_2O)
MOLECULAR DILUTION	1:1	$1:10^2$	$1:10^4$	$1:10^6$	$1:10^8$	$1:10^{10}$
HOMEOPATHIC POTENCY	Mother Tincture	1C	2C	3C	4C	5C

INCREASING POTENCY OF REMEDIES

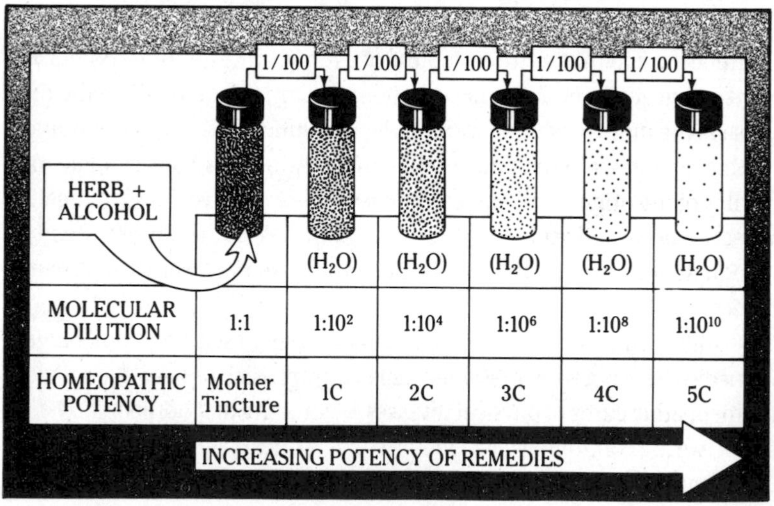

One drop of this dilution is removed and added to 10 or 100 parts of water (again depending on the system of concentration one is utilizing). The same ratio of dilution is always utilized. The mixture is again succussed and the process of dilution repeated again and again. This technique is referred to as "potentization." The reasoning behind the terminology is that homeopathic medicines which are increasingly dilute are considered more potent in their curative powers. Homeopathic remedies that are prepared in this fashion are said to be "potentized."

A solution that has been diluted 10 times using the 1:10 ratio is called 10X. A similar solution diluted 10 times using the 1:100 ratio is called 10C. (The true molecular concentration of a 10X strength is 10^{-10} or one ten-millionth. A 10C potency is actually 10^{-20}.) The resulting liquid is added to a bottle of sac lac (or milk sugar) tablets for administration to patients.

If one is using the 1:100 dilution method, then, after 12 series of dilutions, the homeopathic pharmacist arrives at a mixture with a concentration approximating 10^{-24}. Since the number of atoms in a mole (the molecular weight of a chemical substance in grams) is approximately 6×10^{23}, this means that the 12th dilution (or 12C potency) is unlikely to have even a single atom of the original substance present. Most homeopathic remedies go from the 10th to the thousandth dilution (from 10X or 10C to 1M, in homeopathic vernacular) utilizing the aforementioned potentization process. Homeopathic practitioners find that the higher the dilution, the more potent the remedy. In other words, a 100X potency is felt to be stronger than a 10X potency remedy. Paradoxically, the higher the homeopathic potency, the less likely one is to find even a single molecule of the original substance. (This point aggravates drug-oriented thinkers to no end, for how can one atom of drug have any significant physiologic effects on the human body?)

Let us examine the process of homeopathic remedy preparation from what we have just extrapolated about the subtle-energy properties of water. We know that water is able to extract and store certain types of subtle energies which have measurable effects on living systems. Grad's studies with healer-treated water showed this quite elegantly. In the process of homeopathic potentization, the progressive dilution removes molecular elements of the physical plant and leaves only the subtle energetic qualities of the plant within the water. The active part of the remedy is, in fact, not even physical, as our mathematical argument has demonstrated. Homeopathic remedies are subtle-energy medicines which contain the energetic frequency or "vibrational signature" of the plant from which they have been prepared.

How then do these "vibrational remedies" have their effects upon sick individuals? In order to understand that, we must re-examine what comprises sickness from an energetic standpoint. Hahnemann had reasoned that homeopathic remedies worked by creating an artificial illness (similar to the one he wished to treat) within the body in order to stimulate the natural defenses. A purely physical extrapolation of this technique underlies the process of immunization, whereby trace amounts of a virus or viral component are given to an individual to stimulate their immunity against a particular illness. Instead of causing a physical cellular reaction as in the case of immunization, homeopathic remedies may act by inducing a vibrational mode of illness. How can this vibrational mode cause a sick person to move from a state of illness to wellness? To comprehend the rationale behind this type of energetic therapy, we must explore the concepts of illness and wellness from principles gleaned about the energetic structure of the human body as discussed in the first chapter of this book.

As you will recall, the physical body is associated with a holographic energy template known as the "etheric" body.[9] This energetic matrix contains structural data that encodes information about the morphology and function of the organism. Our etheric template is a growth pattern that directs cellular processes from a higher energetic level. Certain lines of research, to be discussed in greater detail later, suggest that changes in the etheric body *precede* manifestations of disease in the physical body.[10]

Abnormal structuring in the etheric template eventually leads to disruptive changes at the cellular level of the physical body. Therefore, physical illness may begin first at the etheric level before physical cellular changes have even started. Impaired host resistance to infections, and cancer, may be partially due to subtle energetic weakness of the system at the etheric and higher levels.

Based upon this assumption, a truly preventative medicine would be based upon analysis of dysfunctional changes in the etheric body *before* they became crystallized as physical illness. Medicine will only assume this direction when science has developed acceptable diagnostic tools that will allow doctors to accurately observe and characterize changes in the etheric body. Kirlian photography and its derivatives may yet express this futuristic diagnostic potential in medicine. Since diseases of the physical body begin at the etheric level, might not also therapy begin at that level too? It may be possible to treat physical illness by correcting abnormal etheric patterns.

Because it is composed of matter, the physical body has both particle and wave-like properties. The light-like properties of matter confer unique frequency characteristics to our physical and etheric bodies. For the sake of simplicity, let us assume that an individual's physical body, when healthy, resonates with one dominant energetic frequency or vibration. As an example, let us assign a frequency of 300 Hz (cycles per second) to John Q. Public. When Mr. Public is sick, it is reasonable to assume that his energetic homeostatic mechanisms will try to return his system to normal if at all possible.

Assuming that Mr. Public has been infected with a dose of pathogenic bacteria, he may exhibit fever and chills. Over the years, doctors have had mixed opinions as to the positive or negative significance of symptoms such as fevers. At one time, fevers were felt to be beneficial in allowing the patient to discharge the toxicities of illness in a type of healing crisis. (Some misguided doctors have even given malaria to individuals with other illnesses in hopes of inducing a febrile healing crisis!) Later, fevers were felt to be bad for the system, and drugs such as aspirin were given to take away the fever.

From a purely cellular/physiologic standpoint, it now appears that fevers can be good for an individual with a bacterial illness. It has been shown that the white blood cells, our immunologic defenders, eat and destroy bacteria more efficiently at higher body temperatures. (White blood cells have recently been found to release a substance called "leukocyte pyrogen" which *induces* high fevers.) The point of this discussion about fevers is that such symptoms may be produced by the body as an adaptive strategy toward returning the system to a state of homeostatic balance and health.

From an energetic standpoint, one might consider that an individual such as John Q. Public, afflicted with his "cold," would be resonating at a different frequency than the one to which he is normally attuned (300 Hz). Let us assume that the frequency Mr. Public "vibrates at" when trying to throw off his cold is 475 Hz. If he were able to produce more energy at the 475 Hz level, he might be able to throw off his illness more quickly and return to good health.

Hahnemann, with his homeopathic reasoning, assumed that the remedies were producing an illness similar to the one that the body was trying to throw off. He tried to empirically match the symptoms produced by a remedy's proving with the illness he was attempting to treat. Is it possible that when a healthy individual is given a particular homeopathic remedy, the proving (or symptoms exhibited) is caused by an induction of the individual's energy field to resonate at the dominant frequency of the plant substance used to prepare the remedy? According to this rationale, each species of plant should have its own particular energy signature. This energetic signature may be complex, formed by a multiplexing of various frequencies. Different parts of the plant, such as the bark of a tree, may have different energetic signatures than either its roots, leaves, or flowers. *In giving homeopathic preparations of the plant, the physical drug properties of the herb are removed, leaving the subtle-energy qualities that are absorbed into the water to predominate.*

What Hahnemann may have actually been doing is empirically *matching the frequency of the plant extract with the frequency of the illness.* He did this by matching the physical and emotional symptoms of the patient's illness with known symptoms produced by the remedy. Physical observation of the patient was, after all, the only diagnostic maneuver available to doctors in Hahnemann's time, prior to the advent of modern blood counts and multiphasic screening profiles. Matching the *total symptom pattern* of the patient with the complex of symptoms produced by a particular remedy was an ingenious method, albeit unknown to Hahnemann, of energetic frequency matching. Using the Law of Similars, Hahnemann was able to give the patient a dose of the needed subtle energy in the exact frequency band needed. That is why in classical homeopathy one cannot mix different remedies to treat many different symptoms. The remedy that best expresses the patient's unique symptom complex will be curative. Comparison of the patient's symptom complex with a remedy's symptom complex allows the homeopathic physician to make an empirical frequency match that will neutralize the illness.

Homeopathic energy theory suggests that humans are somewhat like the electrons of an atom. Electrons within an atom occupy energy shells or spatial domains which are known as orbitals. Each orbital possesses certain frequency and energetic characteristics depending upon the type and molecular weight of the atom. In order to excite or move an electron into the next highest orbital, one needs to deliver to it energy of a specific frequency. Only a quantum of the exact energetic requirements will cause the electron to jump to a higher orbital. This is also known as the principle of resonance, in which tuned oscillators will only accept energy in a narrow frequency band. Through the process of resonance, energy of the proper frequency will excite the electron to move to a higher level or energy state in its orbit around the nucleus.

Human beings may be similar to electrons in that their energetic sub-components occupy different vibrational modes, which we might call health orbits and disease orbits. For the human being whose energetic systems are in an orbit of dis-ease, only subtle energy of the proper frequency will be accepted to shift the body into a new orbit or steady-state of health. Homeopathic remedies are able to deliver that needed quantum of subtle energy to the human system through a type of resonance induction. This ethereal energy injection moves the system from the sickness vibrational mode to the orbit of health.

Homeopathy's energetic frequency boost is the probable reason behind the initial exacerbation of symptoms seen by physicians when the proper remedy is given. (This so-called "healing crisis" usually occurs prior to complete resolution of the illness.) Patients are given a frequency-specific dose of subtle energy that will help their bodies to resonate in the needed mode in order to return their systems to a state of health or wellness. The healing vibrational mode, enhanced by the remedy, causes the exaggerated symptoms of the illness which are experienced by the patient during the healing crisis. Homeopathy uses the diverse frequency spectrum of nature to discharge the toxicities of illness. This method allows order and equilibrium to be restored to the human energetic system. *From the frequency specific viewpoint of homeopathy, it has been stated that "there exist the treatments for ALL of our ills within Nature."*

This also brings up an interesting point alluded to earlier in the chapter when we referred to the conflicts between homeopathic and allopathic Medicine. It was Hahnemann who originally coined the terms allopathy and homeopathy.[11] As we have seen, homeopathy, from the Greek meaning "like treatment of disease", is based upon the Law of Similars, whereby an individual is given a treatment that produces symptoms "similar" to the illness. Allopathy, from the Greek "allos" meaning "other" treatment of disease, refers to giving remedies not based upon the homeopathic rationale. Allopathy, although truly meaning "systems of healing other than homeopathy," has come to be synonymous with drug-oriented "establishment medicine".

From a simplistic perspective, let us examine the difference between the allopathic and homeopathic treatment of the common cold. Because colds are frequently associated with fevers, coughs, and runny noses, an allopathic physician would prescribe a fever-reducing antipyretic (such as aspirin), a decongestant (such as Actifed), and a cough suppressant (such as a codeine-containing syrup). Of course, each of these modern remedies are, in fact, combinations of many individual drugs in a single mixture. The homeopathic physician, on the other hand, would prescribe a single agent: in this case Allium cepa (latin for "red onion"). Provings of Allium cepa have indicated that, in healthy individuals, it produces a dry cough, watery eyes, sneezing, runny nose, and other familiar cold-related symptoms. However, if Allium cepa is given to an individual who already has those cold symptoms, the patient experiences an almost immediate relief and abatement of the cold.

One sees obvious differences between the multiple-drug approach or "polypharmacy" of contemporary allopathic medicine, and the succinct single agent treatments of homeopathy. *Homeopathy aims to match the correct single remedy with the totality of the patient*. This includes not only *physical*, but *emotional* and *mental* symptoms as well. This allows for the closest "vibrational match" between illness and cure. Because of its attention to disturbances of both mind and body, homeopathy could be considered one of the first truly holistic approaches in medicine. This example of the treatment of the common cold highlights the philosophical differences between giving multiple drugs that work at the cellular level and single vibrational agents that work at a subtle energetic level.

From the perspective of the physical and etheric body, it is not entirely clear at what level the homeopathic remedy has its initial or primary effect. Certain sources of information suggest that homeopathic remedies are somewhat "physical" in their direct energetic effects upon the molecular structure of the physical body. It is possible that Kirlian and other electrographic techniques may eventually prove useful in studying the effects of homeopathic remedies on the etheric and physical bodies.

Homeopathic remedies represent an alternative evolutionary pathway in the application of medicinal plant therapies. Where pharmacologists chose to isolate single, active molecular agents from herbs, homeopaths worked with the vibrational essence of the whole plant substance. The homeopathic preparation process liberates from the plants the subtle energetic qualities to charge water, from which they are then transferred to milk sugar tablets for individualized dosage. Thus homeopathic remedies differ from pharmacologic agents in that they are "etherealized" medicines. The gross molecular nature of the physical plant has been separated from its subtle energetic or ethereal qualities using the intermediate storage medium of water. This is why the higher the dilution the more potent the homeopathic remedy. The higher the homeopathic potency the lower the molecular content and, thus, the more ethereal the characteristics of the remedy.

Another vibrational approach which represents a radical offshoot from herbal medicine is based on the administration of flower essences. As with homeopathic remedies, the preparation of these essences is dependent upon the subtle energetic storage properties of water. Flower essences also utilize the subtle properties of sunlight to imprint upon the medium of water the vibrational qualities of the flowers. The essences are used in a different manner than homeopathic remedies and have energetic effects at much higher levels than we have examined thus far. (Flower essences and their effects will be covered in a separate chapter at the end of the book.) Practitioners who use flower essences prescribe according to different principles of vibrational medicine than the Law of Similars which guides the judgment of homeopathic practitioners. Because they may work at higher energetic levels, flower essences of a given plant often have very different therapeutic effects than homeopathic remedies prepared from leaves of the same plant. This tends to confirm the hypothesis that different parts of the same plant may contain different energetic qualities.

A key concept to remember when discussing homeopathic remedies and flower essences is that the diversity of nature holds many healing agents which we have yet to discover and fully research. Drug therapy has become the more scientifically acceptable offshoot of herbal medicine because it is based on a Newtonian rationale of molecular interactions. The problem with validating energetic mechanisms of homeopathic agents is that the subtle energies which are responsible for their therapeutic effects are difficult to measure with present-day medical technologies. Also, in order to understand the effectiveness of homeopathic remedies in treating illness, one must accept a subtle energetic philosophy of dis-ease and health. The fact that orthodox medicine can only accept hard medical data and conventional models of pathophysiology makes it difficult for modern physicians to understand how microdoses of anything can be therapeutically effective.

Utilizing the principle of potentization via dilution and succussion, one can make homeopathic remedies from nearly any substance, either organic or inorganic. The subtle-energy absorption properties of water make it possible to extract specific vibrational qualities that may be used to coat milk sugar tablets for later administration to patients. Many remedies in use by homeopathic physicians are actually derived from inorganic substances. Each remedy contains the specific vibrational qualities of the primary material in a potentized form for homeopathic treatment. The Law of Similars is used by physicians to match the patient's complaints with a remedy producing the same symptoms. In this manner, the homeopathic physician is able to empirically obtain the best vibrational frequency match between patient and cure. Only the correct frequency match will be effective in homeopathy. By supplying the proper frequency of subtle energy, the homeopathic remedy causes the energetic systems of the body to resonate in the correct vibrational mode. When the body is thus energetically activated, it is assisted in discharging the toxicity of illness.

> Homeopathic remedies usually come from denser inorganic material, while flower essences have a much higher concentration of the life force. Homeopathic remedies often vibrationally duplicate the physical disease in a person to push that imbalance out of the body. Homeopathy integrates into the subtle bodies but still functions upon the vibrational level of the molecular structure. Homeopathy is a bridge between traditional medicine and vibrational medicine.[12]

What is important is that a model for understanding "alternative" medical therapies is beginning to evolve. The spiritual scientist's comprehension of the functioning of these systems of healing will be dependent upon a working knowledge of human subtle energetic anatomy. The etheric body is only one of many levels of input into our subtle-energy systems. Because these subtle components are intimately linked with the physical body, therapies that impact at higher energetic levels will eventually funnel down to affect the physical cellular structure.

The Newtonian model of medicine does not account for, nor believe in, these other energetic systems. It is much easier to deny the effectiveness of alternative systems of healing because they do not make rational scientific sense, than it is to extend an outdated model of understanding to incorporate higher energetic phenomena. The Einsteinian model of matter as an energy field gives us a framework in which we may realistically view and comprehend these subtle-energy systems. Phenomena such as laying-on-of-hands healing and homeopathic medicine present science with repeatable observations that cannot entirely be explained away. They cannot all be hoax and delusion as the scientific critics would have us believe.

One cannot evoke the placebo effect to explain every unscientific healing interaction. The placebo effect demonstrates hidden healing powers of the mind (dependent upon belief) that are vastly underrated by physicians. Dr. Grad's work showed that the effects of belief could be separated from actual subtle-energy events taking place between healer and patient. Although not known by many, Grad's work on laying-on-of-hands healing was recognized, and Grad was given an award by the CIBA Foundation: paradoxically, a scientific organization funded by a major pharmaceutical company!

It is only within the last few decades that technology has evolved to the point where enlightened scientists such as Dr. Grad have begun the process of validating and measuring the energetics of these subtle-energy systems. With time and effort, they will be able to dispel the aura of delusion that enshrouds practitioners of these vibrational therapies. It will be the task of the remainder of this book to provide that framework of understanding by which homeopathy, and even stranger systems of healing, may be accepted and acknowledged for their contributions to the greater understanding of humans as multidimensional beings.

Key Points to Remember

1. The pharmacokinetic approach utilizes measured doses of drugs to influence the physical/cellular systems of the body. The pharmacokinetic model is based on Newtonian mechanistic interactions at the molecular level, as typified by dose-related drug-receptor binding at the cell membrane.

2. The homeopathic approach utilizes minute quantities of medicinal substances to create therapeutic physiological changes through subtle-energy field interactions.

3. In homeopathic remedies, the energetic signature of the medicinal substance is first transferred to a solvent, such as water, then to a neutral pill of milk sugar. It is the vibrational signature of the substance and not its molecular properties which are utilized for healing benefits.

4. In homeopathy, the more dilute a remedy's molecular concentration, the greater its potency. This is in direct contrast to the phar-

macokinetic/drug model, in which there is a greater potency with higher molecular concentrations.

5. Homeopathy is based upon the Law of Similars, whereby a remedy is chosen for its ability to reproduce the symptoms of the sick person in a normal healthy individual. By matching the symptom complex of the patient with the known "drug picture" of the remedy, a correct vibrational match between patient and remedy is achieved.

6. In homeopathy, a remedy is chosen for its ability to stimulate and rebalance the physical body through supplying a needed frequency of subtle energy. If the remedy's frequency matches the patient's illness state, a resonant transfer of energy will allow the patient's bioenergetic system to effectively assimilate the needed energy, throw off the toxicity, and move to a new equilibrium point of health.

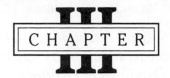

CHAPTER III

*The Earliest Beginnings of
Medical Energetic Approaches:*
THE BIRTH OF
VIBRATIONAL MEDICINE

Within certain subspecialties of conventional medicine, the groundwork for a shift from the Newtonian pharmacokinetic approach to an Einsteinian view of pure energetic healing is presently being formulated. This permutation from conventional drug and surgical therapy to electromagnetic healing represents the beginnings of a revolution in consciousness for the medical profession. In the New Age that is nearly upon us, healer / physicians will begin to comprehend that the human organism is a series of interacting multidimensional energy fields.

Energetic perspectives on living systems will provide the necessary evolutionary impetus for great strides in medical understanding of the higher dimensions of human health and illness. New methods of faster diagnosis will become available. Specialized systems of energetic healing will be designed that will prove more effective and less toxic to the human body than presently accepted drug and surgical approaches. Doctors have moved slowly and cautiously in advancing the medical understanding of human beings from old Newtonian "nuts and bolts" models to an electromagnetic appreciation of life. To appreciate the transition in medical thinking from the Newtonian to the Einsteinian viewpoint, we must trace the historical development of electromagnetic applications in medicine.

The Discovery & Development of X-Rays: Early Medical Models of Using Energy for Diagnosis & Treatment

One discovery that aided modern medicine, and opened new windows on a more penetrating observation of human anatomy, was the diagnostic application of x-rays. X-rays provided a critical look into a previously unseen world within the human body. Along with the development of diagnostic x-ray equipment has come the evolution of our understanding of electromagnetic radiation biophysics. Early experimentation with electromagnetic fields caused researchers to shift their focus from a world of physico-chemical cellular reactions to one of biological systems in continuous interaction with a radiational environment. The application of x-rays in diagnosis made the utilization of electromagnetic fields in medicine a commonplace procedure. X-rays allowed us to extend our vision into a new frequency realm, thus extending the sensitivities of our perceptive abilities beyond their normal ranges.

Yet along with this tremendous gift for peering into the human structure came the destructive side effects of radiation. Ironically, Madame Curie, who first gave the world radium, died from radiation poisoning. Eventually, though, x-rays were put to therapeutic use and have become a powerful tool against diseases such as cancer. A whole new world of therapeutic radiology (and its subspecialty, radiation oncology) has evolved from these early beginnings. Therapeutic radiology is a discipline which is based on the knowledge of how electromagnetic radiation affects living cells. In such applications as the treatment of cancer, the question of cell damage is a critical one. For physicians to deliver a therapeutic dose of radiation to a malignant tumor, they must know not only the effects of the energy on the cancer, but also the radiation tolerance of the surrounding normal tissue cells.

The search for ways of targeting this energy specifically to abnormal cells has pushed radiation oncologists to look for more exotic systems of energy delivery. From the simple cobalt machine to the linear accelerator, new ways of delivering therapeutic doses of energy to the body have become more and more sophisticated. But x-rays are only a part of the transition in medicine toward utilizing energy in healing. An exploration of the therapeutic uses of electricity furthers our model of the understanding and treatment of human beings from an energetic perspective.

Electrotherapy:
From Suppressing Pain to Healing Fractures

The use of electricity for therapy is not new to medicine. People have attempted to use electricity for healing since ancient times. Several old medical texts, for example, listed the use of electrical fishes and eels as accepted forms of medical therapy. Prescribed treatment involved applying the electrical fish directly to the patient's body. The crude but effective delivery of an electrical discharge to the human body was felt to have therapeutic value in a variety of conditions. Only within the twentieth century has electricity become so readily available that its therapeutic applications could be extensively explored.

One application of electrotherapy which has recently come of age is the use of electrical stimulation for the relief of pain. Early devices such as Dorsal Column Stimulators, designed by Dr. Norman Shealy,[1] a neurosurgeon in Wisconsin, were implanted within the spinal cords of patients with intractable pain syndromes. One might consider this a combined Newtonian (surgical) and Einsteinian (energetic) approach. The dorsal columns are long nerve tracts within the spinal cord that transmit pain and sensory information from the body to the brain. The generally accepted reasoning behind the effectiveness of these spinal electrostimulators relates to a theory proposed for the understanding of acupuncture analgesia. The so-called "Gate Control Theory," proposed by Melzack and Wall,[2] suggests that acupuncture stimulation of peripheral nerves, at a level *above* the entry of the pain impulse into the spinal cord, causes the closing of a pain-relay gate. Electrical nerve impulses traversing this "gate" carry ascending pain and sensory information to the brain. By shutting the gate, the pain impulses are blocked from making their normal ascent to the central nervous system where they are interpreted. The Dorsal Column Stimulator, when placed on the spinal cord at a level above the entry of the pain impulses, was said to close the gate electrically and block further ascension of pain messages to the brain.

Spinal cord electrostimulation was carried one step further with the creation of therapeutic systems known as TNS devices or Transcutaneous Nerve Stimulators. Based on the same principle as the Gate Control Theory, these electrical devices produce weak electrical pulses that go to skin electrodes, stimulating cutaneous nerves that carry sensory information, via the spinal cord, to the brain. Rather than interacting with the gate mechanism through a spinally-implanted system, the TNS devices accomplish pain-gate closure through stimulation of cutaneous nerves which enter the spinal cord at levels above the entry of the noxious pain impulses. Applying external electrical currents to the skin presents a safer and simpler procedure for pain control than having to perform a neurosurgical procedure. The TNS electrostimulators provide purely energetic treatment for symptoms of physical pain in a way that goes beyond conventional drugs and surgery.

A curious discovery arose from basic research into TNS control of pain. Researchers reported that the weak electrical currents which were applied to the skin could give more efficient pain control if the electrodes were applied to specialized areas of the skin. These special areas turned out to be classical acupuncture points where traditional acupuncture needle stimulation similarly produced analgesia or pain relief. It has since been demonstrated that acupuncture analgesia is at least partially mediated by the release, within the nervous system, of natural pain-killing substances known as *endorphins*.[3]

Endorphins, or endogenously generated morphines, are the brain's own opium-like pain killers. These chemicals, only discovered in the mid-1970s, were found to have powerful effects in suppressing pain. The reason that drugs like morphine and heroin have pain-killing effects on the nervous system is that they bind to specialized "opiate" or endorphin receptors within the brain. Many opiate receptors are found along pathways in the brain that carry pain messages. Activation of these receptors by internally generated endorphins or externally administered narcotics will have the same effect of inhibiting the transmission of pain signals to the central nervous system. Narcotic antagonists such as naloxone are, in turn, able to inhibit the effects of endorphins by blocking their ability to bind to these opiate receptors. Experiments have shown that endorphin-blocking agents like naloxone reduce the effectiveness of acupuncture needle-induced analgesia as well as the pain-relieving effects of *low frequency* electrostimulation of acupuncture points. This would suggest that pain relief achieved by classical needle acupuncture and electrostimulation of acupuncture points involves the release of endorphins within the nervous system. Endorphins do not tell the entire story, however. Interestingly, *high frequency* electrical stimulation of acupuncture points for pain relief seems to be relatively *unaffected by naloxone,* but is inhibited by the administration of serotonin antagonists.

Spinal gate mechanisms and manipulation of neurochemicals, such as endorphins and serotonin, add further pieces toward solving the complex puzzle of electrotherapy's success in suppressing pain. Such electrical approaches attempt to activate the body's unique mechanisms for self-healing and pain control. Whatever the explanation, specialized modulation and targeting of electricity through TNS systems demonstrates physicians' growing ability to manipulate a wide spectrum of electromagnetic energies for healing and relief of suffering.

Perhaps the most revolutionary application of electrotherapy is in stimulating the body's innate capacity for tissue regeneration. Research pioneered by Dr. Robert O. Becker, an orthopedic surgeon in New York, has revealed fascinating information about how electrical currents within the nervous system mediate tissue repair and regeneration. The most widespread application of this research has been in the area of accelerated healing of bone fractures by externally applied electromagnetic fields.

Becker's original work dealt with a phenomenon known as the "current of injury." An example of this current of injury is the electrical potential that can be measured across the stump of an amputated limb in an experimental animal. Becker found that he could surgically remove a limb from a test animal and measure changes in the electrical potential on subsequent days of wound healing and repair. In studying the complex process of tissue regeneration, Becker examined the differences in repair mechanisms between salamanders and frogs. Because frogs and salamanders are an evolutionary stage apart, salamanders can regrow whole new limbs from the remaining amputated stump, whereas frogs cannot. Frogs appear to have lost this evolutionary potential somewhere along their genetic ascendance on the amphibian family tree. Becker was intensely interested in slight electrical differences between the current of injury measured in stumps of salamanders that could regrow new arms and in the frog counterparts that could not.

Becker surgically amputated the arms of salamanders and frogs and then used electrodes to measure the electrical potential at the point of tissue healing. The frogs showed a positive electrical potential which gradually drifted with time to a neutral or zero potential as the stump healed over. The salamanders, however, after producing an initial positive potential similar to the frogs, *showed a reverse in polarity to negative potential.* This negative injury potential gradually drifted back to zero over a period of days as the salamander regrew an entirely new limb.

Diagram 8.
MONITORING THE CURRENT OF INJURY
IN EXPERIMENTAL AMPUTATION

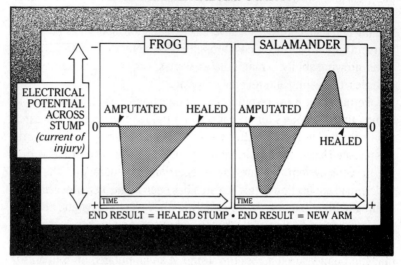

The only apparent difference between the two injury currents was that the salamander, who could regrow a new limb, showed a swing in potential from positive to negative. Becker wondered if artificially delivering a negative potential across the frog's healing stump would affect the outcome. This he did, and, to his surprise, *the frog grew an entirely new limb!*[4]

The idea of using electrostimulation to regrow new limbs or organs is a revolutionary one. Whether the electrical stimulation primarily affects cellular-based repair mechanisms or whether it is possibly releasing the holographic potential of the etheric body cannot be said for certain at this time. Becker has attempted to utilize Kirlian recording techniques to photograph the animal analogue of the Phantom Leaf Effect in animal limbs following amputation. Unfortunately, his attempts in this area have been unsuccessful to date. Possible reasons for this will be explored later in this book when we take a closer look at the implications of Kirlian photographic systems.

Becker's work has also uncovered new mechanisms of information transmission within the nervous system that may be part of a healing feedback loop. This system seems to involve the glial and Schwann cell network that surrounds most of the nerves throughout the body. The Schwann cells form an insulative sheath around most peripheral nerves. The bodies of the

Schwann cells are separated by tiny gaps at regular intervals (known as nodes of Ranvier) along which action potentials are propagated. (Action potentials are the electrical nerve impulses which travel along nerve fibers, or axons, to relay messages.) Glial and Schwann cells were originally thought to be strictly nutritive to the nearby nerves. But Becker's work suggests that both types of cells may be information transmitters. Becker's studies also indicate that the information is transmitted along the glial and Schwann cells via slow analog changes in direct current rather than via rapid changes in the digital pulse code of action potentials as traditionally observed in nerve transmission.[4,5]

The significant research findings of Dr. Becker, and more recently Dr. Andrew Bassett,[6] have resulted in the widespread application of electromagnetic devices to accelerate the healing of fractured bones. Early animal studies utilized surgical implantation of electrodes into the limbs of horses with broken bones. The bone electrodes, connected to special power supplies, pulsed weak electrical currents across the fracture site. The resulting remarkable healings of difficult fractures in animals have led to successful human applications, especially in situations where amputation of a limb for nonunion of fractures (lack of bone mending) was the only alternative. As in the case of the Dorsal Column Stimulator, the surgical implantation of electrodes was shown to be unnecessary. The external application of weak electromagnetic fields across the fracture site (actually placed over the plaster cast) appears to be all that is needed to get the desired healing outcome. Specialized electrodes are worn over the cast, usually during sleep, for periods of weeks to months until x-rays show complete healing.

Some of the remarkable findings which have emerged from these studies in tissue regeneration have shed new light on "energetic" cellular mechanisms of healing and repair. Becker has been a pioneer in the newly developing field of "bioelectronics." He looks at cellular mechanisms from the perspective of electronics and cybernetic systems, and has found that at the level of the single cell, microcrystalline and other cellular sub-elements may be involved in the modulation of intracellular electrical currents in a way similar to semiconductor circuitry. Certain cellular elements, such as membranes, can be seen to act as capacitors. Other internal structures, including mitochondria with their electron transport chains, can be viewed as tiny batteries or electrical power sources. The implication is that there may be electronic switching and transmission systems within and between cells.

Under present biological conditions, development in living bodies from earliest inception follows unicellular semiconductivity, as a living piezoelectric matrix. Primitive basic tissues (glia, satellite and Schwann cells) are supportive to the neurons in the human system where the primary source is electrical. This has been especially shown in bone growth response to mechanical stress, and to fractures which have been demonstrated to have characteristics of control systems using electricity.

The stimulation of cartilage regeneration by current-magnetic injection, the restoration of partial limb regeneration by small direct currents, the stimulation of bone growth by electrical fields, the inhibition of growth of implanted tumors in mammals by electrical currents, are all a part of Electromedicine. Electromedicine is the science which harnesses the cellular electrophysiological energies by using the right electromagnetic field.[7]

The controls for cellular replication may also involve these bioelectronic switching mechanisms. Cancer is a prime example of a disorder in which cellular replication has gone awry, with massive overproduction of abnormal tumor cells. Studies of electrical effects on implanted tumors (melanoma B-16) in mice at Mount Sinai School of Medicine have suggested that electrical currents may enhance cancer-killing effects of conventional chemotherapy. Mice with melanoma that were exposed to special electrical currents and chemotherapy survived nearly twice as long as cancer-ridden mice given chemotherapy alone.[8] Albert Szent-Gyorgyi, the discoverer of Vitamin C, is exploring the implications of the bioelectronic model in understanding cancer. Szent-Gyorgi feels that the problem with cancer is not that cells are replicating themselves, since replication is natural. The abnormality of cancer cells may lie within faulty electronic switching mechanisms which cannot turn off the replicating process. The mouse melanoma experiments suggest that electrical currents and electromagnetic fields may be able to manipulate these abnormal electronic switching mechanisms in an energetic approach to treating cancer.

Another researcher of electrotherapeutic approaches to cancer is Dr. Bjorn Nordenstrom, head of Diagnostic Radiology at Stockholm's Karolinska Institute. Over the last several decades, Dr. Nordenstrom has been exploring the use of specially applied electrical currents to treat cancer. In a limited number of patients, Dr. Nordenstrom has been successful in producing complete remission from various types of cancers metastatic to the lung.[9,10] Additionally, Nordenstrom is recognized as one of the world pioneers in x-ray guided needle biopsies of the lung. He utilizes similar x-ray techniques to assist the placement of platinum needle electrodes into isolated lung tumors. Electrical currents up to ten volts are then delivered to the platinum electrodes for varying periods of time. Utilizing this system of electrotherapy, Nordenstrom has been able to produce tumor regression and complete remission in a significant number of cases considered untreatable by other cancer therapies.

Nordenstrom has postulated a number of mechanisms to explain why electrotherapy may be successful in destroying tumors. He discovered that white blood cells carry a negative electrical charge. These tumor-fighting lymphocytes, he suggests, are drawn to the site of the cancer by the positive electrical charge of the platinum electrode in the center of the metastatic lesion. A second negative electrode is placed into normal tissue adjacent to the tumor. The resulting electrical field induces ionic tissue changes and buildup of acids in the local environment of the tumor which are detrimental to the cancer cells. These effects are similar to the acid buildup on the electrodes of a car battery. The increased acidity also locally destroys red blood cells, or damages their hemoglobin, thus depriving the cancer cells of life-giving oxygen. Additionally, Nordenstrom postulates that the positive electrical field moves water out of the tumor, shrinks it, and swells the surrounding tissue. This swollen tissue puts pressure on local blood vessels and blocks the flow of blood to the tumor.

Dr. Nordenstrom feels that bioelectrical circuits are part of an undiscovered circulatory system in the body. These natural electrical circuits become switched on by injury, infections, tumors, and even by the normal activity of the body's organs. Electrical currents course through arteries and veins and across capillary walls while drawing white blood cells and metabolic compounds into and out of surrounding tissues. Nordenstrom has built up his theories around a sophisticated look at the current of injury, a phenomenon that has also interested Dr. Becker and others. Nordenstrom, like other bioenergetic researchers, agrees that disturbances in the bioelectrical network of the body may be involved in the development of cancer and other diseases.

New models for understanding illness, such as the bioelectronic model, may provide unique new ways of reversing the processes of disease by intervening at a primary, causative, cellular level. Although it is somewhat similar to the allopathic model of drug/receptor interaction, the bioelectronic model may provide purely energetic methods of treating illness at the cellular level. Is it possible that electromagnetic fields, as applied to healing bone fractures, killing tumor cells, and regenerating tissue, may work by invoking the naturally existing bioelectronic mechanisms of defense and repair within cells? At least at a physical tissue level, this is likely to be the case.

Interestingly, the frequency of energy utilized for treatment appears to be a critical element for successful therapy. Regarding the healing of fractured bones, researchers have found that the frequency of the pulsed electromagnetic fields to which the bone is exposed is a key factor. Even a tiny shift in frequency can mean the difference between having the osteocytes in a bone lay down new calcium matrix or reabsorb and remove bone. Thus, a slight shift in the energetic frequency delivered can either strengthen or break down bone tissue.

In addition to using electromagnetic fields for reducing pain, shrinking tumors, and accelerating the mending of broken bones, there are additional treatment approaches which utilize pure magnetic fields for healing. Recently, medical researchers in Poland have documented the effectiveness of using high-frequency magnetic fields to treat rheumatoid and degenerative arthritis.[11] Studies conducted at Sniadecki Hospital in Wloszczowa, Poland have confirmed that magnetic field therapy is an important new addition to the available physiotherapeutic methods for the treatment of arthritis. In most cases, magnetic field therapy was able to decrease pain intensity, reduce swelling, and improve joint mobility.

Over a two-year period, rheumatologists and rehabilitation specialists treated 189 patients with rheumatoid arthritis (RA) and degenerative joint diseases (DJD) using high frequency magnetic field pulses emitted by a Polish-made Terapuls GS-200 apparatus. The dose was varied from patient to patient, depending on the size of the joint, thickness of the fat overlying the joint, and the particular disease process. Patients received one to two treatments per day for 20-25 minutes, and ten to fifteen sessions constituted a course of treatment. Researchers found that 73 percent of patients with RA and 67 percent of patients with DJD had significant improvement following magnetic therapy, compared with a control group treated with only short-wave diathermy in which only 44.6 percent improved. Other European, Indian, and American researchers have reported successes in using different variations of magnetic-field therapy to treat a variety of disorders. As we shall see in later chapters, the effectiveness of magnetic fields for healing has unique implications for less conventional forms of energy therapy.

The advent of electromedicine and magnetic-field therapy has provided new ways of treating pain and illness, but it has also given us new insights into the cellular mechanisms of healing. It is but a gradual shift away from the traditional allopathic model of drugs (and surgery) for the treatment of human illness toward a more energetic approach. The aforementioned applications of electromagnetic energy to treat human illness may begin to open up the scientific minds of the medical establishment to the possibilities of healing with energy. As we begin to extend our understanding of the wider spectrum of known energies, it will be seen that many of the so-called "fringe areas" of medicine are, in fact, applying slightly different principles of "energy medicine." *The energies being applied here, however, are the subtle energies of the life-force itself and its many octaves and harmonics.*

The key to convincing scientists of the existence and application of these subtle life energies may well lie in the considerable problem of rendering them visible for study and diagnosis. Although Kirlian photography may hold diagnostic potential in this direction, it is far from being widely accepted by mainstream medicine at its present point of development. Within the conventional medical field there are evolving tools of diagnosis that are leading the way toward this eventual realization. To understand how this is happening, we will need to return to the starting point of this chapter, and the discovery and application of x-rays.

X-Rays Revisited: The Development of the CAT Scanner

The earliest methods employing x-rays to visualize bones within tissues used simple x-ray tubes placed above the body with a fluorescent screen or photographic plate held behind. With further apparatus development and fine-tune control of the x-ray source, physicians had greater flexibility and control over radiation dosage than was previously possible. Also, the initially weak fluorescent screen images could be brightened by electronic image intensifiers, enabling the practical use of the fluoroscope for real-time observation of motion. Still, the images seen of bone against nearly transparent tissue remained the same except when used with special contrast media to highlight soft tissues such as blood vessels and gastrointestinal tracts.

Perhaps the most revolutionary development in diagnostic imaging came with the marriage of computer technology to x-ray sources. The CAT

Scanner, short for Computerized Axial Tomography, operates by sending a thin beam of x-rays into the subject in question. The beam slowly rotates 360 degrees around the subject and takes a brief "photograph" at every angle. A computer within the scanner mathematically analyzes and sums up the separate "photos," then reconstructs an image which looks like a cross section through the human body. The more advanced CT (Computerized Tomography) Scanners produce images that look like a thin slice through the scanned area of the body. The images produced include that of soft tissue, at one time nearly invisible to the x-ray eye. The CT Scanner has revolutionized diagnosis in neurology. Previously, there existed only indirect methods of visualizing the brain and, at times, exploratory neuro-surgery was necessary. Because of the CT Scanner's ability to see into the tissues of the brain and body, earlier and easier diagnosis of various tumors and structural tissue abnormalities is possible.

What appears of even greater importance than the x-ray CT Scanner is the mathematical and computer methodology that has evolved from its construction. It is now possible to transform analytical data from different types of scanning devices into three-dimensional reconstructions of body parts such as the head.

Whereas the x-ray CT Scanner was able to miraculously display only detailed bone and soft tissue structure, the newer scanners are able to demonstrate physiological and cellular function. Of the scanners developed from this new technology, the first to give insight into the basic cellular function of brain tissue was the PET Scanner. PET stands for Positron Emission Tomography. The PET Scanner is the product of a merging of two previously separate and distinct diagnostic technologies: nuclear medicine and computerized tomography. In nuclear medicine, short-lived radioactive substances with the property of being actively concentrated into a specific organ of the body (like the thyroid gland or liver) are intravenously injected into patients undergoing the scan. The patient is then placed next to a scintillation detector that measures the emission of radioactive particles from the tracers localized in the organ in question. The detector produces a flat, two-dimensional picture of the outline and form of the organ, giving size, location, and any focal filling defects, etc.

The PET Scanner is primarily used for studying the function of the brain. Radioactively labeled glucose (the primary fuel of the brain) is intravenously injected and taken up by the brain. The radioactive glucose is a positron emitter, hence, the source of positrons in PET Scanning. An array of scintillation detectors is strategically placed around the patient's head. By adapting the mathematical computer programs of CT-technology, the PET Scanner is able to recontruct a cross-sectional view of the brain based upon the positrons emitted by the radioactive glucose which has been actively taken up by the cells of the brain. Depending upon how active particular areas of the brain are, greater or lesser amounts of glucose fuel will be utilized. *What the PET scan displays is a picture that looks like a CT scan of the head based on the cellular activity of different parts of the brain.* Using this scanner, scientists are currently studying differences in regional brain activity between normal individuals and those with mental illnesses like schizophrenia and manic-depressive illness. In some cases, a switch in drug treatment based upon the PET scan has resulted in clinical improvement where previously there had been none. Scientists are also studying the areas of the brain involved with certain skills like reading, listening to speech and music, and handedness. Whereas the CT Scanners provide useful insights into structural defects of brain tissue, the PET Scanner allows scientists to probe the dynamic, functional qualities of human consciousness itself.

Although initial results point toward great value of the PET Scanner, cost limitations, such as the need for a linear accelerator to produce the radioactive glucose, will limit widespread diagnostic applications of this device in the psychiatric community. Pure research using this type of scanner may, however, confirm the effectiveness of certain drug and other treatments for healing mental illness.

Since the first work with the PET Scanner, new radioactive substances have been developed. There is now a tracer, for example, which binds to dopamine receptors. For the first time in medical history, cellular components, such as the dopamine receptors involved in schizophrenia and motor disorders like Parkinson's disease, have actually been visualized within the living brain. Previously, cellular components were studied via microscopic analysis of specially treated brain tissue that had been taken from the cadavers of patients exhibiting a specific disease. The PET scan promises to bring wondrous new information to our understanding of the brain. Yet, there is another new scanner in the horizon that promises to bring even more unique insights into the human body.

Beyond the CAT Scanner: The Body According to MRI

As you will recall, the x-ray CT Scanner gave us a cross-sectional view of the structure of the human body for the first time. In the last several years, we have been witness to the slow incorporation of a new tool into the hospital radiology department: the MRI Scanner, also known as Magnetic Resonance Imaging. Three times as expensive as the CT Scanners it may replace, the device has only recently obtained FDA approval. A tremendous undercurrent of excitement and interest is beginning to build within the medical community as preliminary studies of MRI's diagnostic potential slowly find their way into the medical literature. The reason for the mounting excitement lies in the nature of the body images that the MRI Scanner is able to produce. From a purely physical diagnostic standpoint, MRI has been able to visualize tumors in the body that were previously undetectable by conventional CT scan.

MRI is unlike anything that we have discussed thus far in that it involves no x-rays nor injected radioactive substances. Magnetic resonance imaging is a system which utilizes the now familiar CT computer programs to produce pictures of the human body based on their reaction to high intensity magnetic fields. Of interest is the fact that current MRI images are based on the distribution and structured qualities of water within the tissues of the human body. How MRI is able to accomplish this trick involves quite an explanation. Magnetic resonance imagers produce their pictures by exploiting the phenomenon of Nuclear Magnetic Resonance (NMR), an analytical technique which has been known to organic chemists since the 1960s. It was not until the 1970s that it became adapted to medical imaging systems.

To visualize living tissue, MRI capitalizes on the magnetic properties of protons (hydrogen atoms in water). Protons appear to behave like tiny spinning, magnetic earths. Protons have axes forming north and south magnetic poles. In the strong magnetic field of MRI, the random distribution of "N" and "S" poles becomes changed. All the protons align their axes in the direction of orientation of the magnetic field. A second stimulus, a radio frequency beam, is then applied. This beam is attuned to the inherent frequency of the proton. When the beam is switched on, the magnetically aligned protons begin to rotate slowly about their axes. The radio beam is then suddenly switched off. Energy is now released from the stimulated protons in the radio frequency range and is picked up by detectors situated in a circle around the patient in the MRI scanner. The mathematical analysis of data received utilizing the CT computer programs allows an image to be reconstructed based upon the multiple detector measurements. The

MRI Scanner is able to create a thin slice or cross-sectional image of the human body unparalleled in detail by any previously existing scanner. The quality of information revealed by thin "MRI slices" of living individuals approaches the fine anatomic detail seen in sections taken from human cadavers. Using magnetic resonance imaging, we are able to get a noninvasive glimpse of organ structure in the living human body from a viewpoint previously available only to the surgeon and the pathologist.

Current MRI scanners are using stimulated protons as their emitting source. They are dependent upon the body's water (the largest source of protons). Water, as you will recall, makes up 99 percent of the molecules composing the human body. Water is also generated by chemical processes going on within the metabolic machinery of cells.

The key principle behind magnetic resonance imaging is the fact that the atoms under study (hydrogen) are being stimulated by the transfer of energy of a specific frequency. In this case, the energy lies in the realm of radio waves. *The energy is only absorbed by the atom if it is of a particular resonant frequency.* Again, we have a situation analogous to the model of electronic orbitals, or energy shells, of the atom. In order to shift an electron from a lower to a higher orbit, only energy of specific frequency characteristics will be accepted. If the electron descends from the higher to the lower orbit or energy shell, it will release a photon of a similar frequency as that taken to move it from one level to the next. The character of energy required to shift the electron is its resonant frequency. MRI does something similar with the hydrogen atoms in delivering energy of a frequency resonant only to the protons.

Because of this principle of "resonance specificity," researchers are trying to apply MRI's electronic window to studying other atoms, including sodium and phosphorus. Phosphorus is a component of ATP (adenosine triphosphate)—the energy currency of the cell. Phosphorus is also a component of CPK (creatine phosphokinase)—a muscle-specific enzyme. MRI researchers hope that by utilizing an energetic source resonant with the phosphorus molecule, they may be able to actively visualize chemical energetic exchanges at the cellular level. Additionally, doctors may learn to diagnose disorders of muscle (such as muscular dystrophy) without having to biopsy muscle tissue. Magnetic resonance systems may prove to be a tool by which we can measure cellular metabolism in a noninvasive manner.

MRI is able to use magnetic fields to visualize the cellular distribution

and structural qualities of water. Therefore, it would be interesting to speculate as to the diagnostic possibilities of MRI in observing subtle energy
changes of healing in the human body, knowing now what we do about the
"special energetic" properties of water. Bernard Grad's studies on psychic
healing (Chapter 2) noted that healers could alter the molecular and energetic qualities of water and affect the ability of water to promote plant
growth under adverse conditions. If the molecular properties of water were
shifted by the healer's etheric fields, MRI might be used to study the subtle
magnetic effects of healers on the human body and on the inherent structure of water within living tissue. More will be said about the energetic
changes brought about by psychic healers in Chapter 8.

Magnetic resonance imaging promises to bring forth much new diagnostic information about the human body. Yet another new window on the
body has been opened, this time yielding even more detailed cellular pictures of structure and function. But we are still stuck at the level of physical
molecular imaging, a sophisticated Newtonian analysis. Although the information obtained from this approach is highly significant and useful,
there is still a further bridge to be crossed in viewing the human framework
from its true energetic perspective. The principles learned from MRI combined with insights taken from Kirlian photography may soon yield one of
the greatest breakthroughs in diagnostic imaging of human subtle energetic
anatomy.

A Step Beyond—EMR Scanning & Electrography: On the Threshold of the Etheric

The next great step in diagnostic scanner development may lie in the
extrapolation and application of the key principles found in each of the
aforementioned systems. As mentioned previously, one of the most significant breakthroughs in cross-sectional imaging has been the CT mathematical
computer program. The computer allows us to summate a tremendous
amount of data in seconds. It reconstructs large volumes of information into
one pictographic gestalt which can then be interpreted by the human eye
and brain. The human mind is still the most important ingredient in meaningful pattern recognition. It is the physician, not the computer, that makes
the diagnosis. Computers can only create sophisticated images. Yet it is the
ability of the computer to compress hours of boring mathematical calculations into useful pictures that makes it so valuable to diagnostic scanner
development.

In the near future, scientists will capitalize on the groundwork set down by developers of the CT and MRI scanners. Soon, perhaps, computerized electronic imaging systems will allow physicians to study the etheric body in great detail. Biological resonance will be the key which will open up this door into the largely unseen world of life processes. Resonance is the most important principle utilized by creators of magnetic resonance imaging systems. MRI systems broadcast energy of a specific (resonant) frequency. This energy selectively excites cellular components, which in turn emit energy that can be used to create images of the cellular structures. By examining different molecular, cellular, and bodily components which are illuminated by this energetic process, one can literally turn people into "transparent beings." The ability to stimulate only one molecular system allows scientists to be selective about what they wish to examine. As mentioned earlier, resonant stimulation of phosphorus atoms may prove of greater interest to neurologists studying muscle disorders. Similarly, resonant imaging of hydrogen (and thus structuring and distribution of water within tissues) may be more valuable to oncologists looking at normal organ structure vs. cancerous growths.

Although MRI is a revolutionary application of the principle of resonance, doctors are still limited to studying the physical and biochemical components of the human cellular framework. MRI is basically a tool for examining the distribution of molecular structure and biochemical function in the human body. What is needed now is an imaging system that allows physicians to look to the level of energetic causes of illness and not merely the biochemical abnormalities accompanying established disease. The inevitable successors of already existing imagers will ultimately enable doctors to find the true precursors of health and illness and not just the aftermath of a ravaging disease process. Truly preventive medicine awaits the development of an imaging system which will prove to doctors that there is more to human beings than mere flesh and blood, membranes, and receptors.

Kirlian photography holds tantalizing clues to ways that scientists in the New Age may eventually detect precursors to illness by studying the unseen patterns of life energies that bring order or disorder to the minds and bodies of human beings. At the present level of Kirlian research, electrographic fingerprints have hinted at the presence of certain illnesses such as cancer and cystic fibrosis. However, Kirlian fingerprints do not yet carry the weight and accuracy of disease detection that is needed to convince doctors that there are energetic precursors of illness. What is needed is a system based on Kirlian diagnostic technologies which can image the entire body and not just the fingers. Indications are that some Soviet and Rumanian researchers are making headway in this direction. The key that will allow researchers to view the subtle bioenergetic fields of human beings may lie in the phenomenon of resonance. With MRI scanners, physicians are using energetic resonance principles to image physical organs of the body in disease states. A marriage of MRI, CT, and Kirlian systems may make it possible to go beyond present resonance technologies to look even deeper into the subtle energetic makeup of human beings.

To understand how Kirlian systems may hold the key to imaging etheric and other subtle energetic systems, it is necessary to examine the electrographic process in greater detail. For the purposes of our discussion of subtle energetic fields, we will focus on the most important phenomenon that Kirlian systems demonstrate, i.e. their ability to capture the Phantom Leaf Effect. The Phantom Leaf Effect, seen via Kirlian photography, repeatedly demonstrates a holographic energy-field component of living systems. The missing leaf that appears in Kirlian electrographs appears identical in structure to the physical leaf. This phantom is a part of the etheric body of the leaf (a growth template or wave guide) that assists in the expression of the life-force through the genetic potential of the plant. We must, for a moment, ask ourselves how Kirlian photography is able to reveal the etheric phantom. It is a feat which literally makes the invisible visible. What follows is an interpretation of the mechanism by which Kirlian photography is able capture this phenomenon.

The basic principle behind Kirlian photography's ability to produce images on film is the corona discharge phenomenon. Most scientists who have studied Kirlian systems have agreed upon this fact. In the simple electrographic apparatus there is a high-frequency power source connected to an electrode beneath a sheet of film. A high-frequency current, sent to the hidden electrode, creates an electrical field which bathes the photographic film. The film surface becomes charged at a high electrical potential. When a finger or other grounded object is placed upon the film, it provides a pathway for electrons of high potential (on the film surface) to travel to low potential (ground, or earth . . . the ultimate electron sink).

Energy always flows from high to low potential. The electron trails, created by torrents of electrons jumping from the film to the grounded object, create the beautiful electrical corona discharge which is captured (in total darkness) on the photographic film. The image produced by this technique is called a Kirlian photograph. The pattern of electron streamers around the object, as well as the colors captured on film, appears to contain varying amounts of diagnostic information about the photographic subject.

Diagram 9.
TYPICAL CORONA DISCHARGE
OF KIRLIAN FINGERPRINT

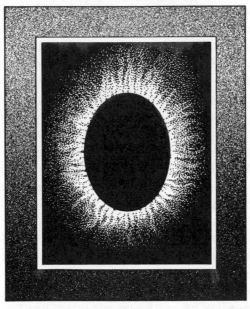

Different researchers have attempted to demonstrate physiologically meaningful information in their Kirlian photos with variable degrees of success. The reason for different success rates between researchers is a key factor in understanding why the Kirlian technique is able to obtain biologically significant information. Many amateur Kirlian researchers have assumed that any electrical device that is able to create a spark discharge, and hence a "Kirlian" photograph, should be able to reproduce the effects reported by other Kirlian researchers. This is a gross oversimplification that has led to much confusion and many mistaken conclusions by workers in this complex field.

It is known, for example, that some Kirlian devices will record images of fingerprints which correlate with the presence of cancer in the body. Many researchers have attempted to reproduce this effect with varying degrees of success. Those who find only random results have often concluded that all Kirlian systems are worthless except in examining moisture content. Whereas some units may produce attractive yet meaningless fingerprints, a persistent researcher may switch to a different Kirlian system and be surprised to find images that reveal meaningful information about the presence of disease. Why is one Kirlian unit able to diagnose cancer while another is not?

The reason behind Kirlian photography's variable success rate appears to lie in the frequency characteristics of the power source. When a person has a fingerprint taken on a Kirlian unit, there is some degree of resonance between the equipment and the subject being photographed. Although nearly any high-frequency voltage source will produce a spark discharge on film, *only those systems which produce frequencies that resonate with natural biological frequencies will display images with significant diagnostic information.* This situation is analogous to the resonance of energy necessary to visualize structures in MRI imaging. Because the quantitation of these inherent cellular frequencies has never been fully explored, probably due to ignorance of their existence, the success of frequency matching in Kirlian units has largely been the result of trial and error.

Most Kirlian researchers are unaware of the necessity for biological resonance between their power source and the subject under study. Many have oversimplified a complex subject by lumping together different frequency systems producing spark discharges as Kirlian units with equivalent diagnostic capabilities. Because Kirlian researchers tend to compare diagnostic results obtained with diverse frequency-producing devices, there have been difficulties in replicating certain findings. There is a tremendous lack of standardization within the field. Differences in frequency characteristics of power sources may explain why there is such a variability among researchers in reproducing significant electrographic effects such as disease detection and capturing of the phantom leaf.

Those Kirlian systems which produce frequencies that resonate with the biological phenomena being studied have the greatest chance of successfully imaging indicators of disease. This same principle is paramount to understanding the success of MRI imaging techniques. Only those MRI devices which transmit radio frequencies that resonate with hydrogen atoms in the human body will capture images that have biological meaning. Similarly, other magnetic resonance systems which broadcast radio frequencies that resonate with sodium versus hydrogen atoms will reveal different, yet meaningful, levels of biocellular information in MRI imagery. Different frequency energy probes are allowing scientists to create selective windows to observe specific biochemical phenomena, as long as the frequencies emitted by the scanners are key resonant frequencies. If the MRI radio frequencies are in a range that do not resonate with integral cellular components of the body, one cannot obtain biologically significant images. The same resonance principles are likely to apply to Kirlian diagnostic systems as well. As in MRI, there are many different resonant frequencies that may allow Kirlian systems to best observe particular bioenergetic phenomena.

In attempting to image the Phantom Leaf Effect, we are working with slightly different variations of these same principles of biological resonance. Instead of trying to produce frequencies that resonate with the physical atoms of the leaf, Kirlian photographers are attempting to resonantly stimulate the etheric atoms of the leaf's etheric template. Although the etheric structure is in a higher frequency spectrum than physical matter, etheric fields are able to affect the behavior of subatomic particles of physical matter such as electrons. The primary imaging phenomenon in Kirlian photography is due to corona discharge, the patterns of electron flow around a grounded object. By causing changes in the electron streamer patterns around the electrographic subject, *Kirlian photography uses etherically stimulated electrons to trace delicate outlines associated with the etheric body of the leaf.*

In a successful phantom leaf image, electrons are deflected by lines of force from resonantly stimulated etheric fields in a manner similar to particles of spray paint adhering to the surface of the invisible man. The phantom leaf is a picture of stimulated electrons mapping out the spatial pattern of the etheric template. In order to consistently reproduce this phenomenon, one must have a Kirlian power source that is able to emit frequencies of energy that resonantly excite the etheric body. *The energies employed in Kirlian are not of the identical frequency of the etheric body, but they consist of lower harmonics or octaves of these higher vibrational energies.* This is one of the primary differences between MRI and what we shall call EMR (Electromagnetic Resonance) imaging systems such as Kirlian photography.

Subtle energies at the etheric level are merely at a higher octave than the physical. As an example, let us compare the differences in octaves along a piano keyboard. The first set of keys at the lower end of the piano produces a musical scale consisting of the low notes. The keys adjacent to these produce a musical scale at a slightly higher octave. Side by side, these keys might represent the two octaves of frequencies that make up the physical and the etheric domains. On the piano, there are higher octaves going further to the right on the keyboard. It is the same with higher octaves of the subtle energy composing our higher frequency bodies, including our astral and mental vehicles. Our subtle energetic anatomy is made up of many such bodies working in unison. They are a unique orchestration of lower and higher frequency energies composing multidimensional symphonies of expression for each unique human being. These higher frequency bodies will be discussed in further detail in the next chapter.

There are harmonies and rhythms which permeate all of creation. This idea is as fundamental to ordinary mathematics as it is to electricity. There are octaves of energy, definite waves and rhythms that can be measured, frequencies and amplitudes and so on. From these simple elements are produced an almost unlimited number of variations. . . from the very subtle to the very dense. . . from pure energy to a dense physical form. . . . Because there are various octaves of energy in creation, there are subtle counterparts to everything existing in the physical octave. . . .

By applying a charge of external energy to a relatively closed system, you can selectively energize a given octave of energy. . . . It's the basic principle of resonance. By selectively applying a specific vibration, you strike a resonance in one of these subtle bands of energy, and this then stimulates the lower octave, which stimulates a lower octave yet, until a simulation of the subtle energy of the higher octave—normally invisible to the human eye—becomes visible. *This is what happens in Kirlian photography,* although the energy is only being stepped down one level. A certain type of energy is being applied to an aspect of the etheric energies. . . . It stimulates the etheric energies so they can be photographed.[12] *(italics added)*

One can better understand this process of resonant stimulation of different energy octaves by re-examining the piano analogy. When one strikes a key on the piano, the metallic string vibrates at a particular frequency in a single octave of notes. At the same moment that the string is vibrating, the sonic energy causes corresponding vibrations to occur in that same key but in other octaves. In other words, striking a low "C" note on a piano will result in a resonant stimulation of the higher "C" notes as well.

This type of resonant harmonics is the same basic process that occurs in Kirlian photography of the Phantom Leaf Effect. The electrical energy vibrates in the octave of physical matter but strikes a resonant note in the higher etheric octave as well. Kirlian differs from MRI in this respect in that magnetic resonance imaging seeks only to stimulate the atoms of the physical body through the process of resonance. Kirlian goes one step beyond by resonantly stimulating the atoms of the etheric body and allowing them to be imaged by their interaction with the electrical fields produced by the Kirlian camera. By utilizing this same basic principle of resonance, it may be possible to find frequencies that will allow us to image octaves of matter and energy that go even beyond the etheric.

While utilizing the Kirlian technique in its present state of development, one can occasionally capture these etheric energies on film. The problem with Kirlian at the present level of understanding is that there are so many physical factors that can interact with the final image that it is hard to separate the physical from the etheric effects. Each Kirlian image, even a fingerprint, represents a summation of many physical and nonphysical factors. Present systems provide no simple way of determining which effects are physical vs. nonphysical (i.e., etheric). The only clear way of doing this at present is to eliminate all physical effects entirely by removing the physical body (as in the case of cutting away the upper portion of the leaf to obtain the phantom). There is another method of getting around this sometimes meaningful (as in cancer detection), but unintentional, physical interference. To understand how, we must first explore a little-known application of the Kirlian technology.

Harry Oldfield, a Kirlian researcher in England, has done successful fingerprint studies in cancer detection. During his studies of Kirlian equipment, he found that the electromagnetic pulse that was carried to the hidden electrode beneath the film was also transmitted to the body of the individual whose finger rested on the photographic plate. Energetic frequency patterns transmitted from the Kirlian power source to the skin could be picked up at a distance of several inches from the patient's body utilizing electromagnetic detectors in the radio frequency and ultrasonic range. A detector probe known as the Kirlian gun was developed and attached to an oscilloscope in order to display the energies it was picking up around the patient's body. Oldfield used a modified Kirlian power source with a stepped-down voltage that was connected directly to patient's body by a wrist electrode. He then passed the Kirlian gun over the patient's body (at a distance of several inches) to scan for energy emission while the patient was connected to the Kirlian power source. Whenever the probe passed over normal tissue, the frequency and polarity of the signal seen on the oscilloscope perfectly matched the signal coming from the Kirlian generator.

What Mr. Oldfield discovered was that if the probe passed over an area of the body where there was a tumor beneath, the frequency and polarity characteristics of the signal would become noticeably distorted. This happened repeatably enough that a pilot study of cancer patients was conducted at Charing Cross Hospital in London to assess the diagnostic value of this system. Preliminary results suggested that the Kirlian gun was highly accurate in pinpointing the presence and specific location of cancerous tumors within the human body. By utilizing several probes at different angles around the body, Mr. Oldfield found that he could mathematically triangulate to calculate tumor tissue depth and the exact three-dimensional location of the cancer.

Oldfield's discovery was an important one. He found a way to use the Kirlian-frequency power source to obtain remote diagnostic measurements at a distance from the body. The results were unaffected by factors such as moisture and pressure. It is likely that Oldfield's studies in cancer detection were successful because the frequency of his power source produced a resonance with some natural cellular frequency. (This frequency factor is perhaps the main difference between successful and unsuccessful Kirlian research protocols. Unfortunately, the discovery of such a power source is often serendipitous, and the reasons for success are often poorly understood by the investigators themselves.)

Oldfield's work provides an impetus for Kirlian technology to evolve beyond the simple fingerprint stage to a level where it may be more valuable in disease detection. The applications suggested by Mr. Oldfield's work are numerous. The most obvious diagnostic application is in the field of cancer detection. But let us utilize this discovery and take it one step further. If Oldfield was able to take multiple measurements around the body and mathematically calculate tumor depth and location, just think of what could be done if this type of detector were to be combined with the technology of the CT mathematical computer programs!

There are interesting similarities behind Oldfield's work and the principles behind MRI imaging. Oldfield used electrical energy of specific frequency characteristics to excite bodily tissues to emit secondary signals in the radio frequency and ultrasonic range. Energetic signals resulting from such stimulation of the body revealed strikingly different emission characteristics for normal and cancerous tissue. Oldfield analyzed energy emitted from patients using a handheld probe (the Kirlian gun) and an oscilloscope. By taking multiple measurements from different angles around the body, he was able to calculate the approximate position of the tumor within the body. Adapting the Kirlian technology to a computerized system would allow one to take many individual measurements and to instantaneously calculate distortions in signal emission at different angles from the body. By employing software developed for CT-type scanners, it would then be possible to create a cross-sectional image of the body and to visually display the information as a single picture. MRI devices and CT scanners employ similar principles in utilizing computers for image generation.

Just as MRI scanners can image sodium or hydrogen depending upon their frequency of resonant stimulation, a scanner appropriating the principle of EMR (electromagnetic resonance) could selectively image different molecular components. Instead of imaging physical molecular structures as in NMR, is it possible to image etheric molecular structures using EMR? Extrapolating data from phantom leaf experiments, it appears that certain Kirlian power sources can capture etheric images because they create electromagnetic resonance (EMR) effects which stimulate etheric matter. *The electrical frequencies of these Kirlian systems seem to be lower harmonics of etheric frequencies.* If one were to use similar frequencies in an EMR scanner of the type derived from the Oldfield experiments, it might be possible to produce a cross-sectional image of the etheric body.

Recent developments in computer imaging of CT data have allowed doctors to add together the many cross-sectional images of internal structures to create three-dimensional pictures of organs and skeletal structures. This new computer technology could be coupled to EMR scanning to generate three-dimensional images of the etheric body, which could be studied as a whole, as well as examined in detail, to observe for disease-related and other changes.

The etheric body is a holographic energy template that guides the growth and development of the physical body. Distortions of the healthy pattern of subtle-energy organization in the etheric template may lead to abnormal cellular growth. From what is known about the etheric body, diseases appear to be seen in the etheric field weeks and months prior to their becoming manifest in the physical body. *The potential for a truly preventive medicine lies within a scanner that could detect illness at the etheric level prior to it becoming manifest in the physical body.* By studying etheric images representing pre-illness stages, it might be possible to utilize various types of subtle energetic therapies to correct the tendencies toward dysfunction in the system. Correction of illness at a pre-physical level could prevent the need for costly, physical, allopathic methods of treatment. The subtle energetic actions of alternative or homeopathic therapies could also possibly be verified through direct observation of the etheric body via the ideal body energy scanner. Physicians could study the etheric bodies of patients to learn the energetic effects of vitamins and nutrition, of light and color, and many other vibrational modalities which would need such technologies for scientific verification of efficacy. Another application might lie in studying long term effects of conventional drug therapies on the etheric and physical bodies.

The potential for building an EMR Scanner exists today. But individuals with the knowledge to create an etheric-body energy scanner need to coordinate and unify their efforts. The EMR Scanner will be the first truly open window into the realm of the etheric energies that is part of our extended subtle-energy framework. By allowing subtle energies to become more easily and repeatably visualized for study, we will begin to see a greater acceptance of the "science of subtle energies" into the greater scientific community. We will have extended medicine beyond its simple Newtonian roots into the future of diagnosis and healing that vibrational medicine holds for us.

Key Points to Remember

1. Orthodox medicine has begun to gradually explore the uses of energy for treating illness. These include the uses of radiation to treat cancer, of electricity to alleviate pain and shrink tumors, of electromagnetic fields to stimulate fracture healing, and of magnetic fields to alleviate the pain and inflammation of arthritis.

2. The physical body has certain self-healing electrical feedback loops, such as the "current of injury," which tend to promote cellular repair and reorganization after the body has been damaged. There may be semiconductor-type electronic systems within and between cells that participate in the normal aspects of growth and cellular replication.

3. Science is rapidly developing new imaging technologies, such as

the CT Scanner, the PET Scanner, and the Magnetic Resonance Imager which give physicians a new window into the structure and function of the brain and body.

4. Certain Kirlian photographic systems have been able to repeatably demonstrate a phenomenon known as the Phantom Leaf Effect. The Phantom Leaf Effect is perhaps the best candidate for a photograph of the etheric body of a living organism.

5. Both Kirlian and MRI systems are able to visualize important cellular and bioenergetic phenomena because they produce frequencies that resonate with the natural cellular and energetic components of the bodies they are used to study.

6. It may one day be possible to create a whole body imager that can create CT-Scanner-like pictures of the etheric body. These cross-sectional slices could then be added together by computer to create a three-dimensional picture of the etheric body. The basis of such a system would be a frequency source that would stimulate the etheric body via a subharmonic resonant frequency of energy that could excite the etheric body to produce electromagnetic resonant effects. Such an etheric body imager could demonstrate disturbances in the etheric body before they became manifest as significant cellular disease changes in the physical body.

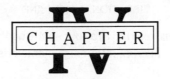

CHAPTER IV

Frequency Domains
& the Subtle Planes of Matter:

AN INTRODUCTION TO HUMAN MULTIDIMENSIONAL ANATOMY

One of the prime differences between the approaches of Newtonian and Einsteinian medicine is their viewpoints of the human body. Newtonian mechanistic thinkers, albeit sophisticated in the molecular biological approach, see the human body as a series of intricate chemical systems powering a structure of nerve and muscle, flesh and bones. The physical body is viewed as a supreme mechanism, an intricate physical clockwork down to the very cellular structure. We have discussed in Chapter 1 the considerable evidence suggesting that the distinction of the physical nature of matter becomes lost on a subatomic level. The solid nature of physical matter is but an illusion of the senses. The new perspective describes matter as a substance composed of particles which are themselves points of frozen light. The wave/particle duality of matter suggests new, previously unconsidered qualities of human physical structure that allow a new model of the physical body to be constructed.

What we will explore within this chapter is the continuity of our physical system with higher energy systems. These subtle-energy systems play an integral part in the total functioning of human beings. The physical system, far from being a closed system, is only one of several systems which are in dynamic equilibrium. What might appear to be a radical departure from conventional thinking is that all of these systems are physically superimposed upon one another in the very same space. These higher energy systems, referred to as our subtle bodies, are actually composed of matter with different frequency characteristics than that of the physical body.

As discussed in Chapter 2, it is likely that since matter is a kind of frozen light, it must therefore have particular frequency characteristics. The difference between physical mattter and etheric matter is only a difference of frequency. It is an acknowledged principle within physics that energy of different frequencies can coexist within the same space without destructive interaction. This principle is demonstrated daily by the manmade electromagnetic soup in which we work and live. We are constantly bombarded by radio and TV broadcasts which pass through our houses and bodies. This electromagnetic energy is invisible to our eyes and ears because it exists at a threshold of energy beyond the energetic frequency sensitivity of our physical organs of perception. If, however, we happen to turn on the TV set, these normally invisible energies become translated into energies of visible light and audible sound which are within our perceptual range of sensitivity. When we turn on the TV set, we do not see Channel 2's image mixed with Channel 7's. Because the energies are of slightly different frequencies, they can exist within the same space without interfering with each other. It is only because of the interjection of our TV set as an extension of our senses that we can even tell that these energies are present.

This principle of energies of different frequencies occupying the same space, nondestructively, has theoretical implications for matter of different frequencies. Because of their differing inherent frequencies, physical and etheric matter can coexist in the same space, just as radio and TV waves can pass through the same space without interference. The energetic matrix of the etheric body, or holographic energy-field template, is superimposed upon the structure of the physical framework. This is why the Phantom Leaf Effect always appears in the space formerly occupied by the physical portion of the leaf. This same principle of matter of different frequencies applies to even higher frequency matter than the etheric body. Bodies of higher energetic frequencies are interconnected and in dynamic equilibrium with the physical body. It will be the purpose of this chapter to illustrate the nature and principles of these higher subtle bodies and their interconnections to the physical body. They synergistically combine to form the greater part of our extended energy framework.

The Physical-Etheric Interface:
The Next Greatest Discovery in the Development of Vibrational Medicine

As discussed in Chapter 1, there is considerable evidence to suggest that there exists a holographic energy template associated with the physical body. This etheric body is a body which looks quite similar to the physical body over which it is superimposed. Within the etheric energetic map is carried information which guides the cellular growth of the physical structure of the body. It carries the spatial information on how the developing fetus is to unfold in utero, and also the structural data for growth and repair of the adult organism should damage or disease occur. It is the template of the salamander limb which allows a new foot to grow if the present one is severed. This energetic structure works in concert with the cellular genetic mechanisms that molecular biology has elaborated upon over the last several decades of medical research. The physical body is so energetically connected and dependent upon the etheric body for cellular guidance that the physical body cannot exist without the etheric body. If the etheric field becomes distorted, physical disease soon follows. Many illnesses begin first in the etheric body and are then later manifested in the physical body as organ pathology.

As mentioned above, the etheric body is, in fact, a body of matter. The matter of which it is composed is called "etheric matter" or "subtle matter." It is the substance of which our higher energetic bodies are composed. Subtle matter is used as a general term referring to types of matter associated with our unseen, higher energetic counterparts. The only difference between the etheric body and those higher bodies (which will shortly be discussed) is that of frequency characteristics. The higher energy bodies are unseen only because the technologies which render these energies visible to the naked eye are still mostly in the developmental stages. The world of radio and x-ray astronomy was also an unseen universe until the appropriate technologies could be developed to extend our senses in those energetic directions. So, in the case of subtle energies, a similar research effort in rendering the invisible visible is greatly needed at this time.

The etheric body is not completely separated from the physical system with which it interacts. There are specific channels of energy exchange which allow the flow of energetic information to move from one system to another. Although these channels have not been known or discussed in Western science until recently, there is much that has been written about these systems in esoteric Eastern literature.

One system which has been explored only recently by Western scientists is the acupuncture meridian system. Ancient Chinese theory has it that the acupuncture points on the human body are points along an unseen meridian system that runs deeply throughout the tissues of the body. Through these meridians passes an invisible nutritive energy known to the Chinese as "ch'i." The ch'i energy enters the body through the acupuncture points and flows to deeper organ structures, bringing life-giving nourishment of a subtle energetic nature. The Chinese believe that there are twelve pairs of meridians that are connected to specific organ systems deep within the human structure. The Chinese also feel that when the flow of energy to the organs becomes blocked or imbalanced, dysfunction of the organ system will occur.

Much has been written recently in the West about the use of acupuncture to treat pain disorders. Western physicians have only recognized acupuncture for its ability to treat various types of pain or for its use as a surgical analgesic. Because of this limited recognition of acupuncture, the theories used to explain acupuncture's analgesic effects, such as the Gate Control Theory of Wall and Melzack, rely heavily on models involving nerve stimulation and, more recently, endorphin release within the central nervous system. Most Western physicians have dismissed the idea of these meridians through which ch'i energy flows in favor of more anatomically and physiologically familiar models. Part of this dismissal stems from lack of anatomical evidence in the Western medical literature for the existence of these meridians within the human body.

There were a series of studies on the anatomic nature of the meridian system in animals which were carried out in Korea during the 1960s by a team of researchers headed by Professor Kim Bong Han.[1,2] Kim did experimental work with the acupuncture meridians of rabbits and other animal models. He injected radioactive P^{32} (an isotope of phosphorus) into a rabbit acupoint and followed uptake of the substance into the surrounding tissue. Utilizing the technique of microautoradiography, he discovered that the P^{32} was actively taken up along a fine duct-like tubule sytem (approximately 0.5-1.5 microns in diameter) which followed the path of the classical acupuncture meridians. Concentrations of P^{32} in tissue immediately adjacent to the meridians or near the acupoint injected were negligible. When P^{32} was deliberately injected into a nearby vein, little to none could be detected in the meridian network. This finding suggested that the meridian system was independent of the vascular network.

More recent studies by French researcher Pierre de Vernejoul and others have confirmed Kim's findings in humans.[3] Radioactive technetium 99m was injected into the acupoints of patients, and the isotope's uptake was followed by gamma-camera imaging. De Vernejoul found that the radioactive technetium 99m migrated along classical Chinese acupuncture meridian pathways for a distance of 30 cm in four to six minutes. Injection of the isotope into random points on the skin, as well as deliberate venous and lymphatic channel injection, were unable to demonstrate similar results, suggesting that the meridians were a unique and separate morphological pathway.

Kim's histologic studies of the ductule system in rabbits showed that this tubular meridian system appeared to be divided into a superficial and a deep system. The deep system was further subdivided into various subsystems. The first of these deep meridian systems was called the Internal Duct System. These tubules were found free-floating within the vascular and lymphatic vessels, penetrating the vessel walls at entry and exit points. Fluids within these internal ducts were usually found to travel in the same direction as the blood and lymph flow of the vessel they were discovered in, but in certain circumstances, ductal fluids were noted to flow in the opposite direction. The fact that these internal ducts penetrate and leave the vessel walls, as well as have their fluid flow sometimes opposite to that of their "carrier vessels," suggests that the formation of these ducts is different (and perhaps earlier in time) than the origin of the vascular and lymphatic system. In other words, the meridians may have been formed earlier in embryogenesis than the arteries, veins, and lymphatic vessels. The meridians may act as spatial guides for the growth and development of the newly forming blood and lymphatic circulatory network. As the blood vessels developed, they would grow around the meridians and leave the appearance that the meridians entered and exited the vessels.

A second series of tubules was characterized and called the Intra-External Duct System. These ducts are found along the surface of the internal organs and appear to form a network which is entirely independent of the vascular, lymphatic, and nervous sytems. A third series, known as the External Duct System, was found to run alongside the outer surface of the walls of blood and lymphatic vessels. These ducts are also found in layers of the skin and are known there as the Superficial Duct System. It is this latter superficial system which is most familiar to classical acupuncturists. The fourth series of tubules, known as the Neural Duct System, are distributed in the central and peripheral nervous systems.

All the ductules were eventually found to be interconnected (superficial to deep systems) so that continuity of the system was maintained. The various duct systems are interlinked together via the connection of the terminal ductules of the different systems. This linkage is similar to the arterial-venous link at the capillary tissue-bed level. Interestingly enough, Kim discovered that *the terminal ductules reach the tissue cell nuclei.* Also, spaced at intervals along these meridians, Kim found special small corpuscles. *Those corpuscles in the Superfical Duct System seem to lie beneath, and correspond with, the classical acupuncture points and meridians of the human body.*

Fluid extracted from these tubules revealed high concentrations of DNA, RNA, amino acids, hyaluronic acid, sixteen types of free nucleotides, adrenaline, corticosteroids, estrogen, and other hormonal substances in levels far different from those ordinarly found in the bloodstream. The concentration of adrenaline in the meridian fluid was twice that of the bloodstream. In an acupoint, over ten times the blood level of adrenaline was found. The presence of hormones and adrenaline within ductal fluids would certainly suggest some link between the meridian system and the endocrine glands of the body. Kim found that the terminal ductules of the deeper meridian system also reach the tissue cell nuclei, which are the genetic control centers of the cells. In view of the presence within meridian fluids of nucleic acids and hormones such as corticosteroids and estrogen, it would appear that there are important interrelationships between the acupuncture meridian system and the endocrine regulation of human beings.

Kim did a number of experiments to confirm the importance of continuous meridian flow to particular bodily organs via the deep meridian systems. He severed the meridian going to the liver in a frog and studied subsequent microscopic changes in the liver tissue. Shortly after severing the liver meridian, the hepatocytes enlarged and their cytoplasm became very turbid. Within three days, serious vascular degeneration took place throughout the whole liver. Repeated experimentation of this nature confirmed the results. Kim also studied changes in neural reflexes when perineural meridian ducts were severed. Within 30 minutes of severing the perineural ducts, reflex time was prolonged by more than 500 percent and this persisted beyond 48 hours with only minor fluctuation. These studies would tend to confirm the classical Chinese acupuncture theory stating that the meridians provide a specialized nutritive flow to the organs of the body.

Based on many experiments, Kim concluded that the meridian system not only interlinked within itself but appeared to interconnect with all cell nuclei of the tissues. In order to find the point at which this nuclear/cellular link was formed in embryogenesis, Kim began to study, in different species, the time at which these meridians were formed. In embryological studies reminiscent of Dr. Burr, Kim found that within the embryonic chick *the meridian ducts were formed within fifteen hours of conception!* This is most interesting because even the most rudimentary organs have not yet formed at this stage. In view of the fact that the completed spatial orientation of the meridian system occurs earlier than organ formation, *this would suggest that the functioning of the acupuncture meridian system exerts an influence upon the migration and spatial orientation of the internal organs.* Because the meridians connect to each cell's genetic control center, the acupuncture meridian system may also play an important role in both replication and differentiation (specialization) of all cells in the body.

We can integrate the research of Kim with parallel studies of Dr. Harold Burr.[4] It will be recalled that Dr. Burr carried out experiments mapping the electrical fields around developing salamander embryos. Through his research, he discovered that an electrical axis developed in the unfertilized salamander egg which corresponded to the future orientation of the brain and central nervous system in the adult organism. The creation of such an electrical axis or wave guide in the unfertilized egg suggests that some type of directional energy field cooperates with and provides spatial orientation to the rapidly dividing and migrating cells of the newly forming embryo. Burr also discovered that in plant seedlings, the contour of the electrical field surrounding the new sprouts followed the shape of the adult plant. If we combine our knowledge of Kirlian photography's ability to capture the phantom leaf phenomenon with the aforementioned data, we come to the conclusion that *the spatial organization of growth from embryogenesis through adulthood is guided by a holographic energy-field template known as the etheric body.*

Kim discovered that the formation of the acupuncture meridian system preceded the development and placement of rudimentary organs in the embryo. He also found close links between the meridians and the nuclei of cells. His work suggests that some type of information flows through the meridians to the DNA control centers of the cells, providing additional modulation of the embryologic developmental process. Because the meridians become spatially organized within the embryo prior to the cells and organs finding their final positioning within the body, this would suggest that the meridian system provides a type of intermediate road map or informational guidance system to the developing cells of the body. Synthesizing from the embryological research of Burr and Kim, *it would appear that the meridian system forms an interface between the etheric and the physical body. The meridian system is the first physical link established between the etheric body and the developing physical body.* Thus the organized energetic structure of the etheric body precedes and guides the development of the physical body. The translation of etheric changes into physical cellular changes occurs in both health and illness. This theory is consistent with data from other sources, such as Dr. Shafica Karagulla's work with clairvoyant diagnosis,[5] that have described dysfunctional changes in the etheric body of people occurring prior to the appearance of overt disease in the physical body.

The acupuncture meridian system forms what might be called the "physical-etheric interface." Bioenergetic information and vital ch'i energy move from the etheric body to the cellular level of the physical body via this specialized meridian network. To quote one psychic source:

> There is a direct link between the nervous, circulatory, and meridian systems partly because ages ago, the meridians were originally used to create these two parts of the physical body. Consequently, anything that influences one of these systems has a direct impact on the other two areas. The meridians use the passageway between the nervous and circulatory systems to feed the life force into the body, almost extending directly to the molecular level. *The meridians are the interface or doorway between the physical and ethereal properties of the body.*[6] *(italics added)*

The meridian system is not just a physical system of tubules transporting hormones and nucleotides to cell nuclei, but is also a specialized type of electrolytic fluid system that conducts certain types of subtle energies (ch'i) from the external environment to deeper organ structures.

The implication that certain types of energies are communicated through the acupuncture points of the superficial meridian system is supported by measurements of electrical skin resistance in and around the acupoints. Quantitative measurements by various researchers have demonstrated that there occurs a nearly twenty-fold drop in electrical resistance at the acupoints.[7] It is well known that energy tends to follow the pathway of least resistance. Water, which makes up the greater part of the human body, is known to be a good conductor of not only electrical but also subtle energies (as discovered in the Grad studies). Kirlian photographic studies have also confirmed that acupuncture points have distinct electrographic characteristics. Of even greater importance is the fact that electrographic researchers, such as Dumitrescu, utilizing abdominal electronographic body scans, have found that changes in brightness of the acupuncture points precede the changes of physical illness in the body by hours, days, and even weeks.[8]

This is in agreement with the supposition that changes in the etheric structure precede pathological changes of illness in the physical body. It also supports the Chinese theory that illness is caused by energetic imbalance within the meridians supplying the nutritive ch'i energies to the organs of the body. The meridian changes reflect dysfunction that has already occurred at an etheric level. These changes gradually filter down to the level of the physical via the acupuncture meridian system. An illustration of this principle, whereby acupuncture meridian changes precede physical organ dysfunction, can be seen in Kim's study of the meridian system of the liver. When Kim experimentally interfered with the nutrient flow of the meridians going to the liver, abnormal changes in liver cells were not seen until three days later.

Thus, the integrity and energy balance of the acupuncture meridian system is crucial to the maintenance and health of the organism. The meridian system holds the key not only to therapeutic routes of disease intervention, such as needle manipulation of acupoints, but also early disease detection as well. Because of their ability to record changes in the subtle energies of the meridian system, Kirlian electrography and various other acupuncture-related electronic systems may have great diagnostic potential for future physicians. Such devices may eventually provide us with tools which can measure subtle physiological imbalances in the body associated with illness much earlier than existing methods.

The acupuncture meridian system will be discussed in greater detail in a separate chapter. This meridian system is not, however, the only link between our physical body and our higher energetic systems of functioning.

The Chakras & the Nadis:
An Indian Subtle Energetic Anatomy Lesson

Information from various ancient texts of Indian yogic literature speaks of special energy centers which exist within our subtle bodies. Let us describe these energy systems and then ask whether there is any modern scientific evidence to support their existence. These energy centers, referred to as "chakras," from the Sanskit meaning "wheels," are said to resemble whirling vortices of subtle energies.[9] The chakras are somehow involved in taking in higher energies and transmuting them to a utilizable form within the human structure. Recently, Western scientists have directed their attention toward the understanding and validation of these previously unrecognized structures. In the past, the chakras and meridians have been largely ignored by Western scientists as magical constructs of unsophisticated and primitive Eastern thinkers. But the chakras, along with acupuncture meridians, are now finding their eventual validation with the evolution of subtle-energy technologies which can measure their existence and functions.

From a physiologic standpoint, the chakras appear to be involved with the flow of higher energies via specific subtle energetic channels into the cellular structure of the physical body. At one level, they seem to function as energy transformers, stepping down energy of one form and frequency to a lower level energy. This energy is, in turn, translated into hormonal, physiologic, and ultimately cellular changes throughout the body. There appear to be at least seven major chakras associated with the physical body.

Anatomically, each major chakra is associated with a major nerve plexus and a major endocrine gland. The major chakras are situated in a vertical line ascending from the base of the spine to the head. The lowest, called the root chakra, is near the coccyx. The second chakra, variously referred to as the sacral or splenic chakra, is located either just below the umbilicus or near the spleen. In actuality these are two different chakras, although both have been referred to as the second chakra in different schools of esoteric thought. The third or solar plexus chakra lies in the upper middle abdomen below the tip of the sternum. The fourth, also known as the heart chakra, can be found in the midsternal region directly over the heart and thymus gland. The fifth or throat chakra is situated in the neck near the Adam's apple. The throat chakra lies directly over the thyroid gland and larynx. The sixth or brow chakra, known as the ajna chakra in

Diagram 10.
THE SEVEN CHAKRAS
& AUTONOMIC NERVE PLEXUSES

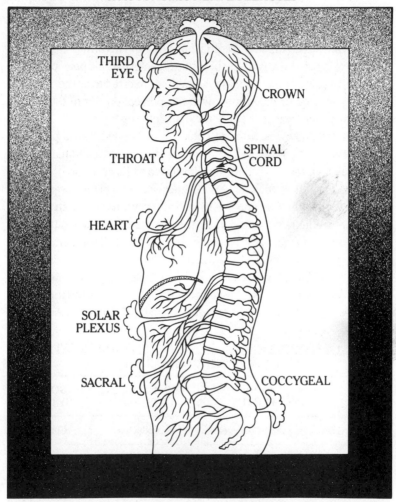

yogic texts, is in the region of the mid-forehead, slightly above the bridge of the nose. The seventh or crown chakra is located on top of the head.

In some esoteric literature there are twelve major chakras discussed. In addition to the aforementioned seven, there are two on the palms of the hands, two on the soles of the feet, and one associated with the medulla oblongata coordinated with the midbrain (sometimes referred to as the alta major chakra). There are also many minor chakras associated with the major joint structures of the body like the knees, ankles, elbows, etc. If one looks at all of the major and minor chakras, then there may be slightly more than 360 chakras in the human body.[10]

Each of the seven major chakras is also reported to be associated with a particular type of psychic perceptual functioning. This brings up the other function of the chakras as a type of subtle organ of psychic perception. For instance, the ajna or brow chakra, sometimes referred to as the third-eye center, is actively involved in clairvoyant perception. From the French vocabulary, clairvoyance literally means "clear seeing."

As noted above, each major chakra is associated with a particular nerve plexus and endocrine gland. The particular associational scheme listed here is based upon both the Western and Eastern races. There is some data suggesting a different endocrine association of the lower chakras for those born in the East and the West. This is because there are actually two different chakra systems. It is further suggested that when these two chakra systems merge, a new chakra system is created. Easterners have the coccyx and gonads, respectively, associated with the first and second chakras, and also the thymus associated with the fourth chakra. Westerners have first and second chakras associated with the gonads and the spleen, respectively, and the fourth chakra is associated with the heart. Also, some

Diagram 11.
NEUROPHYSIOLOGICAL & ENDOCRINE ASSOCIATIONS
OF THE CHAKRAS

CHAKRA	NERVE PLEXUS	PHYSIOLOGICAL SYSTEM	ENDOCRINE SYSTEM
COCCYGEAL	Sacral-Coccygeal	Reproductive	Gonads
SACRAL	Sacral	Genitourinary	Leydig
SOLAR PLEXUS	Solar	Digestive	Adrenals
HEART	Heart Plexus	Circulatory	Thymus
THROAT	Cervical Ganglia Medulla	Respiratory	Thyroid
THIRD EYE	Hypothalamus Pituitary	Autonomic Nervous System	Pituitary
HEAD	Cerebral Cortex Pineal	CNS Central Control	Pineal

sources associate the first chakra with the gonads and the second chakra with the hormone-producing leydig cells within the gonads and adrenal glands.[11] Diagram 11 gives only relative information regarding the endocrine associations of the first and second chakras. For specifics, various reference texts listed at the end of the chapter may be consulted.

The chakras translate energy of a higher dimensional (or higher frequency) nature into some type of glandular-hormonal output which subsequently affects the entire physical body. The chakras, as discussed in the esoteric literature, appear to be centers within the etheric body. There are corresponding energy centers in the higher frequency vehicles (i.e. the astral body). The primary chakras originate at the level of the etheric body. The chakras are, in turn, connected to each other and to portions of the physical-cellular structure via fine subtle-energetic channels known as "nadis."

The nadis are formed by fine threads of subtle energetic matter. They are different from the meridians, which actually have a physical counterpart in the meridian duct system. The nadis represent an extensive network of fluid-like energies which parallel the bodily nerves in their abundance. In the Eastern yogic literature, the chakras have been metaphorically visualized as flowers. The nadis are symbolic of the petals and fine roots of the flowerlike chakras that distribute the life-force and energy of each chakra into the physical body.

Various sources have described up to 72,000 nadis or etheric channels of energy in the subtle anatomy of human beings. These unique channels are interwoven with the physical nervous system.[12] Because of this intricate interconnection with the nervous system, the nadis affect the nature and quality of nerve transmission within the extensive network of the brain, spinal cord, and peripheral nerves. Dysfunction at the level of the chakras and nadis can, therefore, be associated with pathological changes in the nervous system. This dysfunction can be not only quantitative, in regards to the absolute amount of subtle energetic flow to the physical nerve substance, but also qualitative, in terms of coordination between the chakra-nadi and nervous system. In other words, there is a special alignment between the major chakras, glands, and nerve plexuses that is necessary for optimal human functioning.

In addition, the hormonal linkup between the chakras and endocrine glands suggests even further complexities of how a subtle energetic system imbalance can create abnormal changes in the cells of the entire body. A decreased flow of subtle energy through one of the chakras can give rise to underactivity of any of the key endocrine glands. For instance, decreased energy flow through the throat chakra might give rise to hypothyroidism.

Having presented here the most basic aspects of the chakra-nadi system, we must ask whether any convincing evidence exists to substantiate the existence of such a subtle energetic network. Research by Dr. Hiroshi Motoyama of Japan[13] has presented experimental findings which tend to confirm the presence of the chakra system in human beings. As mentioned previously, the chakras are felt to be energy transformers. The energy flow through the chakras can be in two different directions, that is, from the subtle energetic environment into the body, or vice-versa, from within the body projected out. This latter ability appears to be a property of the level of activation of the chakras. The ability to activate and transmit energy through one's chakras is a reflection of a rather advanced level of consciousness development and concentration by the individual.

Motoyama reasoned that if an enlightened subject could indeed activate and direct energy from the chakras, then it might be possible to measure some type of bioenergetic/bioelectrical output from these centers. Even though the primary energy conducted though the chakras might be of a subtle energetic nature, secondary reverberations of energies in a lower octave harmonic, such as electrostatic fields, might be measureable. A similar line of reasoning has been used to help explain how lower octave electrons in Kirlian photography can be used to visually capture higher dimensional etheric phenomena such as the Phantom Leaf Effect. *The electrostatic fields are only secondary effects produced by the higher octave etheric energies, but they are more easily measureable with conventional electronic recording equipment.*

Motoyama created a special lead-lined recording booth that was electrically shielded from outside electromagnetic disturbance. Within the booth was a movable copper electrode that was positionable opposite the various chakras of a subject being tested. The electrode measured the human bioelectrical field at a distance from the surface of the body. Motoyama took multiple electrical recordings from the chakras of a number of individuals over time. Many of his test subjects were advanced meditators and individuals with a previous history of psychic experience. When the electrode was placed in front of a chakra that the subject claimed had been awakened (usually through years of meditation), the amplitude and frequency of the electric field over the chakra being concentrated upon was significantly greater than the energy recorded from chakras of control subjects. Motoyama found that certain individuals could consciously project energy through their chakras. When they did so, Motoyama could detect significant electrical field disturbances emanating from their activated chakras. This phenomenon was found to be replicated many times in Motoyama's lab over the course of a number of years of testing. Itzhak Bentov, a researcher of physiological changes associated with meditation, has also duplicated Motoyama's findings regarding electrostatic energy emission from the chakras, utilizing similar equipment.[14]

Another interesting study, conducted by Dr. Valerie Hunt at UCLA,[15] used somewhat more conventional measuring equipment in a study of the chakras and human energy field. Hunt utilized EMG electrodes (ordinarily used to measure the electrical potential of muscles) to study bioelectrical energy variations in areas of skin corresponding to the positions of the chakras. The electrodes were connected to telemetry equipment that transmitted data to a recording booth, where various types of physiograph systems recorded energetic fluctuations from these points on the body. Most interestingly, Hunt found regular, high frequency, sinusoidal electrical oscillations coming from these points that had never previously been recorded nor reported in the scientific literature. The normal frequency range of brain waves is between 0 and 100 cycles per second (cps), with most information occurring between 0 and 30 cps. Muscle frequency goes up to about 225 cps and the heart goes up to about 250 cps. The readings from the chakras usually lay in a band of frequencies between 100 and 1600 cps, figures far higher than what has been traditionally found radiating from the human body.

Her original study was conducted to learn the therapeutic and energetic effects of a physical manipulative technique, known as Rolfing, on the human body. In addition to electrical recording, Dr. Hunt procured the talents of Rosalyn Bruyere, a trained psychic observer, who could clairvoyantly see the changes occurring within an individual's auric field. Bruyere was to make observations of the subject's subtle energetic field while the chakras were being electronically monitored. During her period of auric observation, she was denied immediate feedback as to the electrical activity coming from the EMG electrodes attached to the chakra points.

The results of her study were most unexpected by Dr. Hunt. She found that Bruyere's auric observations, relating to color changes in the subject's energetic field, correlated *exactly* with the EMG electrode recordings. Over time, Hunt discovered that each color of the aura was associated with a different wave pattern recorded at the chakra points on the skin of her subjects. The wave patterns became named after the auric colors with which they were found to be associated. When Bruyere would describe red in a subject's aura, unbeknownst to her the recording equipment always displayed the wave pattern later associated with red, and so on with other colors. Most interestingly, when colors such as orange were seen in the auric field, the recording equipment picked up the wave forms of yellow and red—two primary colors that when mixed form orange—from different chakras at the same time. When colors such as "white light" were seen in the auric field, the frequency signal measured was over 1000 cps. Hunt has hypothesized that *this high frequency level is actually a subharmonic of an original frequency signal which is in the range of many thousands of cycles per second: a subharmonic of the original chakra's subtle energy.*[16]

Data from experiments such as those carried out by Motoyama and Hunt would seem to confirm the existence of the chakra system. The energies measured coming from the chakras in each of the experiments were, as mentioned, composed of lower harmonics of the original higher frequency subtle energies. All of these energies are merely octaves of the electromagnetic spectrum. The subtle energies appear to occupy an extended frequency range not formerly addressed by Western scientists.

What is important is that there are various intricate systems, such as the meridian and chakra-nadi networks, which integrate the etheric body with the physical body. Although the specifics of these systems have been described for many years in the literature of healing modalities and meditative practices in the Far East and India, they have been ignored for lack of conclusive supportive evidence by Western physicians and researchers. To quote one psychic source:

> The outgoing forces from a center (chakra) play upon the etheric counterpart of the entire intricate network of nerves which constitute the nervous system. These counterparts of identical subjective correspondences are called in the Hindu philosophy, the "nadis"; they constitute an intricate and most extensive network of fluid energies which are an intangible, interior, paralleling system to that of the bodily nerves, which latter system is in fact an externalization of the inner pattern of energies. There is as yet no word in the English language or in any European tongue for the ancient word "nadi," because the existence of this subjective system is not yet recognised, and only the materialistic concept of the nerves as a system built up

in response to a tangible environment yet holds sway in the West. The idea of these nerves being the dense physical result of an inner sensitive response apparatus is still undefined and unrecognised by modern Western science. When recognition is accorded to this subtle substance (composed of threads of energy) underlying the more tangible nerves, we shall have moved forward in our approach to the entire problem of health and disease, and the world of causes will be that much nearer.[17]

The technology has now moved to the point where validation of these previously described subtle energetic links with our physical anatomy may be confirmed and elaborated upon. The beginning confirmation of these ancient subtle energetic systems, described in texts of esoteric literature, brings us now to a discussion of that part of human subtle anatomy which extends just beyond the etheric body.

The Astral Body:
The Seat of Our Emotions & a Mechanism for
Disembodied Consciousness

Up to now we have only described systems which link with the physical body in order to energize, stabilize, and provide mechanisms of cellular growth and repair at a primary level. We have discussed the new frontier of exploration and understanding through an Einsteinian or energetic approach to medicine. Through the acceptance and comprehension of what has been described as the physical-etheric interface, we may discover a new extended viewpoint of human physiological systems. By recognizing these parts of human anatomy, medicine can try to understand and apply unique and effective subtle energetic methods of healing disease. In addition to the meridian system which forms the physical-etheric interface, we have looked at other systems originating primarily at the level of the etheric body. In health and illness, the chakra-nadi system is equally important to the meridians in maintaining the proper physiologic and endocrine balance of the physical body.

In its total expression, the etheric body is an energetic form which underlies and energizes all aspects of the physical body. *A more complete understanding of how the etheric body interrelates with and affects disease expression in the physical body will provide valuable information to a new breed of physicians who are attempting to evolve beyond traditional medical dogma in their attempts to create new and more effective approaches toward healing human illness.* The medical establishment will benefit by beginning to learn the true underlying causes of health. The gradual acceptance of this new information will eventually foster the creation of an energy medicine approach to "preventive medicine."

We must now proceed to the discussion of what can only be referred to as a large "grey area" in the minds of most Western scientists. The reason for the lack of acceptance of this particular dimension of our subtle anatomy stems largely from a conflict between Eastern and Western belief systems and from the separation of religion and science thousands of years ago.

Our examination of human subtle energetic anatomy brings us to a discussion of what has been called, in the esoteric literature, the Astral Body. This astral body is composed of astral matter, which is a subtle substance of even higher energetic frequencies than etheric matter.

Diagram 12.
PIANO KEYBOARD ANALOGY OF
HUMAN FREQUENCY SPECTRUM

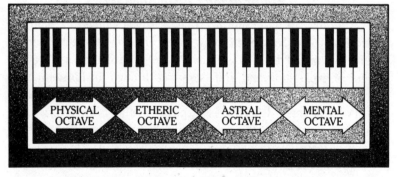

Referring back to our piano keyboard analogy, it was noted that octaves of musical notes could be seen as similiar to octaves of electromagnetic energy. The lowest keys on the left side of the keyboard were compared to the physical spectrum of frequencies. The next set of keys to the right formed the energetic musical scale of the etheric realm. Still further to the right, beyond the frequencies of the etheric, lies the next higher octave, comparable to the realm of astral matter and energies. Although this analogy extends still further, encompassing a full seven octaves of higher frequency vehicles, we will stop here briefly to examine the phenomenon of the astral body and the realm of astral matter.

There is much information in the esoteric literature about the astral, or emotional, body. Knowledge of this part of subtle human anatomy has been known and taught since the earliest Egyptian dynasties. The astral body is a component of the total multidimensional human being and, like the etheric body, is usually superimposed over the physical frame. These octaves are distinct, but not separate, within our being. The astral body is composed of matter of energetic frequencies well beyond the normal human perceptual range, and it is invisible to all but the trained clairvoyant eye. (As we shall discover later, the trained clairvoyant eye is actually the use of the ajna or third-eye chakra of the astral body, which is already attuned to transmuting and transmitting energies of this particular frequency domain.) We had earlier alluded to the function of the chakras as extended organs of perception. Because astral matter exists in a frequency band well above etheric and physical matter, it is able to occupy the same space as the physical and etheric body. This coexistence exhibits a principle of matter which might be called the Principle of Nondestructive Coexistence. This principle states that matter of differing frequencies can occupy the same space at the same time, nondestructively.

It has been noted that the astral body is "usually" superimposed upon the physical structure. What happens when it is not superimposed upon the framework of the human body? The answer to this question is difficult but not impossible to explain. Before delving into this tantalizing question, we must first deal with some of the more physiological functions of the astral body.

According to esoteric sources, the astral body, like the etheric body, also has seven major chakras. These are referred to as the astral counterparts of the chakras. Like the etheric chakras, they too are transformers of energy and are an integrated part of our extended subtle energetic system. The astral centers are transmitters and receivers of astral energy which is, in turn, stepped down and passed on to the etheric chakras where, through the nadis, the energies become translated into nervous and glandular function. Since the astral body is involved with emotional expression, the astral chakras provide a subtle-energy connection whereby a person's emotional state can disturb or enhance health.

The esoteric literature recognizes that the effects of glandular and hormonal functioning occur at the level of cellular activity and that hormones are also an integral factor in the emotional expression of the personality. Recognition of the astral octave influences on health also exists within conventional medicine. For instance, physicians have long recognized the hyperthyroid, hyperkinetic personality, and its contrast with the asthenic hypoadrenal personality. Endocrinologists have acknowledged particular patterns of emotional expression which relate to specific types of dysfunctional glandular activity. What has been missed by most endocrinologists, however, is the fact that *the hormonal activity of the major endocrine glands is dependent upon the energizing influence of their associated chakras.*

The astral body, sometimes referred to as the emotional body, is considered to be the seat of human emotions. Our emotions have a deeper and more subtle origin than is currently recognized by modern science. In the last several decades, medical science has begun to recognize and elucidate upon the relationships between emotional stress and physical illness. Because the astral body has a strong connection to our emotional nature, there is a powerful, unrecognized link between the mind, the physical body, and the astral body, in the expression of physical and emotional illnesses. Emotional imbalances may be due to neurochemical disturbances in brain activity as well as to abnormal patterns of energy flow within the astral body and its chakras.

> *The centers (chakras) and glands . . . basically determine the state of health—good, indifferent, or bad—and the psychological equipment of a man.* The primary effect of the activity of the glands is psychological . . . . A man is upon the physical plane, emotionally and mentally what his glandular system makes him, and incidentally what they make him physically, because that is frequently determined by his psychological state of mind and emotions.[18] *(italics added)*

Another name for the astral body has been the desire body or emotional body. The esoteric literature describes the astral as the seat of our sensual appetites and desires, longings, moods, feelings, appetites, and fears. Surprisingly, fear is one of the dominant astral energies which affects us at this time. *The degree to which people are affected by these desires and fears governs the extent and nature of one's personality expression upon the physical plane.*[19] Although most physicians and Western scientists consider human emotional expression to be a characteristic of neural activity of the limbic system[20] within the brain, this is only a subsidiary system to higher dimensional energies which also have input into the system. The physical brain is viewed by Newtonian mechanists as a complex neurochemical biocomputer. Mechanists see the brain as something akin to a sophisticated servomechanism. The living brain is actually an interface for the expression of the soul into active, physical life. If the nervous system becomes impaired through disease, the personality can become trapped in a nonexpressive vehicle (i.e., the Locked-In Man Syndrome). For instance, stroke victims who suffer a severe isolated motor impairment without cognitive loss may be fully aware yet unable to communicate to those around them.

Programming for this biocomputer system can come from many levels of input. Western scientists, at present, recognize only physical inputs into the nervous system. The astral energies have their impact upon the physical brain and nervous system through their subtle linkup with the etheric body and its interconnections with the physical body. Unlike the etheric body, which supports and energizes the physical body, the astral body also functions as a vehicle of consciousness which can exist separately, yet connected to, the physical body. The mobile consciousness of the individual can move and interact with its environment via the astral body while the physical body is inactive or asleep. Although it might seem strange, this function of the astral body has important implications for explaining an important and only recently recognized human phenomenon: the NDE, or Near Death Experience.[21]

Descriptions of experiences related by individuals who were temporarily clinically dead have been the subject of a number of books by Dr. Raymond Moody[22] and, more recently, by Dr. Kenneth Ring.[23] Interviews with hundreds of individuals who have been temporarily classified as clinically dead have produced similar descriptions of experiences in this eerie state. One of the most common experiences shared by the near dead has been the sensation of floating above the physical body and looking down. Individuals frequently describe accurate details of resuscitation attempts by paramedical personnel down to the clothing of the team members, words spoken, and drugs given. Contemporary physicians, bereft of logical explanations, have attempted to invoke biochemical mechanisms of cerebral anoxia (lack of oxygen to the brain) to explain these apparent hallucinations. While floating above the table and looking down at their own bodies, many describe being drawn upwards toward a light at the end of a tunnel. The near death experiences are representative of a state known as an OOBE, or Out-Of-Body Experience. The OOBE is perhaps a more accurate description of what happens to the individual because, during the NDE, the individual is, indeed, out of his/her physical body. If he or she is out of the physical body, then through what perspective is the person viewing the scene? The answer to this question is that he or she is viewing the world through the eyes of the astral body!

Another term for the OOBE, and perhaps a more accurate descriptor, is the phenomenon known as astral projection. Astral projection involves the projection of the consciousness of the individual outside of his/her physical shell via his/her astral vehicle of expression. During life, it is said the astral body is connected to the physical body through a type of umbilical cord sometimes referred to as the silver cord. Supposedly, at the point of physical death, this cord is severed, leaving behind the decaying physical-etheric shell. The esoteric literature states that during sleep all humans leave their physical bodies, and travel through and interact with elements and inhabitants of the astral realm. Of course, because most humans do not remember what happens to them during sleep, it is most difficult to prove that any astral experiences have occurred. In most cases, people would tend to relegate these experiences to dreaming, a state of consciousness which itself is poorly understood by many. The usual times that individuals have remembered astrally projecting are during traumatic ejections from the physical body, as in violent accidents and Near Death Experiences. In these circumstances, it would seem that the dissociation of the astral form from the physical body is a manifestation of some type of primitive energetic reflex which protects our consciousness from traumatic experience. However, some gifted individuals have been discovered who are able to repeatedly self-induce these out-of-body experiences and project their astral selves to distant locales. After returning to waking consciousness, many of these OOBE explorers are able to bring back unique insights and valuable information about their astral journeys.[24,25]

There have been a number of research attempts, past and present, which have attempted to validate the existence of the astral body and its experiences in the realm of the astral plane, the plane of matter from which the astral body is composed. Early experiments at the Psychical Research Foundation in Durham, North Carolina, carried out by Dr. Robert Morris, tried to gather physical evidence supporting the presence of the astral body at remote locations.[26] Morris worked with Keith Harary, an undergraduate psychology student, who claimed to be adept at projecting his consciousness out of his physical body and into his astral body.

Morris designed an unusual approach to measuring the presence of Harary's astral form, or what was referred to as "the second body" in the study. His first attempt utilized a living detector, i.e., Harary's pet kitten. It was discovered that whenever Harary's astral form was present within the room, the kitten, normally rambunctious and wandering, would settle down and be quiet. In order to quantitate the kitten's activity, it was placed in a special open field container divided into 24 numbered ten-inch squares. The number of squares the kitten traversed over time could be used as a measure of movement. The kitten was filmed during control periods and during experimental times when Harary attempted to project his consciousness into the special experimental animal chamber. During non-OOBE control periods, the kitten was very active and meowed frequently. The kitten would cross a large number of squares and attempt to get out of the container. Conversely, it was found that whenever Harary's "second body" was purportedly present, the kitten was extremely quiet and calm. This effect was repeated during four experimental sessions.

As seemingly inconsequential as this data might seem, the results suggest that the kitten could distinguish the presence of Harary's seemingly invisible astral body. Another experiment using a snake as a living detector produced similar meaningful changes in the animal's behavior during Harary's successful OOBE attempts. Unfortunately, the animals tended to rapidly adapt to their experimental surroundings and later became unreliable as indicators of astral projection.

Another interesting approach described by Dr. Karlis Osis at the American Society for Psychical Research in New York employed the talents of psychologist Alex Tanous, another gifted OOBE subject. Because it is theoretically possible to gain information about a distant location via remote viewing or clairvoyance, by utilizing psychic processes different from astral projection, Osis created a special viewing target that displayed different images to the observer based on the position from which it was viewed. Various figures were placed in a box in such a way that a unique optical illusion could only be seen if viewed from a special peephole at the side of the box. If the arrangement of items in the box was viewed from above or within, a different geometric picture would be seen than the one observed through the peephole. As an additional measure, Osis placed electrical strain gauge detectors in the box to determine if there were any measureable energetic effects in the viewing box at the time the astral body was present and observing. Tanous reported back images during the times he successfully projected which correlated with viewing the optical illusion. Additionally, during these successful projections, significant fluctuations in energy output were picked up from the strain gauge detectors, implying that some type of energetic disturbance, associated with the presence of the astral body, had occurred.

A somewhat more sophisticated approach with similar positive results was carried out at Stanford Research Institute by physicists Targ and Puthoff[27] using a superconductor-shielded magnetometer. This well-shielded apparatus, also known as a quark detector, was actually part of a physics experiment being conducted at Stanford University's physics department. Ingo Swann, one of Targ and Puthoff's gifted OOBE subjects, was asked to try to tune in and project his consciousness into the shielded magnetometer. The apparatus itself was physically inaccessible by virtue of its being buried in a vault beneath the physics building and shielded by layers of aluminum, copper, mu-metal, and even a superconducting shield. Before the experiment, a decaying magnetic field had been set up inside the magnetometer. This provided a background calibration signal that registered as a stable, oscillating, sine-wave-like tracing on a strip recorder. During the periods when Swann felt he was out of his body and looking into the magnetometer, the recorder output showed a doubling of the sine-wave frequency for about thirty seconds. Several other disturbances in the magnetic field were also noted at times Swann directed his attention to the device. In addition, Swann was able to provide accurate drawings of the interior layers of the magnetometer based on his observations during the out-of-body experience. A number of SRI scientists from the physics department felt that this was a very significant observation, although they did not regard it as a carefully controlled experiment.

These experiments, when viewed collectively, suggest that the phenomenon of astral projection is real. Additionally, the evidence implies that the astral body can create electromagnetic disturbances of lower-octave harmonic energies which can be measured by sensitive electronic equipment. There are yet no studies to date which have successfully photographed the astral body, but that achievement may lie with the future development of imaging devices such as the EMR Scanner mentioned in the previous chapter.

If the principle behind photographing the etheric body involves manipulating energetic frequencies in harmonic resonance with etheric energies, then this same phenomenon might be applied to capturing images of the astral body. The only difference between the etheric and astral scanner would be in the frequency of the energy needed to resonantly excite the astral body. If indeed the astral body, like the etheric, is real, are there scientific models which might explain the existence and even the behavior of these higher dimensional phenomena?

A Scientific Model of Frequency Domains: The Tiller-Einstein Model of Positive-Negative Space/Time

Although Western scientists would offer the assumption that no mathematical models currently exist within electromagnetic theory to explain the existence of etheric and astral forms, there are certain pioneering researchers who have taken this matter to closer scrutiny. One such researcher is Dr. William Tiller, a professor at Stanford University and former chairman of the Department of Materials Science at that institution. Over the last decade or more, Dr. Tiller has been working to apply currently existing scientific models to the explanation of certain subtle energetic phenomena without discarding the existing framework of science.

The reason I call this the Tiller-Einstein Model is because its insights are basic to the Einsteinian equation, relating energy to matter, from which it is derived. The most familiar form of this equation is $E = mc^2$, however this is not the entire expression. The shorter equation is modified by a proportionality constant known as the Einstein-Lorentz Transformation. This transformational constant is the relativistic factor that describes how different parameters of measurement, from time distortion to alteration of length, width, and mass, will vary according to the velocity of the system being described. The true Einsteinian equation is illustrated in Diagram 13.

The classical interpretation of Einstein's famous equation is that the energy contained within a particle is equivalent to the product of its mass multiplied by the speed of light squared. This means that there is an incredible amount of potential energy stored within a tiny particle of matter. American nuclear physicists were the first to begin to understand how to utilize the revolutionary information contained within this remarkable equation. Their earliest successful attempts to release this potential resulted in the atomic bombs exploded at the end of World War II. The stored potential energy within a few teaspoons of uranium was all that was necessary to level the cities of Hiroshima and Nagasaki.

A more complex understanding of Einstein's equation has evolved over time which may begin to help scientists comprehend the multidimen-

Diagram 13.
EINSTEIN-LORENTZ TRANSFORMATION

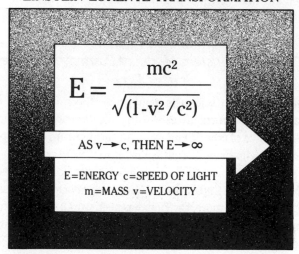

Diagram 14.
RELATIONSHIP OF ENERGY TO VELOCITY

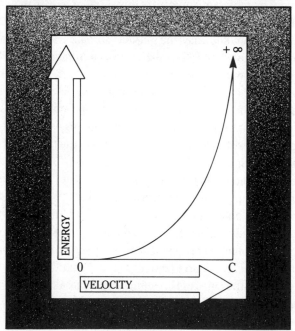

sional nature of the universe. *Einstein's equation suggests that matter and energy are interconvertable and interconnected.* Subatomic matter is actually a form of condensed, particularized energy, i.e. a frozen mini-energy field. The atomic bomb is merely one example which demonstrates how matter can be converted into energy. When one looks at the extended equation above, in which $E = mc^2$ is modified by the Einstein-Lorentz Transformation, new insights into the dimensional aspects of matter, both gross and subtle, can be appreciated. If one accelerates a particle faster and faster until it approaches the speed of light, its kinetic energy increases exponentially as described by the equation: Kinetic Energy $= \frac{1}{2} mv,^2$ where v is equal to velocity. The visual expression of this relationship is displayed in Diagram 14.

This diagram illustrates the exponential relationship between matter and energy at velocities approaching the speed of light. To those interpreting this relationship, it would seem that it is physically impossible to accelerate particles beyond the speed of light. The ascending curve approaches the speed of light (c) but never intersects with it, and continues off into infinity. For instance, high energy particle physicists are aware that as one tries to accelerate a subatomic particle faster and faster, closer to the speed of light, extremely large amounts of energy are needed. The reason for this strange phenomenon is that the relativistic mass of a particle increases exponentially at speeds approaching light velocity, until the energy needed for further acceleration to "c" becomes tremendous. This is, of course, the energy necessary to accelerate a physical particle of matter.

Up until now most physicists have accepted the seeming limitation that one cannot accelerate matter beyond the speed of light. This assumption is partly related to the fact that when one inserts numbers greater than the speed of light into the Einstein-Lorentz Transformation, one arrives at solutions containing the square root of -1, which is considered an imaginary number. Since most physicists do not believe in imaginary numbers, they assume that the speed of light is the maximum velocity at which matter can travel.

Certain pioneering mathematicians, such as Charles Muses,[28] consider the square root of -1 to be one of a category of numbers referred to as "hypernumbers." These hypernumbers, he believes, are necessary to the development of equations which mathematically describe the behavior of higher dimensional phenomena (such as the subtle energetic interactions of living systems that we have been describing throughout this book).

Although at first glance imaginary numbers like the square root of -1 might seem to be impossible to fathom, Muses points out that they are necessary to finding solutions in the equations of electromagnetic and quantum theory. It is perhaps appropriate that so-called imaginary numbers would play a key role in describing the higher dimensional phenomena that conservative scientists have long considered to be imaginary domains themselves.

If we assume for a moment that solutions containing the square root of -1 may be valid in describing higher dimensional phenomena, then we are able to begin to understand the full predictive power inherent in the transformed Einsteinian equation. Diagram 15 is a plot of the energy of a particle relative to its velocity from a theoretical state of rest all the way up to and beyond the speed of light (c). (A lengthier and more complex mathematical description of how this graph is derived can be found in the Appendix at the end of the book.)

Diagram 15.
POSITIVE-NEGATIVE SPACE/TIME MODEL

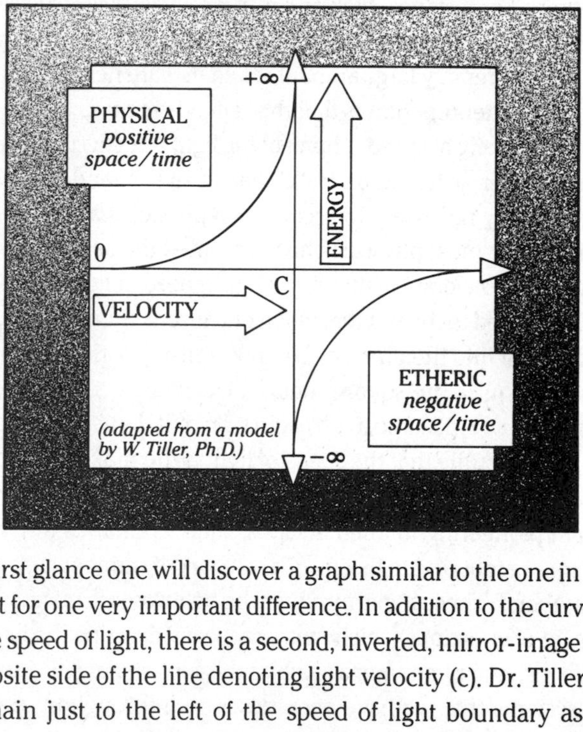

At first glance one will discover a graph similar to the one in Diagram 14 except for one very important difference. In addition to the curve leading up to the speed of light, there is a second, inverted, mirror-image curve on the opposite side of the line denoting light velocity (c). Dr. Tiller refers to the domain just to the left of the speed of light boundary as positive space/time, otherwise known as the physical space/time universe. As the model implies, positive space/time matter can exist only at velocities less than the speed of light. The inverted curve to the right of c, travelling at velocities exceeding the speed of light, describes the domain of *negative space/time* (-S/T). This world of negative space/time, and particles which move faster than light, is an area not unfamiliar to modern physics. A number of physicists have proposed the existence of a particle known as a "tachyon," which would theoretically exist only at speeds exceeding that of light velocity.[29]

The properties of such unusual particles travelling at supraluminal (faster-than-light) velocities are quite interesting. *Whereas positive space/time matter is associated with the forces of electricity and electromagnetic (EM) radiation, negative space/time matter is associated primarily with magnetism and a force which Tiller describes as magnetoelectric (ME) radiation.* We know, for instance, that the particles which make up the physical atom are electrically charged as positive, negative, or neutral. Electromagnetic theory predicts that magnetic monopoles—particles magnetically charged either North or South—should exist in nature. No one has yet successfully captured or repeatably detected magnetic monopoles. It is possible that if the domain of this particle is in tachyonic realms like those in Tiller's negative space/time model, then our present measuring equipment may be inadequate (or insensitive) for the task at hand.

There are other interesting properties of negative space/time particles which have relevance to our discussion of subtle energies. Because all solutions to the Einstein-Lorentz Transformation at supraluminal velocities are negative in character, then negative space/time particles would have negative mass. In addition, *negative space/time matter would demonstrate the property of negative entropy.* Entropy is a term which describes the tendency toward disorder of a system. The greater the entropy, the greater the disorder. In general, most systems within the physical universe tend toward increasing positive entropy and more disorder over time, i.e., things tend to fall apart.

The most notable exception to this entropic rule of the physical universe is found in the behavior of living systems. Biological systems take in raw material (food) and organize these simple components into complex macromolecular structures (such as protein, DNA, collagen, etc.). *Living systems display the property of negative entropy, or a tendency toward decreasing disorder of the system.* They take in substances which are broken down to elements which are less organized, and then build them up into systems which are more organized. Living organisms take in raw material and energy and self-organize them into complex structural and physiologic subcomponents. *One might say then that the life-force seems to be associated with negative entropic characteristics.* (When a body dies and the life-force vacates the physical form, the remaining unoccupied shell returns, via earthly microorganisms, to its raw constituents, in characteristic positive entropic fashion.) *The etheric body, a self-organizing holographic energy template, would also seem to demonstrate negative entropic properties.* The etheric body supplies the spatial ordering properties to the cellular systems of the physical body. This negatively entropic characteristic of the subtle life-energies and the etheric template would appear to satisfy at least one requirement of Tiller's negative space/time matter.

In addition, *negative space/time matter is primarily magnetic in nature.* In Bernard Grad's experiments on the effects of laying-on-of hands healing on living systems, it was discovered that the growth rate of plants could be accelerated by magnet-treated water as well as healer-treated water. A number of other similarities between magnet- and healer-treated water have also been found. Research chemist Robert Miller found that copper sulfate dissolved in regular distilled water forms jade-green monoclinic crystals when it precipitates out of solution. If the copper sulfate solution is exposed to the energies of a healer's hands or a strong magnetic field, it always forms coarser grained turquoise-blue crystals, instead of the characteristic jade-green structures.[30] This may be a property of altered hydrogen bonding and subsequent changes in chemical coordination complexes.

Studies by Dr. Justa Smith[31] have shown that *healers can accelerate the kinetic activity of enzymes in a fashion similar to the effects of high-intensity magnetic fields.* Dr. Smith measured the effects of the energies from healers' hands on test tubes of the enzyme trypsin.

Smith asked a healer to concentrate on sending energy to an imaginary patient—a test tube of enzymes held in his hands. Experimental controls were introduced by having normal individuals also hold test tubes of enzymes in order to simulate the possible activating effects of the warmth of the hands. Utilizing standard spectrophotometric methods, she measured changes in the activity of small amounts of enzymes taken from the healer-exposed and control test tubes over time. Previous work had shown that high intensity magnetic fields could accelerate enzyme reaction rates. Only the healer's energies, as compared to controls, were found to accelerate enzyme reaction rates linearly over time. The experiment was varied utilizing different enzymes. With one enzyme, the healer caused a *decrease* in enzymatic activity; in a third, there was no change. When the enzyme whose activity was decreased (NAD-ase) was looked at from a cellular metabolic perspective, it was found that the decreased activity in this enzyme would result in a greater energy reserve of the cell. *The activity of the enzymes affected by the healers always seemed to be in a direction that was toward greater overall health and balanced metabolic activity of the organism.*

Dr. Smith tried another variation on the experiment. She exposed the enzyme trypsin to ultraviolet light, which is known to damage enzyme activity through protein denaturation (unfolding). High intensity magnetic fields had been previously shown to restore the enzyme's activity. When the healer held the damaged enzymes, they were found to regain structural integrity and become active. After becoming activated, their enzymatic activity continued to increase linearly over time, depending on how long the healer held the test tube of damaged enzymes. Thus, the energetic fields of the healer's hands were able to repair ultraviolet-damaged enzymes in a manner similar to that of magnetic fields. *The energetic fields of healers fit Dr. Tiller's criteria for negative space/time substance, or magnetoelectric energy, in that they demonstrate certain qualitative similarities to magnetic fields, and they also have negative entropic properties, i.e. the ability to reassemble disordered molecules such as enzymes.*

The experimental evidence from the aforementioned studies suggests that the energies of healers appear to be magnetic in nature. However, healers' fields demonstrate properties which are entirely different from what is known about conventional magnetic fields. Both healers' hands and magnets could accelerate the growth rate of plants and cause blue crystallization of copper sulfate. Additionally, magnetic fields and healers hands could increase enzyme reaction rates. Interestingly, early studies with magnetic detectors were unable to register any significant magnetic fields around the healers' hands. However, more recent research by Dr. John Zimmerman at the University of Colorado School of Medicine has added further evidence to suggest the magnetic nature of healing energy. Utilizing an ultrasensitive magnetic-field detector called a SQUID (Superconducting Quantum Interference Device), Dr. Zimmerman demonstrated significant increases in the intensity of the magnetic fields emitted by healers' hands.[32] The increases in magnetic field signals from healers' hands were up to several hundred times larger than background noise. However, these magnetic fields were at intensity levels far weaker than those required to produce enzyme effects in the laboratory. Dr. Justa Smith's experimental work with enzymes used magnetic fields of 13,000 gauss, which are at least 26,000 times more powerful than the Earth's magnetic field. One would certainly expect to find fairly intense magnetic fields around healers' hands if they were palming off magnets to fake their experimental results!

Additionally, healers' energies caused variable changes in the reaction rates of different enzymes, whereas magnetic fields could only cause a nonspecific increase in activity. *The direction of change in enzyme activity always seemed to mirror the natural cellular intelligence.* Also, healers were able to repair damaged enzymes similar to high intensity magnetic fields. *The suggestion here is that the subtle life-energies of healers seem to have primarily magnetic properties.* This is quite a fascinating revelation when one considers that, back in the time of Franz Anton Mesmer's experiments with healing in eighteenth-century France, it was referred to as *"magnetic healing."* Of course, no magnetic fields could be detected then, as now (with the exception of Dr. Zimmerman's recent work with SQUID detectors). The healers' energies differ from conventional magnetic fields in that they are not only qualitatively different in their effects, but also quantitatively different in that the magnetic fields associated with healers are exceedingly weak, yet they have powerful biological and chemical effects. The unusual magnetic nature of these subtle energies fulfills one of Tiller's major criteria for negative space/time substance.

Dr. Tiller theorizes that negative space/time is the domain of the etheric. A third substance called "deltron" has been hypothesized to act as an energy-bonding coupler between the etheric and physical worlds. Tiller feels that the postulation of this deltron intermediary was necessary because there are no resonant vibrational modes possible between etheric and physical energies in view of the fact that there is no frequency overlap between positive and negative space/time. (This may not actually be the case, because we know that there can be interactions between higher and lower octave energies, possibly through resonant harmonic effects, as in the case of photographing the Phantom Leaf Effect.) The important revelation is that we have a theoretical model of matter/energy relationships which begins to give us a mathematical foothold on the physical universe, the physical-etheric interface, and the world of etheric substance. *What is most interesting about the entire positive-negative space/time diagram is that this model is predicted by Einstein's relativistic equation!* I would also suggest that the subtle world of astral matter lies within the domain of negative space/time, vibrates at speeds faster than light and has certain magnetic properties similar to etheric matter. Some of Dr. Tiller's more recent work considers the possibility that astral energies may operate at speeds between 10^{10} and 10^{20} times the speed of light!

The Tiller-Einstein model has interesting significance in interpreting the behavior of etheric and astral matter. The astral domain has certain unique properties, one of which is the principle that astrally or emotionally charged thoughts have a life of their own. At the astral energetic level, certain thoughts, either conscious or unconscious, may exist as distinct energy fields or thoughtforms[33] with unique shapes, colors, and characteristics. Some thoughts, especially those that are charged with *emotional intensity*, can have a separate identity apart from their creator. Certain thoughts may actually be charged with subtle energetic substance and exist (unconsciously) as thoughtforms in the energetic fields of their creators. These thoughtforms can frequently be seen by clairvoyant individuals who are very sensitive to higher energetic phenomena. The fact that our consciousness can influence the energy fields of our subtle energetic anatomy has important implications for both medicine and psychology.

> Subtle matter, especially astral matter, is very magnetic. Movement at this level is relatively fluid, compared to the dense physical plane. There are forms, but they are mercurial. They tend to pulsate, and movement can be in more than one direction at the same time. It is, after all, another dimension of existence and must be understood on its own terms. . . .
>
> One of the discoveries that researchers in psychology and medicine will eventually make some day is that *nonferrous matter also has the magnetic properties which ferrous matter does. This includes the matter which goes into the substance of human thought and feeling*. It is not the type of magnetism which attracts iron filings, of course, but it is most definitely a species of magnetism. It attracts other substances in harmony with it, as well as repelling matter which is not in harmony with it. Experimenters will eventually find that emotions must be dealt with both as highly magnetic nonphysical matter and as an aspect of consciousness. *The difficulty in treating many emotional illnesses stems, in part, from the fact that the emotions which cause these problems tend to be magnetically re-*

sponsive to a kind of astral matter which easily "glues" itself both to our own feelings and to more of its own kind. The magnetic action makes it very difficult to get rid of the "bad" astral matter—and the emotional problem.

Medicine is really at the stage where it needs to take a closer look at some of the remarkable results which have come from. . . unorthodox methods [such as herbal medicine and homeopathy.] Doctors need to learn more about the hidden side of life—the so-called invisible realms and the subtle planes and grades of matter. There is a wealth of material about these subjects which can be investigated scientifically. . . such as the fact that small amounts of vegetable or mineral matter, the essences of flowers or homeopathic remedies, can have a powerful effect in treating human illness.

Certain types of subtle physical or *etheric* matter seem to attract specific illnesses to the physical body. *The right type of magnetism administered as an herbal or homeopathic treatment would be able to dispel or disperse the"'bad" matter, leading to a cure*. . . Indeed, there is a whole science of magnetism waiting to be discovered and applied to physical and psychological health.[34] *(italics added)*

An inferred meaning within this statement is that both etheric and astral matter have higher dimensional or non-physical magnetic properties. If astral and etheric matter are composed of magnetic particles, then the ordered movement of such subtle particles along a linear path would constitute a magnetic current. (Tiller refers to such energy flow as magneto-electric currents.) From what is known about electricity, we find that an electrical current is accompanied by a magnetic field. Conversely, a magnetic current should generate an electrical field. *It is possible, for instance, that the primarily magnetic astral and etheric energies flowing through the chakras would create associated electrical field effects.* This would explain the experimental findings of electrostatic fields over the chakras as measured by Dr. Motoyama's chakra device, and possibly the oscillating electrical currents recorded from the skin at the level of the chakras as detected by Dr. Hunt at UCLA. The electrical fields measured by these different energy-sensing systems constituted a *secondary* effect, *not the primary subtle energetic phenomena*, as was correctly intuited by Drs. Hunt and Motoyama.

Another implication suggested by the aforementioned quote is that various subtle energetic therapies, such as homeopathic remedies, may work by delivering a quantum dose of magnetoelectric or subtle magnetic energy to patients in a way that is able to neutralize abnormal etheric or astral magnetic patterns within the subtle energetic anatomy of the patient. For instance, the Bach flower remedies have been used for many years in England and the United States to treat patients with various emotional difficulties. The vibrational actions of such subtle medicines as homeopathic remedies and flower essences can be highly effective in alleviating the emotional distress and dis-ease of many patients. However, since the energetic effects of such remedies may occur at the level of the negative space/time frame, i.e., at the level of our etheric and astral anatomy, the immediate physiological benefits would be difficult to directly measure with conventional medical testing.

The positive-negative space/time model appears very useful in demonstrating that modern physics may already have within its grasp the mathematical tools available to begin to understand these subtle energetic phenomena. This multidimensional energetic understanding of Einsteinian medicine may ultimately change the way we will view ourselves and the healing arts in the future.

The Mental Body, the Causal Body & Our Higher Spiritual Bodies

Up to now we have described the subtle energetic substance of the etheric and astral bodies with some scientific experimental evidence supporting their existence. In addition, we have looked at a model, based upon Einstein's relativistic equation, that may begin to incorporate these subtle energetic phenomena into the framework of existing physics. As we proceed into matter of higher frequency than the astral, we must unfortunately leave behind the world of scientific measurement, because the tools to examine these phenomena still lie waiting in the minds of their creators. For further information on these far reaches of the unknown, we will call, as before, upon the observant clairvoyant eye and the Theosophical and esoteric literature, where discussion of these phenomena are more commonplace than in the world of hard science.

The first of the subtle bodies which extend into the frequency range beyond that of the astral body is known as the mental body. This body, like the astral, is composed of matter of a higher frequency than the physical. It occupies the next octave of frequencies on the energetic piano scale to the right of the astral. As the astral body is sometimes the vehicle of expression of human emotional aspects, so the mental body is the vehicle through which the self manifests and expresses the concrete intellect. Like the astral body, the mental body also has corresponding chakras which are linked, ultimately, to the physical form. Like its lower vibrational counterparts, the chakras of the mental vehicle are focused at the major endocrine and nervous centers, and surround and enfold the astral and etheric chakras. For energy of the mental realm to have its effects upon the physical, there must first occur a type of cascade effect. The mental energies will have their effects upon that matter of the astral body which is more responsive to the mental energies' particular type of energetic stimulation. Then, through changes in the astral vehicle, energetic changes are transmitted to the etheric, and finally the physical vehicle, through the etheric connections discussed earlier in the chapter.

As discussed earlier, there are energetic forms of subtle substance which are known as thoughtforms. On the astral level, these take the form of emotional types of thoughts. On the mental level, these thoughtforms may represent purely mental ideas that an individual has been (or will be) working on. For instance, a clairvoyant who is adept at observing the auric field of an individual to the level of the mental may see images of ideas, concepts, and inventions the person has been mentally laboring over that will appear to be floating like picture bubbles in that individual's auric field. If the mental body is functioning properly, it allows an individual to think clearly and to focus his/her mental energies in appropriate directions with force, vigor, and clarity. Because the mental body feeds energy into the astral/emotional body, which then funnels down into the etheric and physical bodies, healing a person at the mental level is stronger and produces longer lasting results than healing from either the astral or etheric levels.

At the next highest level of subtle energetic substance, we find the vehicle known as the causal body. In many ways, it is the causal body which is the closest thing to that which we call our Higher Self. The causal body is composed of subtle substance of yet a higher vibrational frequency than the mental body. Its frequency is perhaps one octave higher on the subtle energetic harmonic scale. Whereas the mental body is more concerned with the creation and transmission of concrete thoughts and ideas to the brain, for their expression and manifestation upon the physical plane, the causal body is involved with the area of abstract ideas and concepts.

Causal consciousness deals with the essence of a subject while the mental level studies the subject's details. The lower mental body dwells upon mental images obtained from sensations, and analytically reasons about purely concrete objects. The causal body deals with the essence of substance and the true causes behind the illusion of appearances. The causal plane is a world of realities. On this plane we no longer deal with emotions, ideas, or conceptions, but with the essence and underlying nature of the thing in question. *Unlike the etheric, astral, or mental vehicles, the causal body is much more than an individualized body.* In addition, when we deal with the causal vehicle, we are no longer dealing specifically with the single personality of the individual that is expressing itself through the physical body. Just as the mental body first has its effect upon the astral, and then cascades down to the etheric and the physical, so the causal body has its initial input at the level of the mental, and then moves down the energetic scale. Thus, healing from the causal level will have more powerful effects than integrating at the mental or lower energetic levels of body and personality integration.

Beyond the causal form, there are considered to be even higher frequency subtle energetic dimensions which have their input into the human energetic system. They are involved with higher levels of spiritual energy and essence than the systems we have already described. It is beyond the scope of this text to elaborate upon their specific functions. Suffice it to say that there are other levels of subtle energetic effects of even higher frequency nature than the causal body, which ultimately impact upon the physical and personality expression of the human form in its sojourns upon the physical plane.

A Frequency Model of Our Extended Subtle Energetic Anatomy: A Framework for Understanding the Multidimensional Human

Although the functions of our higher energetic bodies have only been briefly discussed, it would be most productive at this time to examine one working model of how these subtle energetic systems are integrated into the whole person. We are again borrowing from the theoretical models of Dr. William Tiller, Ph.D, who is perhaps one of the leading theorists in the subtle energetic field. Diagram 16 shows in one graphic illustration the entire human energetic spectrum.

In the diagram, we can see a representation of each of our subtle bodies as a bell curve distribution of energies. In Tiller's model, the distinction between different levels of the mind refers to an instinctive (lower) and intellectual (higher) division of the mental body, whereas the spiritual mind represents the causal body. Energetic levels beyond this are referred to as spirit (for simplicity's sake). Each bell curve describes an energetic distribution of the frequencies of matter which make up an individual's different subtle energetic bodies.

Diagram 16.
FREQUENCY MODEL OF
THE HUMAN SUBTLE BODIES

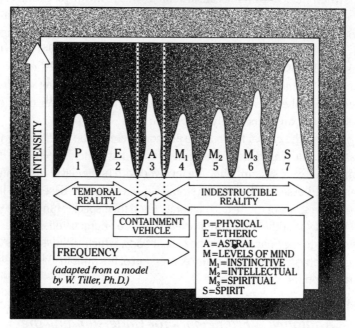

In the case of the physical body, the predominant frequency of the physical form is that frequency directly under the peak of the curve. (The exact shapes of the curves are approximate and hypothetical, especially in reference to specific energetic intensities, as this is, of course, a transitional model of understanding.) In other words, the frequencies of matter which make up the physical body are predominantly of one type of vibration, but others of slightly higher and lower frequency may also contribute to its composition. Similar to the physical, there is a higher and lower astral frequency range. This concept also has relevance to the domain of the astral plane from the perspective of evolutionary trends involving human beings as a group.

To the right of the physical curve, we find the frequency distribution curve of the spectrum of matter which composes the etheric body. Each of the subsequent curves to the right has a similar meaning to that given for the frequency distribution of the physical form, in that the predominant energetic frequency of each particular subtle body lies beneath the peak of the curve.

Because the physical and etheric forms are so intertwined and interdependent, they form what Tiller has referred to as human temporal reality. The physical form cannot exist without the energizing nourishment and spatial guidance provided by the etheric body. When the physical body dies, so the etheric form also dies and, in its dissolution, returns to the free energy of the universe. These two forms combine to create the final physical expression of humanity upon the physical plane (in positive space/time). It is through the physical-etheric interface that we are ultimately influenced by our higher energetic connections.

Due to the perceptual limiting factors of the physical brain, the conscious mind is ordinarily locked into a fixed space/time reference (hence the term temporal reality). Temporal reality refers to our Earth time-frame of reference, and the locked vantage point from our physical perspective of reality. Those subtle energetic bodies beyond the etheric exist at what might be referred to as a non-physical or non-space, non-time level of existence. It is through the unique connections to our subtle energetic counterparts, via the physical-etheric interface coupled with the chakra system, that there occurs a continuous stream of higher energetic input to our final physical expression and consciousness. These subtle-energy bodies also act as multiple vehicles of containment for our mobile consciousness.

Astral projection may be viewed as the transfer of consciousness from the hard-neuronal wiring and fixed time-frame of the physical brain's waking reality into the astral vehicle of consciousness. Although many believe that the sleeping is strictly a time for dreaming, in reality our consciousness moves into the astral body each night for excursions and learning experiences at the astral level. The physical body is able to function quite well without the direction of the conscious mind due to the unique evolutionary development of our autonomic nervous system, a type of sophisticated auto-pilot.

When one is conscious on the level of the astral plane, reality is experienced much differently than one is accustomed to on the physical plane. For instance, the passage of time is experienced differently in the astral realms than in the physical. In Dr. Tiller's positive-negative space/time model, the domain characterized as negative space/time is thought to have negative time flow. (Physicists conceive that tachyonic particles would also flow backward in time.) As negative space/time displays negative entropy, so it is predicted to have negative time flow as well. In actuality, the astral realm exists at some perspective outside of the conventional space/time reference (i.e., non-space, non-time) than the one which we are accustomed to experiencing at the physical level. Whether time flow is negative, or merely different, is perhaps a minor limitation of the positive-negative space/time model at this point in its present development.

There exists a vibrational/frequency relationship to time which is in addition to the particular frequency characteristics of the fabric of matter. The term frequency is said to have slightly different meaning in these two contexts. There is a concept of time which has been referred to as the "eternal now" (or spacious present) whereby past, present, and future may actually exist simultaneously but in different vibrational time frames. It is possible that by shifting the frequency focus of one's consciousness, one may be able to tune into specific time frames outside of the present. In actuality, by shifting one's frequency focus, one may be shifting his/her consciousness from the viewing perspective of the physical up to the astral, mental, causal, and higher energetic levels which are all a part of our total energetic expression.

If there is a cosmic hologram, it might be metaphorically compared to magnetic patterns recorded on a cosmic videotape of the "universal candid camera." One might consider that the videotape of past, present, and future has already been filmed and recorded at some energetic level of subtle substance i.e., a universal magnetic recording media. Because we are hypothetically dealing with a holographic videotape, each individual would theoretically have his/her own cassette copy of the universal movie, i.e., every piece contains the whole. This is basically an extension of the universal hologram concept discussed in the first chapter. The only change is that we have now expanded the dynamically changing photograph to a videotape. The basic hardware of consciousness gives each individual his/her own videorecorder to view the tape, if he or she can only learn to operate the fine-tune mechanism of his/her consciousness properly. The fact that this analogy deals with prerecorded tapes of how the universe will turn out is not to imply predestination and immovable fates, because there are other rationales such as probable universes, free will, and the multiple viewing angles of stored holograms which can easily get us around that limited concept.

That which the conscious mind defines as the present is that part of the tape which is rolling past the magnetic tape head of the brain's cosmic video recorder. Because the neurological wiring of the physical brain is relatively fixed, it can only perceive from the perspective of the tape head. In a metaphorical sense, the ability to tune into past and future might be a function of one's ability to psychoenergetically tap into the holographic interference pattern already stored on the video cassette's reels. Some esoteric sources refer to these archives as the akashic records. The ability to tune into information stored at a sequence on the videotape which is not currently in front of the tape head may similarly be a function of being able to shift the frequency of one's consciousness into a different space/time synchronization (the specifics of which are little understood at this time). *The ability to see the universe from different perspectives may be a reflection of the different vantage points of perception of our subtle energetic vehicles of expression, such as the astral, mental, and causal bodies.*

In addition to its different time perspective, the astral, as mentioned previously, is also the realm of the emotional and desire aspects of human personality. Because of this, one frequently finds that the consciousness of the individual may occasionally take on a more emotional orientation when travelling through astral realms of existence. This depends also on whether one is traversing what has been referred to as the higher or lower astral realms. The fact that there are travellers through these regions suggests that there are both visitors (tourists) as well as local inhabitants of the astral realm.

One of the interesting aspects of Dr. Tiller's model is what he refers to as the "ratchet effect." As discussed previously, energetic interactions which originate at the higher subtle levels, such as the mental level, must first have their impact upon the astral vehicle. The changes in the astral are similarly transmitted to the etheric vehicle and from there, via the physical-etheric interface, to the physical body for its final expression. Similarly, energy inputs from the causal level must first filter down through the mental level and so on to lower energetic levels of substance. This cascade effect down the different curves, from those at the far right in Diagram 16 all the way to the physical curve, is what Tiller refers to as the ratchet effect.

Of course, even though we are dealing with different levels of energetic substance, we must remember that each of the bodies are actually spatially superimposed over the physical form. The clarity and definition with which a psychic may perceive someone's auric field may be a function of the highest level into which their own consciousness may tune. Those psychics who can see only a thin band of energy about the body are probably only able to tune into the etheric level. Those psychics who can see not only the etheric but the extended ovoid forms, colors, and pictures (thoughtforms) in the outer auric field are able to tune their consciousness up to the astral, mental, and higher levels. At these higher levels of consciousness and form, the subtle energetic counterparts of the chakras are able to perceive and process energies relating to their own level of substance.

Diagram 17.
THE HUMAN ENERGY FIELD

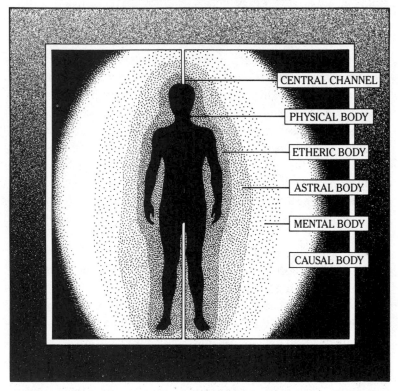

CENTRAL CHANNEL

PHYSICAL BODY

ETHERIC BODY

ASTRAL BODY

MENTAL BODY

CAUSAL BODY

As shown in Diagram 17, we can see the full energetic expression of the multidimensional human being. Although perhaps not all of these higher subtle bodies are photographable, it is quite likely that the etheric and possibly the astral may be captured and measured with sophisticated imaging systems such as the EMR Scanner or its forerunners.

The purpose of this chapter has been to focus on what is known through various channels of information about our extended energetic framework. Those with a more physical-sensory orientation might ask, "What is the purpose of having all these energetic bodies when all that seems to matter is the physical body?"

The etheric body appears to at least have some physiologic rationale in complementing the structure and function of the physical body. When we begin to get into the astral body and higher levels, we move into regions of consciousness that are more difficult to perceive and understand. There is a model which does make sense of these interconnected energy bodies and explains why they have evolved as an intricate part of our personality and physical expression.

Reincarnation & Human Transformation: A Multidimensional Model of the Evolution of Consciousness

Reincarnation would seem to be a rather strange concept to most people. Many would consider it to be a belief system pertaining to only Hindu and Buddhist worshippers. Rather surprisingly, however, a 1982 Gallup poll[35] showed that 23 percent of Americans believe in reincarnation. Reincarnation is a system that explains the function of our many energy bodies and the way we express ourselves upon the physical plane. The physical plane is known as the world of experience. It has been frequently referred to in the esoteric literature as the laboratory of life, where the physical experiments of human personality must be carried out. Physical experiments which explore laws pertaining to our physical form can only be tested upon the physical plane.

Each human lifetime, from a reincarnational viewpoint, is a chance to explore the dimensions of our true inner nature as they are expressed through the physical body. Through our experiences upon the physical plane, we (hopefully) grow in knowledge and stature as we develop various coping strategies for dealing with the life situations into which we have incarnated. Dr. Tiller has a rather appropriate insight into these matters which sums up the purpose of reincarnation from a scientific perspective:

> *Man appears as a being whose primary level of existence is at the non-space, non-time levels of the Universe, and who has placed himself in a space-time vehicle of consciousness for the purpose of growing in awareness of the True Self and of generating coherence in*

the True Self. Our perception mechanisms at the space-time vehicle level lock us into a narrowly restricted view of reality and the Self. *Disharmony created by the ego at the deeper level of self, materializes as error or disease in the space-time vehicle as an indicator that error has been created at a primary level.*

Self-healing or healing by another involves energy coordination at a variety of levels and teaches us that the sensory apparatus of the space-time vehicle perceives only the "World of Appearances" and has no knowledge of Reality. *It teaches us that the space-time vehicle is not Life but only a simulator of Life whose only role is as a teaching tool.* With our thoughts and attitudes, we continuously reprogram the simulator from the Mind level of the multidimensional universe and continuously generate our individual and collective futures by such behavior.[36] *(italics added)*

Dr. Tiller's rather profound statement has many implications and meanings on a variety of levels. The world with which we are most familiar is a picture that we have built up around our limited sensory information. In the first chapter of this book we found that when one observes matter at the subatomic or quantum level, one realizes that the physical universe is composed of orderly patterns of frozen light. The world that we perceive with our five senses and the true nature of reality are actually two different things. The limitation of both our physical senses and the mechanism of consciousness locks us into perceiving only the "world of appearances." What we see on the surface does not always reflect the true behavior of matter at the unseen level of processes and interactions. The world of the physical plane is felt by many in the esoteric literature to be a series of illusions based upon our limited physical perceptual mechanisms. The true nature of reality is beyond the scope of our ordinary sensory channels which piece together information about ourselves and the world around us.

From our previous discussion of the many subtle energetic systems which participate with the physical body and brain, it may be seen how much is unknown or misunderstood about the true (subtle energetic) nature of human beings by the present generation of scientific thinkers. Our various subtle bodies would appear to have evolved for some purpose aside from the maintenance of the physiological functions of the physical body. Although we have approached our subtle bodies as energetic fields associated with the physical, our physical bodies are not the source of these fields. *It is the fields which generate the physical matter and not the other way around!* For many, this will be a difficult concept to grasp, but in discussing the true nature of reincarnation we will have to try and maintain as accurate a picture as possible. The subtle energetic fields precede and organize the formation of the physical form as a vehicle of expression for higher conscious energies.

In support of this concept, whereby the subtle energetic fields support and precede the generation of the physical body, are the aforementioned data from the Kim Bong Han studies of acupuncture meridians. Kim found that the development of the meridian tubule system preceded the organization of the physical organs. Because the meridian system seems to be tied in with the physical-etheric interface, it would seem that energetic input from the etheric level provides the spatial guidance necessary for structural organization of the physical body.

Adding further credence to the idea of an etheric predecessor to the physical body are certain psychic observations made by a renowned English clairvoyant by the name of Geoffrey Hodson. Hodson was a unique clairvoyant investigator in that he worked with many scientists throughout his life in order to test his special psychic abilities under controlled conditions. One of the most unusual studies carried out by Hodson was a clairvoyant investigation of the development of a human embryo from the point of conception to birth. To quote Hodson:

> Clairvoyantly examined, *the prenatal etheric mold, which appears very soon after conception, resembles a baby body built of etheric matter,* somewhat self-luminous, vibrating slightly, a living being, the etheric projection of the Archetype *as modified by karma.*
>
> Within the etheric mold, there is to be seen, in terms of flowing energy or lines of force, each on its own wave length, a sketch plan of the whole body. Each type of tissue-to-be is represented, differing from other types because the energy of which it is an end-product is itself on another frequency. *Thus the bony structure, muscular, and vascular tissues, the nerves, the brain, and other substances are all represented in the etheric mold by currents of energy on specific frequencies.*
>
> The play of the emitted vibrations on the free surrounding matter may possibly be the factor which causes atoms to enter into differing molecular combinations to produce various types of tissue. *These molecules are attracted toward the lines of force and "settle" into their appropriated places in the growing body by virtue of sympathetic vibration or mutual resonance.* Thus, again, every part of the physical body in substance and in form exactly fits the incarnating Ego.[37] *(italics added)*

In the quote from Dr. Tiller, it was stated that humans are beings whose primary level of existence is at the non-space, non-time level. The primary level of mind, for instance, originates at the mental level and filters down through the various subtle energetic shells surrounding and penetrating the physical form. These higher energetic vehicles exist at frequency levels (or planes of existence) which are outside of the conventional (positive) space/time orientation. This is in obvious contradiction to what many believe.

Experiences from each lifetime are processed initially at the astral and mental levels but are more fully integrated at the causal and higher spiritual levels. The causal and higher levels have permanence, whereas the lower energetic vehicles are more transitory learning devices. This is why the causal body is sometimes referred to as the True Self. Tiller refers to the positive space/time vehicle that we call the physical body as the simulator, a teaching tool. Learning acquired by the ego during experiences at the level of the physical simulator are absorbed into and processed at the causal and higher levels, where all previous lifetimes' experiential knowledge is stored. Thus, the causal view of reality allows a wider perspective of life than can be seen at the level of the physical perceptual mechanisms.

One of the primary purposes of the reincarnational system is to allow the soul to undergo a wide spectrum of learning experiences through which the evolving consciousness may become spirtually mature. This is what Dr. Tiller refers to as generating greater coherence in the True Self. The more experiences a soul has to learn from, the more diverse and successful the coping strategies that each soul may develop for dealing with life on the physical as well as the higher planes of existence.

The degree of spiritual coherence and ordered patterning generated within the higher energetic systems is ultimately reflected in the character of the cellular makeup and the personality traits of the physical/mental/emotional vehicles chosen for each successive incarnation. Growth and development of the physical body, from fetus to adulthood, are affected not only by molecular genetic patterns derived from the parents, but also by the higher vibrational patterns of the incarnating soul. Energetic patterns from the causal level are subtly imprinted upon the lower vehicles, which go on to influence the ongoing patterns of cellular expression.

The reincarnational system is not random. It allows the soul freedom to choose the circumstances of each successive incarnation. Physical characteristics as well as social and cultural influences are taken into account when selecting the particular physical vehicle of expression for the soul.

The natural question many people ask when told that an individual has choice as to what body he or she wishes to occupy is, "Why come back as someone with oppressive difficulties such as physical illness or poverty?" Reincarnation is perhaps one of the only philosophies which may make sense of this question. If the soul does survive beyond each individual lifetime to experience life again and again in its many rounds, then the soul would appear to have certain immortal qualities. Its expressions upon the physical plane are only transitory within the full scope of its cyclic incarnations.

A lifetime chosen with a particular obstacle, such as illness or poverty, is actually viewed by some as a gift which the individual may have chosen to use toward the evolution of his or her inner spiritual qualities. Just think about an event in your life where you were successfully able to overcome something very difficult. The process of going through the event was no doubt quite stressful at the time. But the experience and inner strength gained in overcoming the obstacle made you a stronger and wiser person. When again subjected to a similar circumstance, the individual who has been able to successfully overcome a stressful situation is stronger, and better able to handle the challenge. The more we are able to learn and prosper from experience, the greater become our coping mechanisms for dealing with new and unknown situations.

Being born with a particular handicap such as blindness or hearing impairment might seem a cruel punishment, but one need only look at someone like Helen Keller to see that the obstacles may be surpassed to create a unique and talented individual. There is no such thing as a life without stress. Stress is a necessary thing in life. If there were no stress, there would be no growth. Even bone needs some type of stress to maintain its form and strength. If an individual never got out of bed, their bones would begin to reabsorb and weaken so that even the simplest movements would become painful. There is a certain functional amount of stress which might be known as "eustress" (as opposed to distress). From the reincarnational perspective, even periods of distress may have long-term positive learning qualities.

From a similar perspective, let us view another illness such as cancer. Cancer is perhaps one of the most feared and dreaded illnesses of modern times. There is a unique (and rather controversial) form of cancer therapy which uses the power of the mind, through meditation and active visualization, to gain control over the immune system in order to actively remove the cancerous cells from the body. Pioneered by a radiation oncologist named Carl Simonton,[38] this technique has brought hope and successful cancer cures to many individuals who were formerly given up as terminal by their private physicians. A most remarkable thing tends to occur in many individuals who have beaten cancer in this method. They tend to change their lifestyles and mindstyles, and frequently gain a new, higher level and quality of life that is far beyond their precancerous existence. Some go on to become cancer counselors themselves, sharing their new-found strengths and insights with others similarly afflicted.

One might argue that *in these individuals, catastrophic illness has become a transformational point which allowed movement of consciousness and lifestyle to a new and higher level of function.* It is only through learning of such success stories that one can even begin to look upon severe illness as a gift and learning tool by which to gain insight into the deeper questions and issues of life. Frequently it takes a life-or-death issue, such as the threat of terminal cancer, to change people's ingrained beliefs about themselves and others. Death is known as a transformational process for many reasons other than the fact that it involves a transition from life to death. People tend to become so complacent in their worldview that it is only through the intervention of something which threatens to change the very nature of their existence that they are able to stop and re-evaluate their priorities and life tasks.

In the section discussing the astral body, we mentioned the phenomenon of the Near Death Experience, or NDE. This phenomenon has direct relevance to the issue of reincarnation. The majority of individuals undergoing this experience come back with a unique out-of-body perspective as well as a loss of their fear of death. Many individuals report meeting relatives who were previously unknown to them in life or who had died while they were at an early age. The Near Death Experience appears to be a phenomenon we have called astral projection. When death does actually occur, however, the individual does not return to the physical body as in the case of these individuals who undergo a Near Death Experience. Consciousness leaves the decaying physical form to reside at the astral and higher levels.

The astral body is a containment vehicle for the personality beyond the transition of physical death. The consciousness of the individual and his/ her personality are transferred to the astral vehicle, as occurs during life when astral projection takes place. The mental body is still associated with the astral at this point, as is the causal vehicle. *The causal body is the repository of the sum total of lifetime experiences gained through successive incarnations.* The causal vehicle is less like a single bodily form associated with an individual personality, and more like that which has been referred to as a group soul. *The Higher Self, as expressed through the causal body, is the gestalt consciousness of all that the soul has learned and experienced throughout its many lifetimes upon the physical plane.* The causal body might be viewed as a tree trunk of a large oak tree with many branches. Each of the branches of the tree represents a different personality and life experience of the soul. Imagine that a tremendous flood of water has immersed the tree so that only its uppermost branches can be seen poking though the water. To the ordinary consciousness, it would seem that each branch above the water is a separate plant, but beneath the water and beyond the perspective of the superficial observer, each branch is an outgrowth and expression of a common trunk and nurturing root system.

To the positive space/time observer locked within a perspective of linear time flow, each personality and life expression of the soul would seem to live at widely separated points in history. To the true soul consciousness at the causal level, where time is experienced as the eternal now, the past, present, and future are seen to exist simultaneously. There, the branches of the tree are viewed as intimately interconnected. Time, as we know it, is left behind. Alternatively, some have viewed time as being spherical. In spherical time, each of our lifetimes would be seen as points separated upon the face of a ball, similar to cities on the surface of a world globe. The geographical distance between the points would be analogous to the years between lifetimes. When we are experiencing each incarnation, it is as if we are living in the cities represented by points on the spherical time globe. If we can attain a more cosmic or causal consciousness, we can elevate our perspective and observe the globe of spherical time in its totality, and can experience all separate lifetimes simultaneously: past, present, and future.

The experience bank of the causal body carries the memories of all reincarnational lifetimes, stored at a higher energetic level of existence. When an individual dies, his or her personality and consciousness is preserved and lives beyond the dissolution of the temporal physical-etheric vehicle. The purpose of our higher subtle energetic bodies is to preserve that accumulated knowledge of many lifetimes, as well as to allow access to this information bank by the incarnating entity when the proper states of consciousness are attuned to.

As Dr. Tiller said in the opening quote of this section, the physical body is a simulator of life. It is a teaching tool. The physical form is a transitory suit of physico-chemical clothing that we put on to experience and interact with life at the physical plane level. Through our many encounters at the physical level, we grow in substance, knowledge, and purpose, expressing inner qualities that are too numerous to be developed in any one lifetime. Additionally, we choose to experience many difficult trials and tribulations in order that we may test the metal of the soul's ability to adapt to new and unusual situations.

Upon entering each new physical form, a built-in forget mechanism erases all conscious knowledge of previous existences. If we were to have the knowledge and personality of our previous lives, we would have the same prejudices and biases that we had previously left. Each lifetime is a chance to start anew with a clean slate, so to speak, with the mistakes of the past behind us. Actually, the mistakes of our past are forgotten but not erased. Through the mechanisms of karma, our past deeds influence the circumstances of our future incarnations. This is the true meaning of the expression, "as ye sow, so shall ye reap." By incarnating as male and female, white and black, as Indian, Chinese, and Chicano, by experiencing life from all possible viewpoints, the reincarnational scheme allows us to see the world from all possible perspectives. With each succeeding lifetime, the sum total consciousness of the soul is able to benefit from positive learning experiences as we climb the uphill trend of evolution. As we evolve from ignorance, so it is said that the frequency of consciousness moves to higher and higher levels. The frequency of consciousness is proportional to the complexity with which it can respond to its environment.

As we can see in Diagram 18, the evolutionary arrow moves us in a direction further to the right and the higher spiritual levels. Each bell curve in this diagram represents many beings, as opposed to Diagram 17, which described the frequency characteristics of a single individual's body. The darkest curve on the left represents the human spectrum of consciousness. As there are very intelligent, as well as very ignorant, individuals making up humankind, there is a bell curve distribution of the quality of consciousness of the race as a whole. Those who are average fall under the peak of the curve. The more intelligent fall just to the right.

What the succeeding curves represent is the evolutionary trend toward breaking into the higher frequency realms of consciousness by those individuals at the leading edge of the human curve. Gradually, humanity as a

Diagram 18.
QUANTITY VS. QUALITY OF CONSCIOUSNESS

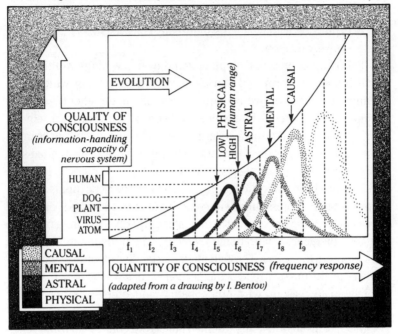

whole will move up the evolutionary scale toward the higher vibrational realms, with greater insight into the multidimensional human reality. It is only though successive rounds of physical lives that the soul may progress to the highest levels of insight which will allow it to move beyond the continuing turns of the reincarnational wheel. What happens when we evolve beyond that cycle is beyond the scope of this textbook, but various reference texts listed at the end of the chapter may give further exposition of this spiritual issue.

Consciousness is seen by many in the esoteric field as a type of energy. The energy of consciousness takes on many forms as it evolves to progressively higher levels of frequency, insight, and cosmic perspective. As consciousness gains experiences from interacting with its environment, it moves forward in expanding its dimensions of creative expression, as well as evolving upward in the frequency dimension of energy. The model above suggests that even the most basic constituents of matter, the atoms (and even the electrons), have some level of consciousness which evolves to progressively higher levels of experiential output and behavioral repertoire. As the energy of consciousness moves its way to progressively higher levels of frequency, it moves upwards into the various life forms. At each new level, there is a proportionately higher degree of complexity of response and fullness of expression with which the indwelling consciousness may expand, create, evolve, and grow.

This chapter presents a type of grand overview of the multidimensional human, in form and consciousness, as something which is in dynamic equilibrium with many levels of subtle energy existing simultaneously. Through that which has been called the physical-etheric interface and the chakra-nadi system, these higher dimensions have input to the physical expression of the human being. Because of the limited sensory abilities of our physical apparatus, scientists working strictly from the physical level have tended to ignore these higher energetic inputs into the human system. Unless these energetic inputs are addressed, orthodox physicians will never be able to understand the diverse range of subtle energetic therapies of vibrational medicine which the remainder of the book proposes to explore. Through an understanding of these energetic influences on the physical field of the human form, it will be seen that there are legitimate reasons why homeopathic and other types of energy medicine have their ultimate physical healing effects.

Much of the information presented here is of a controversial and scientifically unproven nature. It will be left up to the discretion of the individual reader as to what he or she wishes to believe or disbelieve. That which is given can be of much value if humanity will only be open enough to direct further research into proving or disproving the ideas herein presented. One must always remember that the nature of ideas which are beyond their time is that they are often seen as science fiction. However, with increasing frequency, the science fiction of yesterday becomes today's science fact.

We are on the threshold of a revolution in consciousness and healing that has been set in motion by such far-sighted thinkers as Albert Einstein and Dr. William Tiller. Each of the models, research findings, and ideas presented here can be considered as transitional tools. It is hoped that the building of such models may assist us in understanding the concept of humans as multidimensional beings and in comprehending the evolution of consciousness through states of illness and health. It will be up to the rest of us to apply those tools toward developing a new science of healing the mind and body, and hopefully toward broadening the scope of recognized human potential. Through these new scientific insights gained about the true nature of humanity, we will have moved that much further toward recognizing our true spiritual and evolutionary heritage.

Key Points to Remember

1. All matter, both physical and subtle, has frequency. Matter of different frequencies can coexist in the same space, just as energies of different frequencies (i.e. radio and TV) can exist nondestructively in the same space.

2. The etheric and physical bodies, being of different frequencies, overlap and coexist within the same space.

3. The acupuncture meridian system is a discretely organized network of microscopic ducts which connects the physical to the etheric body, forming the so-called physical/etheric interface.

4. The meridian system relays a nutritive subtle energy, known as ch'i, from the environment to the nerves, blood vessels, and deeper organs of the body via energetic portals in the skin called acupuncture points.

5. Energy disturbances in etheric body and the acupuncture meridian system precede the physical/cellular manifestation of illness.

6. The chakras are specialized energy centers in the subtle bodies, each associated with a major nerve and glandular center in the physical body. The chakras act as transformers to step down subtle energies and translate them into hormonal, nerve, and cellular activity in the physical body.

7. The major chakras, especially the crown, brow, and throat chakras, are also subtle organs of perception and are associated with the psychic abilities of higher intuition, clairvoyance, and clairaudience, respectively.

8. The chakras are connected to each other and to various aspects of the physical body through energetic threads known as nadis, together forming the chakra-nadi network.

9. The astral body is another subtle body, like the etheric body, made up of matter of a higher frequency than etheric matter. It is similarly superimposed upon the physical-etheric framework. The astral body is energetically involved in both the experiencing, expression, and repression of emotion.

10. Dysfunction in the astral body caused by emotional imbalances can impair the flow of energy through the chakras, eventually resulting in glandular imbalance and physical illness.

11. Consciousness can move into the astral body and separate from the physical-etheric vehicles. When this occurs naturally it is known as astral projection or an Out-Of-Body Experience (OOBE). When this separation of consciousness occurs traumatically it is often referred to as a Near Death Experience (NDE).

12. Einstein's equation predicts the existence of a faster than light energy referred to by Dr. William Tiller as magnetoelectrical energy (ME). ME energy is analogous to etheric and possibly astral energy or substance. ME energy displays the unique properties of negative entropy and a magnetic nature, and is not easily measureable with conventional electromagnetic (EM) field detectors.

13. Experiments with healers show that they possess energy fields with characteristics that fit the predictions for the behavior of ME energies, i.e. they are magnetic and negatively entropic in nature.

14. There are additional higher frequency vehicles, the mental and causal bodies, which also contribute energies to the physical body.

15. Reincarnation presents a model by which consciousness is repeatedly projected into physical vehicles for the purposes of gaining experience, knowledge, and spiritual maturity.

16. The experiences and knowledge gained from all lifetimes are stored at the level of the causal body, sometimes referred to as the Higher Self.

17. Reincarnation is one of the few models which explains why diseases, as well as physical, emotional, and socioeconomic handicaps, may be viewed as learning experiences and opportunities for soul growth.

18. Viewed from the subtle energetic level, consciousness is a form of energy which continually evolves to higher levels of complexity and understanding.

CHAPTER V

Subtle-Energy Systems
& Their Relevance to
ANCIENT APPROACHES TOWARD
HEALING

In the first four chapters of this book, we have examined the human body and mind from a diverse range of perspectives. By now it should be clear that there must be more to human beings than just their physical body. We know through modern quantum physics that the physical body is actually a unique aggregation of physical particles of matter which, themselves, are points of frozen light. Interfaced with this physical body of light are additional light bodies composed of subtle energetic matter of higher frequency levels than that which the physical eye can perceive. The mechanism of interface between the physical body and these higher energetic systems is a unique part of our subtle anatomy known as the physical-etheric interface. The most familiar component of this interface appears to be formed by the acupuncture meridian system. Therefore, it would seem most appropriate that we begin our analyses of energetic healing approaches by examining the mechanisms of acupuncture.

Acupuncture & the Chinese Philosophy of Healing:
Modern Approaches to an Ancient Method of
Diagnosis & Treatment

Acupuncture is one of the most ancient and, until recently, mysterious methods of healing which is currently in therapeutic usage. The *Nei Ching* or *Yellow Emperor's Classic of Internal Medicine*[1] is the earliest known text

173

on acupuncture. It is believed to have been written during the reign of Emperor Huang Ti between the years 2697 B.C. and 2596 B.C. During the seventeenth century, Jesuit missionaries were sent to China in order to introduce the basic doctrines of Christianity to the Orient. Although their attempts to convert the Chinese were less successful than hoped for, the missionaries did bring back unbelievable accounts of Chinese physicians curing illnesses by inserting needles into the skin.

In 1884 Emperor Tao-Kuang prohibited the practice of acupuncture within the palace on any members of the royal family. Subsequently, the scope of acupuncture practice became confined to the common people and was ministered by the so-called barefoot doctors of China. After a long period of disfavor, acupuncture found new acceptance in the eyes of Mao Tse Tung. During the Long March of 1934-35, Mao's red army found acupuncture of great use in maintaining the health of its vast legions, and in allowing soldiers to avoid major illnesses and epidemics even under the most arduous of living and fighting conditions. Following Mao's subsequent conclusion that acupuncture was a vital step toward the rebirth of a New China, this ancient healing art has been gradually able to find its way back into mainstream Chinese medicine.

Although mentioned as a treatment for sciatica in some early Western medical textbooks, acupuncture was not of interest to America until 1972 when President Richard M. Nixon visited China. Accompanying Nixon to China was a journalist named Reston who brought back unique stories of surgery performed under strict acupuncture anesthesia. After an initial phase of enthusiasm and skepticism among Western physicians, acupuncture research began to establish its place within scientific medicine as an acceptable form of therapy in the treatment of certain pain syndromes.

Acupuncture has grown in acceptance among the scientific community as a direct result of research linking acupuncture analgesia with the release of endorphins within the central nervous system. The endorphin model gave scientific theorists the first conclusive experimental evidence for acupuncture's link with known pain pathways in the brain and spinal cord.

There have been a number of theories attempting to explain why acupuncture is effective in treating pain. Most Western physicians assumed that the analgesic effects of acupuncture had to be mediated through some type of stimulation of pain pathways within the nervous system. The original theories proposed by Melzack and Wall suggested that acupuncture needles stimulated peripheral nerves to close a gate within the spinal cord, thereby preventing ascending pain impulses from reaching the brain. Although the Gate-Control Theory[2] does not accurately describe the true mechanisms of acupuncture analgesia, it provided a first step into understanding the mechanisms of acupuncture. Further refinements of this model have provided new directions in neurological research by detailing other pain pathways in the nervous system which can be manipulated by such modalities as electrical TNS devices (Transcutaneous Nerve Stimulators).

It was suggested earlier that the endorphin model, although successful in explaining certain types of acupuncture analgesia (low-frequency electroacupuncture), was unsuccessful in explaining other acupuncture approaches. For instance, high-frequency electroacupuncture was found to be inhibited by serotonin antagonists but unaffected by endorphin blocking agents such as naloxone.[3] (Serotonin is another one of many neurotransmitters found within the central nervous system). The picture being formed is that acupuncture analgesia is mediated by more than one neurochemical intermediary and is influenced by the type of stimulation applied to the acupoints. Therefore, although it has been popular to attribute all of acupuncture's effects to endorphin release, the data pertaining to the role of serotonin implies that acupuncture analgesia is much more complex than indicated by initial neurochemical models.

The early theories created to explain acupuncture's ability to relieve pain have done much to further scientific inquiry into this unique system of healing. The recent flurry of research within the growing field of neuroendocrinology has done much to add credence to these unusual therapeutic techniques which originated in ancient China. In reality, the acupuncture analgesia models fall short of addressing the true potential of acupuncture as both a multidimensional healing modality (with applications other than the treatment of pain) and as a unique system of diagnosis. In order to develop a greater understanding and appreciation for acupuncture, it will be necessary to examine some of the Chinese philosophy behind this ancient healing art.

Yin/Yang & the Five Elements: The Chinese View of Nature

The ancient Chinese philosophy underlying acupuncture therapy, as well as other aspects of Chinese Medicine, is an outgrowth of viewpoints on our relationship to the universe around us. The Chinese see human beings as a microcosm within a universal macrocosm. The principles demonstrated by the inner workings of humans are reflected in universal relationships of energetic flow. One of the primary concepts of energy flow is that of ch'i or qi, a unique energetic substance that flows from the environment into the body. The Chinese feel that *ch'i is an energy of both nutritive and cellular-organizational characteristics which supersedes the energetic contributions of ingested food and air.* Ch'i is a type of subtle energy which permeates our environment. It has sometimes been referred to as "prana" in ancient Hindu writings. This peculiar type of environmental subtle energy may have partial origin in solar radiation outside the recognized electromagnetic window of visible light. As humans, we are continually bathed by the unseen radiations of a diverse vibrational environment, from the more common radio, television, and radio frequencies, to the more subtle aspects of solar energy. We live in resonance with and can be subtly affected by many different energy frequencies that permeate our local geocosmic setting. As many ancient cultures have worshipped the sun and its healing rays, one wonders whether or not such cultures had knowledge of the subtle energetic influences of ch'i and prana.

In the Chinese model, ch'i energy is absorbed into the human body via portals of entry on the skin. These portals of entry are formed by the acupuncture points, which are inlets along a specialized meridian system running deep below the integument to underlying organ structures. Through twelve pairs of meridians, the Chinese feel that the ch'i flows into the bodily organs to provide life-giving/sustaining energy. Each pair of meridians is associated with a different organ system or function.

Another key concept of Chinese philosophy is the idea of energy polarity, as expressed by yin and yang. In a way, yin and yang represent an ancient Chinese predecessor to the modern-day concept of complementarity. The wave-particle duality of matter is a kind of yin/yang puzzle of modern physics. The *Nei Ching* states that, "the entire universe is an oscillation of the forces of yin and yang." Yang is viewed as the male principle: active, generative, associated with sun, light, and the creative principle of life. Yin is seen as the female element: passive, destructive, associated with the moon, darkness, and death. The dualistic principle of yin/yang extends into all aspects of life cycles and cosmic processes. The two seemingly contradictory aspects of yin and yang reflect an energetic oscillation between polar opposites. Both are necessary to reach a balanced steady state, a dynamic equilibrium within a universe of constant change. In order to have birth, there must also be death. Death, however, is necessary before one can undergo rebirth, as in the cases of reincarnation and stellar evolution.

The many complementary, yet different, dimensions which yin and yang describe are a reflection of the positive and negative polarities of the energies of consciousness. An interesting demonstration of this principle can be seen in the different yet complementary aspects of consciousness as expressed through the right and left cerebral hemispheres. The left brain is the seat of logical thinking. It represents our more analytical, mathematical, linear, and verbal natures. The right brain constitutes the emotional half of the cerebral cortex, expressing our artistic, aesthetic, spatial, and non-linear intuitive qualities. Both sides are necessary to obtain a balanced holistic viewpoint of the universe.

The Chinese philosphy sees a healthy life as one which contains an even balance of the forces of yin and yang. Maintaining a perfect balance between yin and yang is felt by the Chinese to result in perfect health of mind, body, and spirit. An imbalance in these polar characteristics or energies causes a shift in the equilibrium of the organism which ultimately crystallizes into patterns of disharmony and illness in the physical body. *Energetic dysfunction at the physical level may be reflected by imbalances in the paired meridians of the body.* For every organ, there is energetic flow through two sets of meridians. The equal flow of ch'i energies through the right and left meridians of the body reflects the basic yin/yang concept. This principle stresses the necessity for balance in the polarity of energies as applied to individual organ systems. Imbalance in the flow of meridian energies leads to subsequent organ pathology.

Disharmony within the human organism can take place at many energy levels beyond the physical, as our discussion of the etheric, astral, and mental levels has indicated. Imbalance of energies at the mental level filters down through the lower octaves of the astral and etheric energies and finally manifests into the physical body via the physical-etheric interface. The physical mechanism which allows this etheric energy transfer is the acupuncture meridian system. *The meridians distribute the subtle magnetic energies of ch'i which provide sustenance and organization for the physical-cellular structure of each organ system.*

It was noted in Kim Bong Han's research[4] on the ductule system which corresponded to the classical acupuncture meridians, that when the meridians to the liver were interrupted, hepatocellular degeneration soon followed. This example demonstrates how an imbalance in subtle energetic flow (via an artificially induced energy deficit) can result in pathological changes at the physical-cellular level. Although the subtle energies which the Chinese refer to as ch'i are hard to measure, there is indirect evidence for some type of electromagnetic energy circuit which involves the meridians and acupuncture points.

The acupuncture points along the superficial meridians in the skin demonstrate unique electrical properties which distinguish them from the surrounding epidermis. The electrical resistance measured in the skin overlying the acupoints is lower than the surrounding skin by a factor of approximately 10 to 1. The value of this resistance, as measured by a special direct-current (DC) electrical amplifier, shows that the electrical parameters of the acupuncture points vary according to physiological and emotional changes within the organism. Russian researchers have demonstrated that different states of consciousness, such as sleep and hypnosis, can produce significant changes in the electrical conductivity of the acupuncture points. Additionally, disease states produce characteristic disturbances in the electrical potentials of the acupoints along particular meridians. These disease-related electrical shifts in the acupuncture points have important diagnostic significance. It is possible to detect illnesses utilizing instrumentation which can measure these energetic changes in the meridian system.

The meridians can be viewed as electrical circuits which connect the superficial acupuncture points to deeper organ structures. It is essential for the health and well-being of the organism that there be sufficient energy in these circuits and that they all be balanced with respect to one another. There is a characteristic rhythmical flow demonstrated by the ch'i energy as it passes through the twelve meridians which supply energy to the internal organs. This cyclic energy flow reflects innate biological rhythms and cycles of a subtle energetic nature. These well-defined cycles, which describe the flow of energy within the body, are a reflection of the cyclic energy interaction between the five earthly elements (as viewed by Chinese philosophy). The Five Element Theory is a primary relationship in the Chinese system. It relates all energy and substance to one of the five elements: fire, earth, metal, water, and wood.

There are two basic cycles that illustrate the interaction between these elements. In the first cycle, known as the Cycle of Generation, each element generates or produces the succeeding element. This is sometimes known as the Mother-Son Law. One element gives birth to the next and nourishes it by a flow of energy. In the oriental viewpoint, *fire produces earth* by burning wood, and ashes are returned to the earth. *Earth pro-*

duces metal. Metallic ores are found within the earth. *Metal produces water.* The source of flowing water can frequently be found near mineral deposits. *Water produces wood.* Trees grow by absorbing water through their roots. *Wood produces fire and fire produces earth.* Then the cycle begins again. In the creation cycle, fire is considered the son of wood and also the mother of earth. (The connections here seem somewhat more metaphorical than literal, but they demonstrate definite Chinese energetic principles, as will soon be seen.)

In the second cycle, known as the Cycle of Destruction, each element destroys or absorbs the succeeding element. It is really a control cycle in that it represents the process by which the elements check and balance one another. If one element becomes too strong or too weak, it can attack another or be injured. Thus, *wood can injure earth* (roots penetrate the soil). *Earth controls water* (via dams). *Water injures fire* (puts it out). *Fire destroys metal* (metal can be melted by strong fire). *Metal destroys wood*

Diagram 19
THE FIVE ELEMENTS & THEIR RELATIONSHIP
TO ENERGY FLOW BETWEEN THE INTERNAL ORGANS

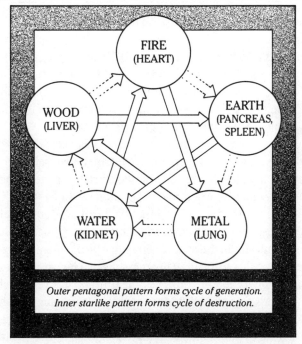

Outer pentagonal pattern forms cycle of generation.
Inner starlike pattern forms cycle of destruction.

(as an axe cuts a tree), and the cycle begins again. The importance of these two cycles of generation and destruction is that they form the rational basis for the application of acupuncture therapy.

The Chinese believe that the individual is a microcosm, a reflection of the surrounding earthly macrocosm. The interactions of our inner bodily functions (and thus, our inner organs) are felt to mirror the cycles of generation and destruction which describe the energetic relationships between the five earthly elements. Chinese medicine identifies each of the bodily organs with one of the five elements. The Chinese also pair hollow viscera, such as the intestine or gallbladder, with their corresponding solid organs.

Diagram 20.
ELEMENTAL ASSOCIATIONS OF
THE ORGANS & VISCERA

ELEMENT	WOOD	FIRE	EARTH	METAL	WATER
ORGAN	Liver	Heart	Spleen/Pancreas	Lungs	Kidneys
HOLLOW VISCERA	Gall-bladder	Small Intestine	Stomach	Large Intestine	Bladder

As noted in Diagrams 19 and 20, in the Cycle of Generation, the heart (fire) supports the spleen (earth). The spleen (earth) energies, in turn, cycle to the lungs and large intestine (metal). From the lungs and large intestine (metal), the flow is to the kidneys and bladder (water). From the kidneys (water), energy flows via the meridians to the liver and gallbladder (wood). From the liver, the subtle energies are recycled through the meridians to the heart and around through the cycle again.

If the ch'i energies within an organ are not balanced, that organ, unable to complete the natural meridian circuit, may adversely affect its adjacent organ in the meridian series. This dysfunctional pattern is reflected in the inner (starlike) cycle depicted in Diagram 19, the so-called Cycle of Destruction. Thus, if the energies within the heart (fire) are unbalanced, the meridian disturbance will adversely affect the lungs (metal). This is actually seen, clinically, in the case of congestive heart failure where a drop in cardiac output due to a failing heart results in adverse changes in the lungs via pulmonary congestion. The lungs (metal), if adversely affected, will cause energetic and subsequent cellular disturbances in the liver (wood). Again, in congestive heart failure, the failing right ventricle, suffering from having to pump blood through congested lungs, creates back pressure in the venous system and leads to passive venous congestion of the liver. From the failing liver (wood), the meridian disturbance causes further imbalance in the spleen (earth).

In chronic right-sided congestive heart failure, continued hepatic congestion ultimately leads to a condition known as cardiac cirrhosis. This cirrhosis of the liver creates further venous obstruction to the portacaval system and leads to portal hypertension, venous congestion, and enlargement of the spleen. It is fascinating to see how modern-day pathophysiology follows ancient Chinese principles of energy flow as demonstrated by the Cycle of Destruction. It is also interesting to note that these principles, which are thousands of years old, may add complementary insights to modern viewpoints of illness causation.

Cyclic interactions between the organs and bowels (hollow viscera), as viewed by the Chinese, mirror the interactions between the elements. This is an ancient demonstration of the principle of "as above, so below." The human microcosm reflects the planetary macrocosm of Earth. These energetic principles allowed the ancient Chinese to form a rational basis (in their eyes) for the acupuncture treatment of illness. For instance, it can be seen from the Cycle of Generation that energy flows in a clockwise circuit. The ch'i energy travels from heart to spleen and pancreas, from spleen to lung, from lung to kidney, from kidney to liver, from liver to heart, and so on, continuing the cycle.

If the lungs are suffering from a disease process, they must subsequently utilize all their energy to sustain function. Because the lungs are unable to allow unobstructed energetic flow along the circuit, the kidneys (the next organ in the Cycle of Generation) must suffer additional impairment since the lungs support the kidneys in this energetic scheme of the five elements. From a Western medical perspective, it is now clear that there are actually homeostatic mechanisms which connect kidney physiology to pulmonary function. For instance, in an individual with emphysema, the ability to absorb oxygen through the lungs is impaired. It has only recently been discovered that the kidneys produce a hormone, known as erythropoetin, in response to lowered blood oxygen levels. Erythropoetin release ultimately results in a higher level of hemoglobin in the bloodstream via an increase in the number of red blood cells in the circulation. Thus, with more hemoglobin, a greater carrying capacity for scarce oxygen is developed as directed by this internal feedback loop between the lungs and the kidney. (It is interesting to note how modern physiology nicely complements ancient Chinese energetic theory.)

Returning to our example, it was noted that kidney impairment would follow energetic imbalance within the lungs because of impaired energy flow within the bodily circuit. In order to revitalize the kidneys, it would be necessary to treat the acupuncture points along the meridians supplying energy to the lungs, thus allowing them to better support the kidneys.

The principles of classical acupuncture therapy frequently involve this type of cyclic, energetic circuitry viewpoint. These principles allow one to visualize the most strategic points for subtle energetic disease intervention in order to get the desired therapeutic response. Energy imbalance, as viewed by acupuncture theory, can be due to either too much or too little energy flow through particular cyclic loops in the body's meridian circuitry. Acupuncture therapy by acupoint stimulation may allow new energy to enter into meridian circuits where an energy deficit exists. Conversely, acupoint stimulation may also release excessive energy by providing a kind of safety release valve which allows excessive flow to be diverted from overloaded meridian circuits.

Chronobiology &
the Acupuncture Meridian System

In Chinese acupuncture theory, the cycles of ch'i energy moving through the organs follow a daily clock-like pattern. The flow of energy through different meridians, and thus different underlying organs, is said to follow oscillating energy cycles with respect to time of day. Each of the main meridians has two, two-hour periods during which energy flow is first at a maximum and then later at a minimum intensity of circulation.

The time at which energy flow is the greatest through a particular meridian may define the time of day at which it is best to treat a disease in the associated organ system. For instance, the peak time for energy flow in the lung meridian is from 3:00-5:00 AM. Asthma attacks are felt to be best treated by acupuncture during these hours because of the peak activity in the lung-associated meridian. Obviously, there are certain practical limitations to this biorhythm theory, even for the most dedicated of acupuncturists.

The idea of optimal treatment relating to time of day is an area only recently explored by Western medicine. The newly developing field of chronobiology is exploring the nature of human inner biological rhythms from a variety of perspectives. There is now significant experimental evi-

Diagram 21.
BIORHYTHM CYCLES OF THE MERIDIANS

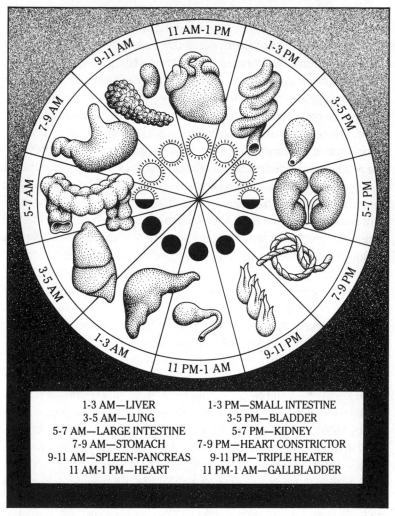

1-3 AM—LIVER	1-3 PM—SMALL INTESTINE
3-5 AM—LUNG	3-5 PM—BLADDER
5-7 AM—LARGE INTESTINE	5-7 PM—KIDNEY
7-9 AM—STOMACH	7-9 PM—HEART CONSTRICTOR
9-11 AM—SPLEEN-PANCREAS	9-11 PM—TRIPLE HEATER
11 AM-1 PM—HEART	11 PM-1 AM—GALLBLADDER

dence to support the concept of an internal biological clock. This internal timepiece which governs many bodily functions, including cyclic enzymatic activity within the brain, also seems to have an effect on the expression of drug toxicity.

Cancer researchers have experimented with chemotherapeutic agents such as cis-platinum to determine if there was an optimal time to give the drug in order to minimize toxic side effects to patients. It was discovered that drug therapy administered during early morning hours had the least toxic effects on experimental animals. Therefore, it appears that drug therapy, as well as acupuncture treatments, may be optimally applied at certain hours of the day. Whether or not cyclic energetic flow through the meridians is responsible for time-related levels of drug toxicity is unknown at this time. This is an idea that will be further explored as the study of chronobiology is pursued at the subtle energetic level of understanding.

It is possible that some of our innate biological rhythms are reflections of higher frequency subtle energetic rhythms. These subtle-energy rhythms are, in turn, in resonant synchrony with the cosmic cycles of the universe. The acupuncture meridian link may be one route by which we are attuned to the energies of the celestial bodies. It is well known that many biological events seem to follow the maxima and minima of solar activity.[5] The meridian system may be the energetic mechanism by which changes in solar activity are translated into cellular and physiological effects. If Western scientists would take into account the time-related energetic flow of cosmic energies through the acupuncture meridian system, it might be possible to understand certain cyclic changes in biological phenomena that are studied by chronobiologists.

Cyclic energy changes in the meridians have importance to acupuncturists attempting to restore balance in diseased organ systems. The acupuncturists see meridian dysfunction as a precursor of organ pathology. The meridian circuit abnormality reflects an imbalance in the polar energies of the forces of yin and yang. Neither force exists alone, but is in relation to the total energetic needs of the organism. Acupuncture's restoration of energy balance in the body's meridian circuitry will result in an improvement in disease states by correcting the energetic patterns which precede cellular dysfunction and disorganization.

Utilizing this type of energetic philosophy, Chinese acupuncturists have been able to successfully impact upon many different organ diseases besides simple pain syndromes. Unfortunately, the Western mind has chosen to focus on that particular dimension of therapy because, until recently, only acupuncture analgesia seemed to make rational scientific sense. This view is the result of identifying the meridian channels with the nervous system instead of seeing them as a unique energetic system. The metaphorical philosophy of organ energy circuits behaving like earthly elements, yin and yang, is too much for most Western physicians to tolerate.

To the majority of Western scientists, acupuncture meridians seem like imaginary structures because there are no published anatomical studies of the meridians in orthodox medical journals to substantiate their existence. They prefer to believe that nerve pathways constitute the true mechanism of acupuncture therapy. The way for Western scientists to conceptualize acupuncture meridians will probably come from new physics instead of medicine, because new physics conceptualizes energy in a similar way.

The acupuncture meridian and nervous systems operate in complementary fashion. Each system works in harmony to translate higher energetic events into cellular patterns of physiology. The work of Kim Bong Han suggests that there are actual tubular meridian structures which run throughout the framework of the physical body. Kim's extensive studies have demonstrated the existence of a separate division of this ductule-like meridian system which is specifically involved with providing energy to the neuronal network of the body. By severing the nutrient meridians supplying the nerves, Kim found that nerve conduction times were significantly prolonged.

One might ask at this point if there is any other experimental evidence besides the work of Kim Bong Han that adds further testimony to the existence of the acupuncture meridian network? Is there further research which substantiates the correspondence of the Chinese system of meridian pathways to the organs of the body? The answer to this question is yes. Research confirming the meridian-organ link has been conducted utilizing systematic measurement of the electrical characteristics of the meridian system. Through the measurement of these electrical parameters, it may be possible to demonstrate not only the existence of the meridians but also the diagnostic potential of the acupuncture system in pinpointing diseased organ systems.

The Acupuncture Meridian System as A Diagnostic Interface

Acupuncture points have unique electrical characteristics which distinguish them from surrounding skin. The drop in electrical skin resistance at the acupoints (a reflection of increased conductivity) can be used to electronically locate these points along the superficial meridians. A number of experimental studies by various Eastern researchers have suggested that the acupuncture points may be useful not only in treatment but also in diagnosis of disease states.

Dr. Hiroshi Motoyama, a researcher in Japan (mentioned earlier as the developer of the chakra machine), has also devised a system which measures the electrical characteristics of the various acupuncture meridians in order to obtain physiological information. The device, called by Motoyama the AMI Machine,[6] short for Apparatus for Measuring the Functions of the Meridians and Corresponding Internal Organ, is a computerized system which can diagnose physiological imbalances within an individual in a matter of minutes. The AMI Machine has 28 electrodes which attach to the terminal acupuncture points of each of the meridians, characteristically located at the ends of the fingers and toes. Acupuncture needles or specialized clips are attached to these acupoints in order to obtain electrical information. The electrical data from the acupuncture points is relayed to a special computer which then analyzes and interprets the information.

The points which are measured by the AMI Machine are the termination points of the paired meridians. The lung meridian, which brings ch'i energy to the lungs, actually exists as a paired set. One of the meridians travels along the right side of the body and the other along the left. The rationale behind measuring electrical data from the paired meridians stems from the Chinese theory of yin and yang. The modern adaptation of this theory suggests that internal organs which are in a state of energetic balance (i.e., health) will have paired acupuncture meridians which are electrically similar in value. Organs which have underlying disease that may be already present or about to manifest will demonstrate a marked electrical difference between the two associated meridian pairs. The AMI Machine is able to register localized skin currents coming from the acupoints at the ends of the meridians.[7]

Motoyama studied over five thousand subjects utilizing the AMI Machine in order to derive statistical reference values for physiological and electrical normality and abnormality. Electrical differences between the right and left meridians of an order greater than two standard deviations from the norm were printed out by the AMI unit in red in order to highlight the organ systems that are out of balance. Meridian pair values that are electrically similar (by computer reference standards) were printed out in black.

Motoyama and others working with the AMI Machine have found strong correlations between meridians that are electrically out of balance and the presence of underlying disease in the associated organ systems. The Bob Hope Parkinson Research Institute in Florida has been working with the AMI Machine in order to study energetic abnormalities and physiologic imbalances in individuals with Parkinson's Disease (a degenerative neurological disorder which affects motor coordination). Early data obtained from the AMI Machine suggests that many Parkinsonian patients have abnormalities (as predicted by meridian imbalances) in the large and small intestines as well as the heart. It is possible that this gastrointestinal imbalance reflects a functional problem with the bowel's absorption of key nutrients involved in neurotransmitter synthesis. Parkinson patients are known to have deficits of dopamine in certain nuclei of the brain known as the basal ganglia. Researchers at the institute hope to use the AMI to distinguish different stages and types of Parkinsonism and perhaps gain information that could help patients and physicians attain greater control over the primary disease process.

One local government in Japan is using the AMI Machine to screen all employees during their annual required medical examination. Only those individuals with abnormal meridian readouts are required to undergo further medical diagnostic testing. A number of other medical practitioners in the United States are also utilizing the AMI with positive results.

The early success of the AMI technology does more than affirm the usefulness of acupuncture-based technologies. The fact that AMI information correlates with the status of deep internal organs confirms the ancient Chinese theory associating particular meridians with specific organ systems. Also, we are now examining acupuncture theory from a diagnostic perspective. The acupuncture merdians are being used not just for therapy but for diagnosis as well.

Western theories on acupuncture mechanisms have tended to focus on neurological pathways of action such as spinal gate mechanisms and on endorphin release in the brain. Although nerve stimulation may be acceptable to scientists attempting to explain acupuncture analgesia, it is less clear how a peripheral nerve in the finger or toe would be able to give valuable information about the status of a patient's liver or lung.

Data from the AMI Machine adds further evidence to support the existence of the meridian system and its predicted organ associations. Through instrumentation like the AMI Machine, the acupuncture meridian system is beginning to find technologic confirmation and value as a model of physiological functioning. In addition, the ability to noninvasively diagnose early disease states or tendencies toward illness via external electrical monitoring of the acupoints has obvious significance for public health screening.

Another system of instrumentation which has brought credence to Chinese acupuncture theory has been Kirlian photography and its technologic offshoots. Initial reports on Kirlian work from the Soviet Union suggested that acupuncture points could be photographed utilizing high-frequency discharge devices. Some replication of this claim has also been carried out by a number of American Kirlian investigators, including Pizzo[8] and others. Perhaps the most sophisticated approach to electrographic imaging of acupuncture points has been researched by Dr. Ion Dumitrescu, a Rumanian physician who has developed a body-scanning process known as electronography.

Dumitrescu's work with electronography is a reflection of his search to develop the Kirlian process beyond the level of the primitive fingerprint devices presently in use by most researchers. Utilizing computers and special scanning electrodes, electronography has allowed electrographic scanning of large body surfaces such as the chest and abdomen. In his early work, Dumitrescu noted particular areas on the body where electrically radiant points appeared. Many of these points, which he referred to as electrodermal points, were found to correlate with the classical acupuncture points along the body. After studying literally thousands of individuals with the electronographic process, Dumitrescu came to a number of conclusions about these electrodermal (or acupuncture) points.

It was found that the points only appeared in electrographic scans of individuals where pathology was present (or imminent) in a particular organ system. The points which were found to glow brightly coincided with acupuncture points along the meridian associated with the diseased organ. The size and brightness of the acupuncture points was later found to correlate with their electrical activity and the acuteness of the disease process. The larger the electrodermal points, the more acute the pathology. The electrodermal points did not appear in electrographic scans if there were no underlying or active diseases within the body. In other words, acupuncture points would only be electrically visible when there was a meridian imbalance reflecting underlying organ dysfunction. Although the meridians themselves were not photographed by this process, the electrodermal points were often found to occur along linear paths mirroring classical acupuncture meridians.

Dumitrescu has concluded that the electrodermal points are "electrical pores"[9] concerned with energy exchange between the body and the surrounding electrical medium. They are a point of communication between the organism and its surrounding energetic fields. Dumitrescu's discoveries on the behavior of electrodermal points complement the electrical meridian data from Motoyama's AMI Machine. Both researchers independently established the link between energetic meridian imbalance and underlying organ pathology. Dumitrescu's research demonstrates in a more graphic fashion the nature of energy exchange between the electromagnetic environment and the meridians via the acupuncture points. Motoyama monitored specific acupuncture points for illness, while in Dumitrescu's electronographic scans of the body the acupoints reflecting energetic imbalance appeared spontaneously as sites of energy disturbance.

The acupuncture meridian system is an interface of energetic exchange between our physical body and the energy fields which surround us. These electromagnetic energies include not only local and cosmic environmental factors but also other types of energetic input from our higher frequency bodies such as the etheric, astral, and higher vehicles.

The phenomena which are measured by these new technologies, such as the AMI Machine and the electrographic scanner, are electrical reflections of higher frequency energetic processes. As we saw in our earlier chapter discussing positive and negative space/time energies, these higher frequency energies are of a primarily magnetic nature. Research suggests that *the etheric body forms a type of holographic magnetic grid which communicates with the electrically based matter and cells of the physical body via the acupuncture meridian system.*

The electrical potentials measured at the acupuncture points reflect subtle internal currents which move throughout the meridian system. These internal currents flow through a specialized meridian circuitry which distributes these vital, organizing, subtle magnetic energies to the organs of the body. The acupuncture meridian system interacts with the nervous system through a series of energy transduction steps which ultimately allow these higher energetic phenomena to influence cellular electrophysiology.

The Meridian-Glial Network: An Electrical Interface with the Human Nervous System

The reason that Western theorists have discovered neural and neurohormonal links with the acupuncture system is not because the meridians are nerves. *It is because a division of the meridian system works closely with and influences the central and peripheral nervous system.* The nervous system communicates by way of electrical action potentials which transmit messages via a special digital frequency language. Information is conveyed by changes in the frequency of action-potential bursts. The brain is able to interpret this frequency information by rapidly decoding the changes in firing rates of incoming action potentials (electrical nerve signals). In other words, the nervous system transmits and receives information through messages that are digitally encoded in the number of electrical nerve firings per second. The same numerical code of nerve firing rates will carry different meanings, depending upon whether a particular nerve is communicating with the area of the brain that processes touch, smell, taste, or another sensory center.

It has been recently discovered that the Schwann and glial cell systems, formerly felt to have only nutritive function to the nerves they surround, also carry out an additional function of an electrical nature. Research has indicated that the glial cell network is able to transmit information via slow shifts in DC-current potentials. This type of information transmission is referred to as analog-based, as opposed to the digital pulse code of neural action potentials. The analog system of data transmission operates by varying the voltage of the cell membrane (the DC-current membrane potential), where an upward or downward shift in cell voltage translates into a particular character and type of information that is relayed along the glial circuit. Analog transmission is known to be considerably slower than digital transmission but is recognized as an effective alternative form of data communication.

The DC-current system of the glial cells appears to be involved in self-healing electrical feedback loops and relates to such phenomena as the current of injury. This was discussed with the work of Dr. Becker in Chapter 3. It is likely that the acupuncture system has some type of input into the nervous system as evidenced by acupuncture analgesia's ability to cause endorphin release in the brain. At one level, this might be accomplished by influencing the DC potentials of the glial cell network which follow the pathways of the nerves. Electrical currents conducted through the acupuncture meridian system may reflect the meridians' role in forming a unique type of energy circulatory system that exists in relation to other established physiologic pathways. It is possible that *the DC-currents associated with the meridian and glial network may influence the production and transmission of action potentials by the nerves.* Certain paraphysical information tends to confirm this hypothesis:

> The direct current potentials, measurable on the intact surfaces of all living beings, demonstrate a complex field pattern that is spatially related to the anatomical arrangement of the nervous system. The surface potentials are directly associated with elements of the various circulatory systems. *The "fifth circulatory system" is one which is connected with an internal energetic current working through the acupuncture lines. It is continually at work and available to shape the action potential system, which is used by the network of nerves.* This action potential system, therefore, exists upon a substratum of direct current potentials which actually precede the action-potential mechanism of data transmission. The preexisting direct current potentials have original functions which govern biological processes, thereby controlling the basic properties of living organisms.
>
> The human form is a grid of magnetic domains which move between the primary blueprint of the Overself (etheric and higher light bodies), and the pattern angles of the human organs, (i.e., the axial relationship). The lines which tie together these magnetic domains are known as "axiatonal lines." Axiatonal grids (formed by intersecting axiatonal lines) interface with the biological activities of the organism. The grids allow interaction of the physical cellular structure with higher or lower vibratory frequencies.
>
> *Man's biological interconnection with the higher frequency energies takes place through the Acupuncture Meridian System,* which is interfaced with the Axiatonal Line and Grid System. *The acupuncture and axiatonal lines are part of a fifth dimensional circulatory system, which are used to draw from the Overself body, the basic energy used for renewing the physical-cellular form.*[10] *(italics added)*

This paraphysical data puts into perspective the neural link between the acupuncture meridian system, the electrical currents measured at the acupoints, and the meridian interface to the higher energetic domains (collectively referred to here as the overself). It is suggested that *meridian energetic inputs influence the action-potential output of the nervous system by varying the DC-currents which are part of the electrical environment in which the neurons function.* This indirect energetic link with the nervous system explains why one can measure neurological phenomena in response to acupuncture stimulation.

Dr. Bruce Pomeranz has done studies on the transmission of action potentials through neuronal pain pathways in the spinal cord as they are influenced by acupuncture analgesia.[11] Pomeranz found that painful stimuli to a mouse's tail were accompanied by a significant increase in the firing rate of neurons along the pain pathway in the spinal cord. Acupuncture analgesia, directed toward desensitizing the tail to pain, resulted in an inability to increase the neuronal firing rate beyond the resting level in response to painful stimuli, but only after a 30-minute interval. Mice whose pituitary glands were surgically removed were unable to demonstrate the same acupuncture-mediated suppression of nerve response to pain. Naloxone, an endorphin blocking agent, also prevented this acupuncture-mediated phenomenon. Pomeranz's conclusion from the study was that endorphins were the mediators of acupuncture analgesia.

Endorphin release is a measureable event in the acupuncture pathway, but Pomeranz's experimental data does not explain how a stimulus to the acupoint travels to the pituitary gland over this delay period. The 30-minute delay suggests some type of slow signal transmission. The mechanism of transmission is likely to involve slow analog DC changes in the glial cell network, as discovered by Dr. Robert Becker in his research on the current of injury. These DC-current changes in the glial cell network are probably influenced by energetic changes in the meridians after the acupoints have been stimulated. The glial DC-current changes subsequently affect activity in the neurons leading to the central nervous system. *Therefore, the glial cell network may function as an interface between the meridians and the nervous system.* Exactly how changes in DC potentials affect nerve firing rates is a rather complex issue. In order to understand how this may take place, we must first understand some of the basic aspects of neurophysiology.

Recent neurochemical research has led scientists to a more complete model of nerve cell functioning. It is now known that neurons do not turn on and off when they transmit signals. The nerve cells exist in a constant state of readiness and activity which allows them to respond to stimuli in milliseconds. The nerve cells are constantly releasing minute quanta of neurotransmitters into the synaptic gaps between themselves and the neurons they contact. At these synaptic sites, the continuous release of micro amounts of transmitters keeps the system quietly active, yet poised for action, in a fashion similar to a car's engine on slow idle. One need only step on the accelerator to speed up an engine which is already in a state of readiness to respond.

When an action potential is initiated in a nerve cell, such as when a peripheral nerve relays sensory information from pressure receptors in the skin, the electrical impulse initiates a sequence of events that ultimately sends a message to the brain. A stimulus to the receptor in the skin initiates this chain of events by starting a volley of action-potential bursts that travel down the axis of the sensory nerve fiber until they reach its synaptic ends. At these synapse relay stations, nerve endings exist side by side, with microscopic gaps between them. The electrical impulse undergoes an energetic translation at the synaptic gap through its conversion into a neurotransmitter release. Each action potential stimulates the presynaptic nerve to release, into the synaptic cleft, tiny packets of neurotransmitter which induce electrical changes in the cell membrane of the adjacent nerve. These electrical changes, in turn, are reconverted into the digital pulse code of action-potential bursts which are rapidly transmitted to the end of that nerve and another synaptic gap. The final synapses occur after spinal cord neurons relay the digitized sensory message to the brain.

The process of neurotransmitter release is affected by the number and rapidity of action potentials reaching the presynaptic membrane in addition to local membrane factors. These local factors have their effects upon the electrical potential of the neuronal membrane. *The cell membrane's electrical potential determines the responsiveness of each neuron to releasing neurotransmitter packets on cue.* The electrical status of the neuronal membrane is affected by many factors. The most significant of these factors, only recently understood, is the effect of other neurochemicals which are in contact with the individual nerve cell. Each nerve cell exists, not in isolation, but in contact with many other nerves in a network. The synaptic foot-processes of many different nerves impinge upon any single neuron. These foot-processes contain many different types of neurochemicals, which have varying effects upon the nerve membranes they synaptically contact.

Although there appear to be many types of neurochemicals, it is now clear that most neurotransmitters function in two general ways. One group is known as the excitatory neurotransmitters. These chemicals increase the responsiveness of the individual neuron to electrical stimulation. The other group is the inhibitory transmitters. They decrease the responsiveness of the neurons they contact by causing opposing shifts in neuronal electrical membrane potential. What happens at the individual neuronal cell membrane is that the many neurochemical influences summate in a particular electrical direction. The electrical status of the neuronal membrane thus changes from moment to moment. *The electrical responsiveness of each neuron is proportional to the balance of inhibitory and excitatory transmitters impinging upon the cell membrane near the synapse at any one moment in time.*

Of the newer transmitters discovered, the endorphins are considered a hot area of research in conventional medicine. They are one of a growing number of newly discovered brain chemicals which are currently under study in the developing field of neuroendocrinology. Of the many neurochemicals under investigation, it is the endorphins which figure most prominently in conventional theories of acupuncture analgesia. *The endorphins belong to a class of neurochemicals which have been referred to as "neuromodulators" or "neuroregulators."*[12] These chemicals modulate the effects of other transmitter systems through their ability to influence neuronal membranes. The endorphins belong to a subclass of transmitters known as peptidergic hormones[13] (or neuropeptides). Other neurochemical divisions of the nervous system include the adrenergic, cholinergic, and dopaminergic systems. In addition, there are many other neurochemical transmitters whose functions are poorly understood at this time. Although there are many different neurochemical substances which may impinge upon nerve cells, there appear to be additional membrane factors, aside from neurochemicals, which modulate the transmission of neural impulses. Specifically, *changes in the electrical field microenvironment of the synapse may influence neurotransmission.* In order to understand how these energetic membrane factors relate to the neurological effects of acupuncture, let us return to Dr. Pomeranz's groundbreaking study.

Dr. Pomeranz discovered that acupuncture analgesia caused the release of endorphins from the pituitary gland. Endorphin release was found to coincide with the inhibition of pain impulse transmission to the brain. Pomeranz found that acupuncture analgesia prevented painful stimuli from increasing the firing rate of spinal cord neurons above basal resting levels, but only after a 30-minute period. Endorphin blocking agents were able to prevent this acupuncture-induced neuronal change. There was found to be a 30-minute delay period from initial acupoint stimulation to eventual endorphin release. The delay appears to be due to slow transmission of the initial signal from the acupoint to the pituitary gland before endorphin release can occur. It is suggested by this author that *the release of endorphins is not the final endpoint, but only an intermediary event along a complex transmission pathway.*

The ultimate pathway of action in acupuncture from acupoint stimulation to final physiologic result must be viewed from the perspective of sequential stages of energy transduction. This principle of stepping down energies from one level to another in a type of cascade effect is seen in many organizational levels of biological function. There are, however, technological limitations in the ability of Western scientists to trace the pathways of expression when causes originate at the subtle energetic level. One's ability to define true cause and effect (as in the case of the neurohormonal effects of acupuncture) may be limited by the sensitivity of the measuring devices chosen to monitor the biological systems in question.

At the physical level, we can easily measure neurohormonal changes, such as increases in spinal-fluid endorphin levels, that are a result of acupuncture stimulation. *These neurochemical changes are secondary by-products of energy signal transduction through the meridian-nervous system link. An energetic signal becomes converted into a hormonal signal.* The path between stimulus and response follows a more circuitous route than the nervous system alone. The nerves form a link in a chain of events. The neurological model of acupuncture is, at present, only partially adequate to fully explain the 30-minute delay in signal transmission. If nerves were the primary mechanism in acupuncture, one would expect a faster response time from needle insertion to analgesic effect. Nerve response time is ordinarily in the range of milliseconds, not minutes. Some theorists have suggested that the time delay between needle stimulation and pain relief is due to the slow release of the endorphins from the pituitary, and their gradual effect upon the pain-relaying nerve fibers in the spinal cord. However, an alternate theory proposed by this author may give greater understanding to both the 30-minute delay in pain relief as well as the complex nature of the acupuncture-nervous system link.

It is likely that part of the delay noted in signal transmission is due to participation of the glial-cell network in meridian energy transduction. The glial cells demonstrate a slower method of analog data transmission via gradual shifts in DC potentials.[14] This perineural transmission system is composed of Schwann, glia, and satellite cells which form an electro-interactive interface with the nervous system. The perineural network participates in one intermediate step in a series of progressive signal transductions whereby primary meridian energies ultimately influence the nervous system.

From initial acupoint stimulation, there occurs a stepwise transformation of the natural energetic currents which flow from the meridians to the nerves. *The primary energetic currents flowing through the meridians are*

of a negatively-entropic magnetic nature (negative space/time energy).[15]
These magnetic currents, flowing through the acupuncture meridians, in-
duce secondary electrical fields at the physical tissue level. It is these secondary electrical field effects, associated with the acupuncture points and
meridian system, which are measured by such instruments as Motoyama's
AMI Machine and Dumitrescu's electrographic scanner.

These induced electrical fields are translated into DC-current interactions between the meridian and glial-cell network. The meridian network
interfaces with the axiatonal grid system, an etheric-energetic structure
which focuses higher frequency energies into the physical body. One entry point for these higher energies thus occurs at the acupoint-meridian
network via its connection to the etheric-axiatonal grid. The grid provides
an access route for the organizing life-energies which provide and maintain coherence within the physical-cellular structure. These subtle magnetic currents create measureable changes in the physical-cellular matrix,
in part through the induction of secondary electrical fields. These electrical
fields go on to affect primary bioelectronic processes which occur at the
cellular level.

The glial-cell network is part of a DC-current/analog-based system
of information transmission which participates in bioelectrical processes

Diagram 22.
ACUPUNCTURE ENERGETICS
& NEUROENDOCRINE MODULATION

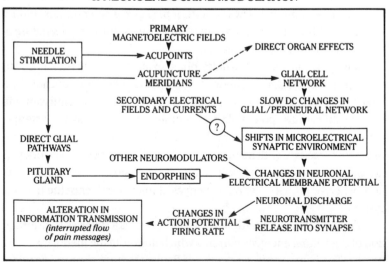

of cellular repair typified by the current-of-injury phenomenon. By modi-fying the energy-field environment of the glial cells, the meridian system is able to directly affect bioelectronic systems of growth and repair. In ad-dition, the meridian-glial network also utilizes DC-current effects to create an electromagnetic microenvironment around the nerves of the body. *The DC potentials carried over the glial and Schwann cells energetically affect the nerves they surround by creating specialized microenergetic influences at the presynaptic sites. These electrical-field phenomena modulate neural responsiveness to stimulation and conduction by varying changes in neuronal membrane potentials.* The DC field effects summate with the chemical neuromodulators and act in concert at the presynaptic nerve membrane. *The total effects of chemical neuromodulators, combined with DC-current influences, act to fine tune the digital transmission of the action potential code.* Thus, both chemical and energetic factors may influence the ability of nerves to transmit pain impulses to the brain.

Through the acupuncture meridian network, ch'i energies are trans-formed into DC-current changes, which are then slowly transmitted along perineural pathways throughout the glial network. At the level of the brain, these changes in DC potentials are also associated with neurochemical mechanisms (i.e. endorphin release) that may precede or coincide with the action-potential changes in individual neurons. The neurochemical release of endorphins, which are known to be widely active throughout the body, suggests a multitude of possible hormonal effects of acupuncture on the entire body, beyond simple changes in neuronal firing rates. Pituitary hormones, such as endorphins and similar peptides, are normally distributed through-out the body via the route of the bloodstream. From there, these potent hormones have their effect on multiple cellular systems.

Thus endorphins are not an endpoint, but are instead intermediate actors in this complex energetic system of the body. They provide one step which can be monitored with conventional drug assays, just as the firing rate of spinal cord neurons may be empirically studied with microelectrodes to measure the indirect effects of acupuncture stimulation. *The neurochemical and electrical changes which occur in the nervous system are secondary effects and not primary events.* They are an objective confirmation of an unseen energetic process taking place, but they are not the final answer to explaining acupuncture's effects. *Acupuncture is mediated by a primary, subtle energetic system that influences the network of physical nerves.* In addition to acupuncture's influence on nerves, it has multiple therapeutic effects on other cellular components of physiology which are less easily measured by present medical technologies.

The Acupuncture
Meridian System as a Therapeutic Interface:
A Return to the Concept of Healing with Energy

The previous studies on acupuncture analgesia have all involved classical needle stimulation of acupoints in order to obtain the sought-after therapeutic effects. This is the most ancient method of acupuncture, and is still practiced throughout China today. In conjunction with the use of acupuncture needles, moxibustion is an adjunctive modality which seems to enhance therapeutic effectiveness. The ancient Chinese discovered that burning a small portion of the native plant known as "moxa" directly on the acupoint, or on the outer end of the inserted acupuncture needle, seemed to improve therapeutic effectiveness of the treatment.

More recent technologic improvements in this ancient system have involved the application of weak electrical currents to the acupuncture needles in order to enhance their efficacy. Various modifications of the pulsed electrical current have been demonstrated to variably enhance therapeutic effects, depending upon the frequency, amplitude, and pulsatile nature of the rhythmic currents applied.

In addition to the conventional application of acupuncture needles to the acupoints, a wide variety of energetic stimuli have proved effective in creating similar therapeutic changes via the meridian pathways. One method which has already been discussed is the pulsing of high or low-frequency electrical currents into the meridians via superficial electrodes that touch the skin overlying the acupoints (also referred to as "electroacupuncture"). In addition to electrical stimulation, simple finger pressure, also known as "acupressure," is somewhat efficacious, although this technique is less effective than needle stimulation.

A number of other energetic modalities have been tried with variable therapeutic success. Dr. Irving Oyle in California has been successful in treating a variety of disorders utilizing a technique he refers to as sonopuncture,[16] which involves the use of ultrasonic stimulation to classical acupuncture points. Dr. Oyle employs the use of the sonicator, a device employing a special *crystalline* transducer which is able to focus *high-frequency sound waves* into a small region of skin overlying the acupoints. Dr. Oyle has claimed to have had success in using sonopuncture to treat a variety of illnesses ranging from anxiety reactions, allergic dermatitis, and dysmenorrhea, to lower back pain. Other practitioners have had similar success with this modality, which is significantly less invasive than needle puncture.

Perhaps the most futuristic approach to acupoint stimulation has been the Soviet work with the technique referred to as "laserpuncture." Laserpuncture involves the focusing of *low-energy laser beams* upon acupuncture points. The beams do not actually cause physical penetration of the skin as the name might imply. Russian researchers are employing this technique to experimentally treat hypertension, inflammatory bowel diseases, and joint and metabolic disorders.[17] Other reports indicate that the Soviets have been successful in aborting epileptic convulsions by focusing the laser beam on an upper-lip acupoint at the onset of a seizure.

Interesting results with laserpuncture have been noted on facial paralysis in children. Researchers compared electrical voltage measurements from acupoints on the right and left side of the face. In facial paralysis, there was an electrical imbalance between the two sides, similar to what Motoyama has measured utilizing the AMI Machine. Following laser treatment to the imbalanced acupoints, normalization of meridian voltages was found to be associated with a cure of the paralysis.[18]

In a more sophisticated approach, some Soviet scientists such as Dr. Victor Inyushin are using Kirlian body scanners before and after stimulation with helium-neon lasers, in order to assess pre- and post-treatment energy states of the acupoints. This research is reminiscent of Dumitrescu's work with electronographic scanning, but the Russians go one step further in utilizing their Kirlian-based technology to assess both diagnosis and treatment.

In terms of therapeutic results, laserpuncture has been found to be even more effective than classical needling or electrical stimulation of acupoints. A number of American and Italian researchers are also beginning to explore the therapeutic benefits of this unique modality.

Laserpuncture and sonopuncture are truly unique therapeutic approaches in that they employ the pure energetic frequencies of light and sound to heal human illness. The energies imparted to the acupoints by these modalities have their ultimate physiological effects by shifting the natural flow of subtle energies through the meridians.

During the process of acupoint stimulation leading to a final physiologic outcome, there is considerable signal transduction along the energetic pathways. The intermediate by-products of signal transduction, from DC-current changes at acupoints to hormonal release, may provide physicians with an avenue for monitoring aspects of organ physiology and pathology.

We have seen that the firing rates of nerves may be affected by acupuncture as well as by the release of pituitary hormones such as endorphins. These are effects which conventional medical techniques are easily capable of measuring. A much more sensitive and useful approach lies in monitoring the electrical fields and currents secondarily associated with the meridian system. *Measurement of changes in the electrical parameters of acupoints, through such technologies as the AMI Machine and Kirlian-based scanners, will ultimately prove to be the diagnostic avenues of the future.* As we shall see in later chapters, these technologies will provide sensitive information about the physiologic status of the human organism, as well as guidelines to follow in monitoring different types of therapy.

Because the primary energies flowing through the meridians are of a subtle energetic nature, the electrical parameters of the acupoints provide the closest indirect information that is possible with our conventional level of instrumentation. Utilizing these new systems of diagnosis, we will be able to understand more about the mechanisms and benefits of many different types of subtle energetic therapies which may be useful in treating human illnesses. It will be through the exploration of the physical-etheric interface, as provided by measurements of the acupuncture meridian system, that medicine will slowly evolve toward a more subtle energetic orientation of diagnosis and treatment.

Key Points to Remember

1. Chinese medicine sees the human being as a microcosm within the universal macrocosm. Therefore, the principles that determine the flow of energy throughout the universe are seen as applicable to the human energetic system.

2. The Chinese consider the state of the universe to be a changing, dynamic equilibrium between polar opposites in nature, which they have characterized in their essence as yin and yang. A correct balance of the yin and yang forces within the microcosm of the human body is critical to achieving and maintaining health.

3. Acupuncture points are access points that allow energy to flow from environmental energy fields into the subtle fields of the etheric and physical bodies. The acupoints can be located on the skin via their characteristic of low electrical resistance, i.e. high conductivity, which is consistent with their role as portals of energy entry into the body.

4. Ch'i, a nutritive subtle life-energy, is absorbed from the environment into the acupuncture points and through the meridian system. The meridian system is largely divided into twelve main sets of meridians that deliver energy to the major organs of the body.

5. According to Chinese philosophy, the flow of ch'i energy through the twelve paired meridians follows certain well-defined cycles that mirror principles in nature. These Cycles of Generation and Destruction demonstrate the patterns by which ch'i energy flows sequentially through the meridians, and thus, to the organs of the body, during periods of both health and illness.

6. The flow of ch'i energy through the meridians follows a biorhythmic pattern. The flow of ch'i through a particular meridian is always highest at a particular time of day or night. Knowledge of this pattern of timing can be helpful to the clinician in knowing which times to treat a particular meridian using acupuncture therapy. Also, this time-related flow of life-energies may be a contributing factor to physiological phenomena which are strongly affected by time of day.

7. The acupuncture system delivers ch'i to the organs through paired meridians on the left and right sides of the body. When an organ is diseased, or illness is imminent, the paired meridians delivering energy to that organ demonstrate an electrical imbalance between the two sides of the body.

8. Such disease-related imbalances in the major bodily organs can be determined by using diagnostic systems such as the AMI Machine, a computerized instrument which electrically measures and compares the terminal acupoints for each of the major paired meridians.

9. Electrographic scans of the body demonstrate that acupuncture points glow brightly when their associated meridian is out of balance, thus allowing an alternative method of disease detection.

10. Stimulation of acupuncture points produces changes in the nervous system (i.e. endorphin release and relief of pain) because the meridians indirectly influence nerve pathways in the body. Such acupuncture-associated nerve changes are probably mediated by energy field

fluctuations in the vicinity of the nerves and the glial cells which surround them.

   11. The acupuncture meridian system is both a diagnostic interface as well as a therapeutic interface. Energy changes in the meridian system can be measured through the acupoints to detect the presence of illness. Conversely, energy can be introduced into the meridian system to promote healing of diseases via a variety of therapeutic modalities, including stimulation of acupoints by finger pressure, needles, electrical currents, sound waves, and laser light.

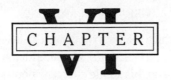

CHAPTER VI

New Windows
On an Unseen World:
THE DEVELOPMENT OF SUBTLE
ENERGETIC TECHNOLOGIES

As we have begun to understand from the previous chapters, humans are multidimensional organisms. Seen another way, many different frequencies of consciousness exist within one self. Human beings have complex energetic interconnections between their observable physical bodies and their invisible higher bodies. Observations by gifted clairvoyants have helped many spiritually oriented researchers to understand the invisible subtle energetic anatomy, but such data is frequently disregarded by the skeptical scientific community. The ability to change the mechanistic viewpoint of present and future physicians will depend upon the development of instrumentation which can extend our physical senses to perceive the subtle energies of this invisible realm. Such tools to understand human subtle energetic anatomy already exist in the world today. Knowledge of the existence and use of this equipment is either disregarded or unknown to the majority of Western scientists. In order to shed greater light on the field of subtle energetic diagnostic systems, we shall begin with a closer examination of the meridian system of the human body.

Meridian-Based Diagnostic Systems:
Hahnemann Updated with New Age Technologies

As mentioned in the previous chapter, the physical-etheric interface is one of our important links to higher dimensional energies. This interface is an energy system which maintains a delicate balance between our physical and subtle bodies. The acupuncture meridians are the conduits of energy flow that make up this subtle energetic network. The acupuncture points are the most physically accessible aspects of the physical-etheric interface. It has been demonstrated that the electrical characteristics of the meridians, as measured through the acupoints, contain important information about the status of the body's internal organs.

The subtle energies flowing through the meridians are not electrical in nature, but they are able to induce electrical fields and currents because of their magnetic properties. This energy, known to the Chinese as ch'i, is actually a manifestation of the life-force which animates and energizes living systems. Ch'i energy is negatively entropic in nature. It moves the organism toward states of increased order and greater cellular energy balance. When the flow of life energy to a particular organ is deficient or unbalanced, patterns of cellular disruption occur. *The ability to measure electromagnetic disturbances in the meridian system and to find imbalances in the flow of ch'i allows one to detect ongoing cellular pathology in a particular area of the body as well as to predict future organic dysfunction.*

In recent years, a number of diagnostic systems have been developed which utilize this energetic meridian information. One unique system which makes use of electrical information associated with the acupuncture points is the Motoyama AMI Machine[1] discussed in Chapter 5. Utilizing electrodes which attach to the terminal (seiketsu) acupoints of the twelve main meridians, the AMI Machine is able to compare the electrical balance between the right and left sides of the body. The AMI computer analyzes electrical differences between the right and left meridians that supply energy to the same deep organ system. By comparing the degree of electrical imbalance between the two meridians, the AMI Machine is able to provide detailed information about energetic imbalance in the physical body. *Electrically unbalanced acupoints, as diagnosed by the AMI Machine, appear to reflect the presence of existing or impending disease in meridian-associated organ systems.*

Motoyama's AMI Machine provides us with an unusual window with which to observe and measure the subtle energetic streams that organize and nurture the physical biosystems of cellular growth and repair. These subtle energies supply information from the etheric body. In addition, these etheric-based energies are an intermediary link in the flow of information from the higher subtle bodies down to the physical cellular level.

It has been previously shown that Kirlian photographic studies of the Phantom Leaf Effect and Dr. Harold Burr's work[2] with electrical fields around plants and animals substantiate the existence of the etheric body. (The etheric body is a holographic energy template which provides structural information for the cellular systems of the physical body.) Although the cells of the body have unique enzymatic control systems for self-maintenance and replication, they are guided by energetic patterns of a higher frequency nature.

The subtle nature of the etheric (and other) energies which influence the physical cellular network makes direct measurement of these energies difficult with present levels of technology. Because these energies have special magnetic characteristics (see Chapter 4 on negative space/time energies[3]), they are able to induce secondary electrical fields and currents. Although measurement of the primary subtle energies has proven difficult, their associated secondary electrical phenomena are easier to monitor. Measurement of the DC-currents at the acupuncture points of the body allows one to gather biologically significant information about the energetic status of the organism. *By electrically monitoring the acupoints and acupuncture meridians, one is able to tap into the specialized internal bioenergy circuit which connects the etheric and physical energy fields.*

Clairvoyant research suggests that illness begins first in the etheric and higher frequency vehicles. If this is so, then signs of illness can be seen in the etheric body earlier than they can be detected in the physical body. Ideally, one would like to find illness at an early-enough stage that the physician's intervention could actually prevent a disease from physically manifesting at the cellular level. We have already established that the meridians are carriers of etherically-based biological information. Because changes in the etheric body precede the onset of physical diseases, *electroacupuncture technologies may allow us to actually measure subtle-energy imbalances which are precursors to illness. In addition, these same technologies can reveal illness in the physical body which may already be present but which is still too subtle to be measured by conventional laboratory tests.*

From a simplistic view, it is possible to *indirectly* monitor the flow of vital energies to the deeper organs via systems like the AMI Machine in order to examine the underlying health of particular organ structures like the heart, lung, and kidneys. The AMI Machine compares the electrical symmetries of right and left meridians to derive nonspecific information about imbalances in the organ systems of the body. Motoyama's computer can pinpoint which organs are affected by illness, but it does not identify the particular disease process. However, there are other meridian-based technologies which may be used to acquire more detailed physiological information about the strengths, weaknesses, and specific illnesses that affect the physical body.

One system, which is beginning to grow in popularity among doctors and dentists, is a device known as the Dermatron or Voll Machine. The prototype of this system was developed by Dr. Reinhard Voll,[4] a German physician. This technique is also known as EAV, or Electroacupuncture According to Voll. Instead of solely monitoring the terminal acupoints of the meridians by remote computer measurement, as in the AMI system, the Voll device allows one to measure the electrical parameters of any acupuncture point in the body. The Dermatron comes with a hand-held electrical probe which the physician presses against the individual acupoint of interest. The patient holds a brass tube in one hand, which is connected by a wire to the Voll Machine. By holding this tube, the patient permits a completed electrical circuit to occur when the metal-tipped probe touches the acupoint. The probe relays microvoltage electrical information from the acupoints to the Voll Machine, where it is displayed on a type of voltmeter readout.

Certain levels of electrical norms for the acupoints have been established by Voll's previous research. Unlike the AMI system, the Voll Machine is used to examine the parameters of individual acupoints instead of comparing paired meridian acupoints for electrical symmetry. The electrical voltage level for a particular acupoint reflects the energy level of its meridian-associated organ(s). The direction of electrical deviation from the norm can have important implications about the nature of the underlying problem in a particular meridian. For instance, an acupoint voltage that is lower than normal may be caused by degenerative disease within an organ system or by conditions which produce a low general vitality. Conversely, higher than normal acupoint voltage readings can be indicative of an underlying inflammatory process. Further information may be derived as to the acute or chronic nature of the disease process by determining the responsiveness of the acupoints to electrical stimulation by the Voll Machine. When the Dermatron is switched to "treatment mode," it is capable of delivering a voltage charge to a particular weakened acupoint and its associated meridian. The ability of a meridian to accept and hold onto a charge is a function of how chronic the condition of illness is. Individuals with mild illness or slightly low vitality can usually be recharged by using the Dermatron's electrical probe to stimulate the low-reading acu-point. Those people with more serious and chronic illnesses are more dif-ficult to recharge in a short period of time.

In addition to being able to discover which organs are affected by ill-ness, EAV systems can detail the type and degree of dysfunction that exists within an afflicted organ. Researchers working with the Voll system claim to have found associations between particular acupoints along an organ's meridian and various aspects of that organ's function. For example, there is a meridian which carries ch'i energy to the pancreas. Among the acu-points that are located on the pancreatic meridian, there are specific points which reflect the functional status of individual pancreatic enzyme sys-tems. One acupoint on the pancreatic meridian reflects the status of the prot-ease (protein-digesting) enzymes secreted by the pancreas. Other acupoints on the same meridian are said to reflect the functional integrity of different enzymes such as lipase (fat-digesting) secretions. By analyzing the electri-cal voltages associated with the individual acupoints along a meridian, detailed data may be obtained about multiple parameters of organ function.

As an example, let us look at how the two meridian-based technolo-gies might be useful and complementary in noninvasively diagnosing the reasons behind a problem of weight loss due to intestinal malabsorption. Conventional x-ray and biopsy studies of the intestine might reveal normal bowel mucosa. Motoyama's AMI Machine would register an imbalance in the functioning of the pancreas by detecting asymmetrical electrical read-outs from the right and left pancreatic meridians of the patient's body. But the AMI system would not tell you what was wrong with the pancreas. Us-ing the Voll Machine to fine tune the diagnosis, one could pinpoint that there was a specific problem in the pancreatic production of lipase, an im-portant component of fat digestion and absorption.

The Voll Machine allows one to carry out an energetic inventory of the functions of the different organs in a very detailed fashion. The energetic information may be in the form of too little or too much meridian electrical energy. This first step may give a clue as to the presence of degeneration or inflammation in the organ in question. One can further investigate the nature and extent of the dysfunction by measuring readings from different points along the same meridian. Although the Voll Machine is more time consuming to use than the AMI system, it is capable of eliciting a more detailed inventory of organ function.

The AMI Machine is perhaps better suited for screening larger populations because it is simpler and faster. It is an ideal noninvasive system that can be used to detect illness, either imminent or established, in the organs of the body. Alternatively, particular organs found to be in a state of energetic imbalance by the AMI Machine might be analyzed in greater detail by the EAV system. The sequential acupoint testing of various organ systems on the Voll Machine is a somewhat time-consuming procedure except to the most experienced of practitioners. The information gained, however, provides deeper insights into the energetic physiology of the human being.

The Voll Machine is capable of going beyond the diagnosis of energetic imbalance levels in particular systems. It is frequently capable of finding the actual *causes* of the energetic dysfunction, as well as potential cures for the disorders. The manner in which the Voll Machine is able to carry out this type of analysis is a function of biological resonance.

Resonance is a phenomenon which occurs throughout nature. At the level of the atom, we know that electrons whirl about the nucleus in certain energetically defined orbits. In order to move an electron from a lower to a higher orbit, a quantum of energy with very special frequency characteristics is required. An electron will only accept energy of the appropriate frequency to move from one energy level to another. If the electron falls from the higher to the lower orbit, it will radiate energy of that very same frequency. This required atomic frequency is referred to as the "resonant frequency." The phenomenon of resonance is the principle behind the imaging systems of MRI and EMR scanning as discussed in Chapter 3. Atoms and molecules have special resonant frequencies that will only be excited by energies of very precise vibratory characteristics. For instance, the singer who is able to shatter a wine glass by delivering a high amplitude note does so by singing in the precise resonant frequency of the glass.

Another definition of resonance has to do with the phenomenon of energy exchanged between tuned oscillators. Let us use as an example two perfectly tuned Stradivarius violins placed at opposite ends of a small room. If we pluck the E string of one violin, a careful observer will notice that the sister violin's E string will also begin to vibrate and "sing" in harmony. The reason that this occurs is because the E strings of the violins are carefully tuned and responsive to a particular frequency. The E strings can accept energy in the E frequency because that is their resonant frequency. The E strings of the violins are like the electrons of the atoms. They will vibrate at a new energy level only if they are exposed to energy of their resonant frequency.

In Chapter 2, we examined the practice of homeopathy from the energetic perspective of resonance. It was postulated that homeopathic medicines contained an energy essence of the plant or other substance from which they were prepared. The energy essence of the homeopathic medicine carries a type of subtle-energy signature of a particular frequency. It is the task of the skilled homeopathic practitioner to match the frequency of the homeopathic medicine with the energetic frequency needs of the ill patient. Illness, from a homeopathic and energetic point of view, is the energetic imbalance of the human organism as a whole. The vibrational mode of the physical body is a reflection of the dominant frequency at which it resonates. Although the energetic level of humans varies from moment to moment and day to day, the physical body tends to vibrate at a particular frequency. There are many factors that contribute to the total frequency expression of the physical (and etheric) body.

The human mind/body/spirit complex is the holistic expression and sum total gestalt of a wide spectrum of interactive energy systems. These energetic factors include the bioenergetic currents of cellular semiconduction, and also the subtle magnetic currents of primary meridian flow. The meridian currents are, in turn, an end expression of many higher frequency energetic influences.

The final energetic expression of illness at the physical level appears to be a function of two central factors. These key factors are *host resistance* and *noxious environmental influences*. Negative environmental factors may vary from viruses, bacteria, fungi, and protozoa to unseen radiation and toxic chemicals. The ill effects of radiation may be due to toxic doses of electromagnetic energies in a wide variety of frequencies (i.e. overdoses of x-rays, microwaves, UV light, and radar beams). Toxic chemicals can include known carcinogens, corrosive agents, and poisonous chemicals, as well as environmental substances which produce idiosyncratic sensitivity reactions within the bodies of certain individuals. This last category is the subject of intensive study by practitioners of clinical ecology.

Host resistance appears to play an even greater role in the causation of illness. A key factor affecting an individual's ability to defend self from attack by the aforementioned noxious agents is the general level of energy and vitality. Someone who is in a weakened, debilitated state from any number of causes will become ill more easily when exposed to negative environmental agents. The general vitality of an individual is an indirect reflection of the level of functioning of the immune system. The immune system is one of the most important factors in the human defense against illness. It is able to recognize molecular elements of self and to distinguish non-self foreign proteins from the body's own membranes. Through the recognition and removal of all substances that are non-self, the immune system surveys and destroys potentially threatening viruses, bacteria, fungi, and even cancer cells. If, however, the immune system is weakened, then the body as a whole becomes more susceptible to illness from exposure to any noxious stimulus. As the body becomes weakened by stress, depression, starvation, and chronic illness, the immune system is also impaired in its ability to function properly. When the body is in a healthy energetic vibrational mode, a small innoculum of virus is easily discharged from the body. In an individual who is energetically imbalanced and thus immunologically weakened, this same viral exposure may allow a serious systemic viral illness to occur. It is well known that emotional depression, physical stress, chemical toxicity, and nutritional deficiencies can adversely affect the body's immune defenses.

From an energetic standpoint, the human body, when weakened or shifted from equilibrium, oscillates at a different and less harmonious frequency than when healthy. This abnormal frequency reflects a general state of cellular energetic imbalance within the physical body. When a weakened individual is unable to shift his/her energetic mode to the needed frequency (which allows their immune system to properly defend the body), a certain amount of subtle energetic help may be needed. If this same individual is supplied with a dose of the needed energetic frequency, it allows the cellular bioenergetic systems to resonate in the proper vibrational mode, thereby throwing off the toxicities of the illness. This frequency-specific subtle-energy boost allows the physical body and associated bioenergy systems to return to a new level of homeostasis. Providing this needed subtle-energy boost through choosing the right homeopathic remedy is one of the key concepts of homeopathic practice.

Homeopathy has grown up around a system of empirical frequency matching based on the techniques discovered by Samuel Hahnemann. Hahnemann's system of homeopathic prescribing has been slowly refined over the years by various innovative homeopathic physicians. In the homeopathic approach the practitioner tries, through careful history taking, to match the total symptom complex of the sick patient with a remedy which induces these same symptoms in normal individuals. If the frequency match is correct and the needed energy is supplied to the patient by the remedy, a healing occurs. Frequently, the final resolution of illness is preceded by an exacerbation of symptoms known as a "healing crisis." This crisis is an indication of the physical body resonating at the needed energy frequency, and the keynote symptoms of toxicity release being transiently intensified. Only the exact frequency match between patient and remedy will cause a healing because, by the principle of resonance, biological systems will only accept certain resonant frequencies that allow the system to move toward a new level of energetic organization and function.

Throughout the history of homeopathy, the idea of frequency matching was unknown. As such, attempts to actually measure the energetic frequencies associated with illnesses and remedies were not considered by homeopaths. Instrumentation has now been devised which actually allows the measurement of such energetic parameters. Meridian-based technologies, including the Voll Machine, allow one to correlate remedy with illness though energetic frequency matching. This match is accomplished on the Voll Machine through utilization of the principle of resonance.

Attached to the Voll Machine is a small, circular, metallic platform (sometimes called a honeycomb) in which cylindrical holes have been drilled. Each hole can hold a small ampule of medication to be tested. This metallic table is attached to the Voll system via an electrical wire connection. EAV researchers have discovered that any substance placed upon the metallic table becomes part of the energetic circuit of the Voll Machine. When the EAV practitioner first touches the probe to the acupoints for energetic reading analysis, he or she does so with nothing on the metallic accessory table in order to examine baseline meridian conditions. Once the initial electrical readings have been taken, the absolute level of microvoltage on the meter tells the practitioner if the acupoint and associated meridian are electrically normal or in a state of energetic imbalance.

If the acupoint is found to be out of balance, the practitioner may then place various homeopathic remedies upon the electrical accessory table in order to observe the changes in the acupoint electrical readout. Any substance that is placed upon the metallic table becomes part of the energetic circuit. It is believed that certain aspects of the remedy's subtle energetic patterns are conducted over electrical wires, in a fashion similar to electricity. For most remedies placed in the energetic circuit, additional acupoint electrical readings will reveal no significant changes from the initial measurement. However, when a remedy is placed on the metallic table which matches the frequency of the energetic imbalance of the patient, a resonance effect occurs, and a significant change in the acupoint reading is observed.

Utilizing the Voll Machine, the patient is linked through his/her acupoint-meridian interface with the needed subtle energetic frequency. A resonance effect occurs between the patient and the circuitry in a fashion similar to that observed between Kirlian equipment and photographic subjects. In the case of the Voll Machine, individual frequencies are tested one at a time by placing a small portion of substance of a particular subtle energetic frequency into the circuit. In Kirlian photography, the energetic frequencies are artificially produced by an electrical frequency generator. In both cases, the patient is exposed to a particular energetic frequency. The only energetic frequency which has diagnostic significance is one which resonates with a relevant biological frequency of the organism being tested. Both systems measure variation in electrical outputs. They differ primarily in their methods of data collection. In the case of Kirlian photography, measurement involves capturing energetic patterns of electron streamer discharge on a piece of film. In the case of the Voll Machine, measurement is in the form of a voltmeter readout from an acupuncture point. Both systems employ the phenomenon of resonance to obtain meaningful biological information about the organism being studied.

It was mentioned earlier that the Voll Machine was capable of demonstrating the *causes* of illnesses. The way in which this is accomplished is through testing different types of homeopathic bionosodes on the Voll Machine platform. Homeopathic remedies can be prepared from any substance, be it plant, animal, or mineral. In the case of the bionosode, a small portion of tissue from a diseased organ is ground up and used to prepare a homeopathic remedy. Because there are no physical molecules left in the final homeopathic remedy, only the energetic essence of the tissue and local pathogens remain. The absence of physical pathogens such as bacteria and viruses in the homeopathic preparation means that the bionosode is incapable of directly transmitting illness to a patient receiving this remedy. (See Chapter 2 on the preparation of homeopathic remedies.) If the illness was caused by a particular bacterium or virus, then only its energetic signature remains in the bionosode.

When a particular bionosode induces a resonance reaction in the acupoint as measured by the Voll Machine, it may be inferred that the cause of the patient's illness has been uncovered. Various types of diseases originating from bacterial infections can be diagnosed utilizing the Voll method. Bionosodes can be prepared from cultures of individual types of bacteria. For example, a bionosode exists for the *Salmonella* bacterium. The way in which a homeopathic Voll practitioner might diagnose *Salmonella* food poisoning without obtaining blood tests or cultures is as follows:

The physician would test the acupoints along the meridians associated with the small and large intestine. If electrical imbalance was discovered, then the practitioner might move on to determine the chronicity of the illness. This is accomplished by trying to transiently correct the energetic dysfunction. The EAV practitioner uses the probe to electrically either charge or sedate the unbalanced acupoint and associated meridian. Acute energetic disturbances in meridian function are more easily affected by electrical stimulation than are imbalances of a chronic nature. (This is somewhat of an oversimplification.) Information gathered by this technique gives the practitioner an idea of the acute or chronic nature of the bowel disturbance reported by the patient.

Next, various bionosodes of suspected pathogens would be sequentially tested by placing them upon the metallic accessory table. EAV researchers have compiled tables of pathogens which list the most frequent causes of energetic imbalance in particular meridians. If indeed the pathogen is *Salmonella*, placing a bionosode prepared from the *Salmonella* bacterium on the metal accessory table would produce a significant resonance reaction in the meridian electrical readout when the probe is again touched to the imbalanced intestinal acupoint. This type of reaction would confirm the presence of pathological dysfunction within the large and small intestine, with the confirmed pathogen being the *Salmonella* bacterium.

If a significant reaction occurs, it is confirmed by examining the acupoint's reaction to particular homeopathic strengths of the bionosode in order to find the perfect amplitude of frequency match between patient and remedy. Having found the exact remedy strength, the bionosode could be given to the patient either as a pill, sublingual liquid, or intramuscular injection. The correct frequency match would be confirmed by the rapid resolution of the patient's symptoms upon taking the homeopathic remedy.

This technique of matching homeopathic remedies with patients via the Voll Machine is the subject of considerable controversy between classic homeopathic practitioners and New Age technology physicians. The classical homeopaths do not believe that this type of technology can replace the old method of matching key symptoms reported by patients with the remedies listed in their *Materia Medica* (as is part of their standard methodology). One of the differences in philosophy revolves around the aspects of acute and chronic homeopathic prescribing. In traditional homeopathy, acute homeopathic prescribing involves giving remedies for acute illnesses and injuries. Chronic or constitutional prescribing has to do with an examination of the entire life pattern of the individual since birth, including specific tendencies, likes, dislikes, and weaknesses. Thus, in constitutional prescribing, the entire life history of the patient, distilled and focused to accentuate specific keynote symptoms, is matched with an appropriate homeopathic remedy. Homeopaths distinguish unique remedy personality types as a reflection of this gestalt pattern of mental, emotional, and physical symptoms.

In reality, the Voll method deals with superficial levels of energetic stratification within the organism. That is, one is able to match homeopathic remedies with an individual's needs based upon his/her most acute symptoms of distress. What has been discovered by a number of Voll practitioners is that sometimes certain remedies will be associated with an acupoint resonance reaction, and at other times the same remedy will not produce this effect. The reasons for this phenomenon may have to do with a type of "onion" or "artichoke" effect.

In treating a patient with an EAV-determined remedy, certain of the patient's acute symptoms will be immediately relieved. Following this resolution, patients may report that older symptoms which seemed to have been previously resolved have returned. Retesting of the patient on the Voll Machine will reveal resonance reactions with remedies that may have previously shown no effect. What is happening is that the EAV practitioner's testing is able to successively peel away layers of the onion. Human beings tend to accumulate small traumas and physiologic insults to their bodies over the course of a lifetime. If these progressive insults are not fully resolved at the time of the initial trauma, they are incorporated into the energetic structure of the individual. Stratification of levels of injury are gradually created by the organism. The energetic depth at which a layering of reactive armor is discovered reflects the timing of the original insult in the life history of the individual. When the Voll Machine uncovers a remedy to neutralize acute symptoms, it peels away the most superficial layer of the onion or artichoke. As the acute symptoms resolve, a slightly older level of energy imbalance resurfaces and brings with it older symptoms of dysfunction. As the Voll practitioner is able to peel away successive layers of disturbance in the individual with repeated homeopathic treatments, he or she is able to get closer to the inner heart and deepest origins of energetic dysfunction within the individual (the so-called heart of the artichoke.)

This therapeutic approach of peeling away the layers of imbalance through successive homeopathic remedies can be accomplished with either classical homeopathic prescribing or EAV testing. Many times the more intuitive classical homeopaths are able to see around superficial symptoms and explore more deeply into the constitutional nature of the individual. In so doing, they are able to go beyond the Voll Machine to get to the deeper origins of energetic imbalance within the individual.

EAV & Environmental Illnesses: A New Look at Clinical Ecology

The Voll device has great value in matching homeopathic remedies to patients, but its value goes beyond this particular facet of application. The meridian-based technologies are able to reveal much about the energetic and physiologic status of the individual from many different perspectives. These systems employ the acupoint resonance effect to examine a wide variety of energetic disturbances in the individual. One area of increasing interest has been the application of Voll techniques to study the ill effects of particular environmental agents. Studies in this direction are part of the growing field of clinical ecology.[5]

Pioneering workers in this developing field have done much research to show that common environmental substances may produce unseen ill effects in humans. If asked about environmental agents which adversely affect human health, most individuals tend to think about toxic waste and industrial chemicals. More recently, it has been shown that the list of substances affecting us includes many more items than those which are by-products of industrial manufacturing. As civilization has become widely industrialized and technologically advanced, humans have come to accept life in a chemical-filled environment. Most research on the adverse effects of hazardous substances in our environment has focused on the carcinogenic influences of long-term chemical exposure. Standardized methods involve giving huge doses of suspected chemicals to laboratory animals over short periods of time in hopes of simulating the biological effects of long-term microexposure. Other tests involve measuring the mutagenicity of similarly suspected chemicals in their ability to cause chromosomal alterations

in bacteria. The relevance of extrapolating this type of data to human beings has been brought into question by a number of different groups.

One problem with studying the adverse physiologic effects of chemicals is the traditional scientist's inability to measure subtle changes in
human beings. Certain chemicals may induce subtle abnormalities in
behavior and mental alertness. Some agents may induce headaches, body
aches, and other nonspecific symptoms which cannot be as measurably
quantified as the tendency toward cancer cell production.

Research by workers in the field of clinical ecology has demonstrated
that many people are adversely affected by exposure to unnoticed factors
in the home and work environment, such as synthetic plastics and natural
gas. Of more recent interest have been the ill effects produced by certain
substances contained in foods. Food dyes, additives, and other controversial agents have received much attention in the news media. It is becoming increasingly evident that there are now many synthetic and naturally
occurring agents in the foods we eat which cause a variety of abnormal
physiological effects. Many of these adverse effects are subtle, and frequently ignored by doctors because of their inexperience in this field.

In regards to food allergies, most physicians only recognize physiologic
mechanisms involving the classical IgE-mediated pathways of the immune
system. IgE (immunoglobulin E) is a special type of antibody which causes
the release of histamine and other allergic mediators from tissue mast cells
when stimulated by specific evocative antigens. The symptoms most commonly produced by IgE-mediated food allergies are the familiar symptoms
of wheezing, itching, skin rashes, etc. These symptoms are among the
common responses evoked by histamine and other immunologic mediators of allergy.

The problem of abnormal physiological reactions to agents in food is
of greater importance than is currently recognized by the medical establishment. One of the reasons for doctors' inattention to this problem is their
lack of understanding. Most physicians cannot comprehend, and thus do
not believe, that substances can evoke adverse physical reactions in the
body without involving the familiar IgE pathways of the immune system.
The wide spectrum of symptoms caused by food allergies is due to classical
allergic phenomena as well as sensitivity reactions mediated by non-IgE
immunologic and other subtle physiologic pathways. One tool which has
been sensitive enough to evoke diagnostic information about these sensitivity reactions has been the Voll Machine.

One of the pioneers in the field of linking EAV technology to clinical ecology is Dr. Abram Ber[6] of Phoenix, Arizona. Working with the Voll Machine, Ber has been able to apply the discoveries of other researchers in the clinical ecology field toward rapid diagnosis and treatment of food allergies. One of the primary sources for Dr. Ber's diagnostic application is the research of Dr. Robert Gardner[7] of Brigham Young University in Utah. Dr. Gardner discovered that many allergies were caused by sensitivities to certain aromatic chemical compounds found naturally in all plant foods and pollens. These plant-associated compounds, which contain aromatic or phenolic groups derived from the benzene ring, were later discovered by other researchers to occur in all foods.

It has been suggested that these compounds are not allergic antigens, but that they act as "haptens." A hapten binds to other naturally occurring substances in the body, thereby changing its appearance to the immune system. The old familiar protein or membrane structure, now combined with the new phenolic hapten, is no longer recognized as a part of self, and thus induces adverse immunologic reactions. A common example of this type of reaction is penicillin-induced hemolytic anemia. In certain sensitive individuals, penicillin, acting as a hapten, binds to the red blood cell membrane and changes its appearance to the immune system so that it is no longer recognized as a familiar component of self. The penicillin/red cell complex induces an antibody response which ultimately results in destruction of the red blood cells via a rupturing of their external membranes by immune attack.

Immunologic changes which occur as a result of exposure to phenolic compounds include reductions in the number of T-cells and T-suppressor cells (a subgroup of T-cells).[8] This reduction in T-cell number is reflected in an altered T to B cell ratio. T-cells are special lymphocytes which attack and remove cancer cells, viruses, and fungi. A particular type of T-cell known as the T-suppressor cell works to keep the immune system from attacking the body itself. B-cells are another type of lymphocyte which produces antibodies. There is usually a particular ratio of T to B cells that reflects a normal proportion of immune components. Immunocompetence is partly a reflection of this special balance in types of lymphocytes. Certain phenolic compounds have been associated with changes in this T to B-cell ratio. Similar immunologic alterations in T and B-cell ratios have been seen in the AIDS syndrome and other immune deficiency syndromes. Reduction in T-suppressor cells has been noted to occur in certain autoimmune diseases. This is not to imply that phenolics are the cause of these diseases, but that the types of alterations in immune function seen in response to phenolic exposure have been associated with significant illness.

Other physiologic changes produced by phenolic compounds include cardiac stimulation and rapid heart rate. This appears to be due to the phenolic compounds' effect on increasing the body's responsiveness to catecholamines (a class of adrenergic neurotransmitters which includes adrenaline and dopamine). Additional changes induced by phenolic compounds include depressed serotonin levels, elevated histamine and prostaglandins, and abnormal immune complex formation. From a clinical perspective, research on food-borne phenolics has demonstrated their ability to induce behavioral disturbances in children, including the hyperkinetic syndrome.[9]

The classical, clinical ecology method of testing for sensitivity to phenolic compounds involves a technique known as sublingual neutralization. In this technique, several drops of a one-percent solution of the suspected phenolic compound are placed under the tongue of the patient. Following the phenolic challenge, various parameters of physiologic and mental function are tested. A positive response is felt to consist of a change of pulse or blood pressure, acute symptom onset, or changes in the mental status of the patient.

Once a reactive phenolic substance is discovered, the compound is presented to the patient in a variety of dilute solutions to find the concentration which will neutralize the induced symptoms. Progressively more dilute solutions are tested until a reversal of symptoms occurs at what is referred to as the "neutralizing dilution." The patient is given a bottle of the phenolic compound, prepared in the neutralizing dilution, and is instructed to place two drops under the tongue three times a day. Retesting is then necessary in the same manner, as the initial potency loses its effectiveness over time. Similar tests at a later date show that the patient needs a change in the concentration of the phenolic compound to achieve the same beneficial effect. The patient is switched to the new neutralizing dilution of phenolic and the process is repeated again and again over the course of many months. There are obvious similarities to classical allergy desensitization, except that the testing methods are different and the patient is given sublingual drops instead of shots.

The inital testing procedure can be quite time consuming and may involve many hours and days to test a large panel of suspected phenolic com-

pounds. Because of this, Dr. Ber sought to improve the efficiency of diagnosis by utilizing the Voll Machine in testing for phenolic sensitivity. The
procedure involved is quite unique in that it allows testing of a variety of
compounds at various dilutions in a matter of 20 to 30 minutes.

The phenolic compounds are prepared in a series of dilutions which
follow a type of homeopathic rationale. The first dilution consists of a 1:5
ratio made from one part of the original phenolic and four parts of distilled
water. The second tincture (referred to dilution number two) is a 1:5 dilution made from the first tincture. The third dilution is prepared by a 1:5 dilution of the second tincture, and so on. This process continues up to the fortieth tincture at which point the dilutions become 1:10 (usually up to the
sixtieth). As the dilutions go up in number, there is progressively less and
less physical substance of the phenolics actually present. A fortieth dilution should contain 5^{-40} (or 1.1×10^{-28}) times the number of phenolic molecules which were present in the original phenolic solution. This is considerably less than Avogadro's number (6.02×10^{-23}, the number of molecules in a mole or gram molecular weight of a chemical), hence there is less
than a single molecule in the fortieth dilution. The phenolic dilutions prepared by Ber are actually homeopathic remedies in that the majority contain not so much the physical material but the energetic signature of the
phenolic compound.

Dr. Ber has created a special EAV testing setup which consists of an
open wooden stand with multiple metal-lined shelves. The metal base of
each shelf has an electrical connector which allows one to plug in a wire
from the Voll Machine. The metal shelf operates in a fashion similar to the
EAV metallic accessory table. Thus, multiple remedies placed on a metallic
shelf can be tested simultaneously. Groups of remedies of the same levels
of dilution are arranged on their own special metallic shelf units. By plug-
ging the wire from the Voll Machine into the metal bases of different shelves
in a sequential fashion, whole groups of remedies can be tested simultaneously for acupoint resonance reactivity. If a shelf of compounds tests positive via an acupoint resonance reaction with the patient, a process of progressive elimination is employed. This consists of individually testing each
substance on the reactive shelf until the guilty substance is identified. Once
the reactive substance is discovered, progressive retesting with various
dilutions of the substance is done via acupoint resonance until the exact
neutralizing dilution is pinpointed.

The types of substances which make up Ber's first group of phenolic compounds include gallic acid (which is found in up to 70 percent of foods), apiol, cinnamic acid, coumadin, indole, phenylalanine, ascorbic acid, and others. The second group includes many neurotransmitters, or precursors to their synthesis, such as choline, dopamine, histamine, serotonin, tyramine, norepinephrine, and a number of others. Regarding reactivity to the second group of phenolics, it is unclear whether patients are sensitive to these agents in ingested foods or whether the Voll Machine is picking up an internal difficulty with these particular transmitter systems. The second hypothesis is probably the more likely, but the symptoms associated with reactivity to these phenolic substances still resolve with sublingual use of neutralizing dilutions.

The remarkable thing that Ber has discovered in using the Voll Machine is that a variety of syndromes found to be untreatable by conventional drug therapies appear to be caused by sensitivity reactions to common phenolic compounds. Confirmation of this hypothesis is suggested by relief of these symptoms following the use of sublingual doses of neutralizing dilutions of the suspected offending phenolic. For instance, reactivity to gallic acid, perhaps one of the greatest offenders, has been linked to lower back pain, sciatica, chronic severe chest wall pain, musculoskeletal aches, and chronic fatigue. As mentioned before, gallic acid is found in nearly *70 percent of all foods.* It has also been linked with hyperactivity and learning disabilities in children, and is found to exist in many food-coloring agents. Removal of food dyes and additives in the diet of such afflicted children, as in the Feingold Diet, may relieve hyperactivity by the avoidance of gallic acid. Ber has found sublingual neutralization to be as effective in decreasing hyperactivity as the avoidance diet, and it is easier for the children to follow.

When the offending phenolic compound is isolated and the proper neutralizing dilution discovered, relief of symptoms following sublingual administration may result in dramatic relief of symptoms. Ber discovered that if patients were experiencing pain-related symptoms at the time of EAV testing, sublingual presentation with the neutralizing dilution frequently caused significant symptom improvement and relief within approximately ten minutes.

Another common phenolic-related problem is found with reactivity to coumarin, a compound found in at least 30 foods—especially wheat, cheeses, beef, and eggs. Ber discovered that the majority of asthmatics tested have coumarin sensitivity. Neutralization of this particular phenolic frequently results in a significant improvement in the patient's asthmatic reactions, as evidenced by a reduction in the need for bronchodilator medications. Coumarin has also been found to contribute to arthritic symptoms, cervical and lower back pain, and digestive disturbances, particularly bloating. Abdominal distention due to coumarin sensitivity can be so severe that patients may be unable to fit comfortably in their clothing within minutes of eating a coumarin-containing meal. (Bloating after meals is a frequent complaint made by patients to their doctors. Physicians currently have little to offer other than gas-absorbing agents, such as simethicone, which are often ineffective in relieving the patient's symptoms. The frequency of the symptom of bloating may suggest how common sensitivity to coumarin may be in the general population.)

Another phenolic substance that Ber has found to be problematic is the amino acid, phenylalanine. Ber feels that although most patients do not have the classical intolerance for this amino acid seen in the newborn disorder of PKU (phenylketonuria—a genetic inability to handle phenylalanine), many people may have a subclinical form of intolerance which is unrecognized. Ber has found phenylalanine sensitivity to be associated with hypertension, headaches, respiratory diseases, and collagen disorders. Most interestingly, he has noted significant lowering of blood pressure in hypertensives with phenylalanine sensitivity when they are presented with neutralizing dilutions of the amino acid.

This list of reactive substances goes on and on. The variety of common, often nonspecific, complaints such as headache, back and neck pains, and chronic fatigue, make one realize how helpless conventional physicians may find themselves when conventional drug therapies do little to relieve these problems. Many of Dr. Ber's patients have found significant relief in his neutralizing drops when other doctors failed to offer even palliative drug effects. The widespread nature of these substances in the food we eat, and the potential unseen ways we are affected, gives greater impetus for the use of energy-sensitive devices such as the Voll Machine, which offer unique diagnostic capabilities.

The meridian-based technologies, though currently unaccepted by the mainstream medical establishment, are slowly beginning to find their way into many physicians' and dentists' offices. In recent years, the Food and Drug Administration authorized at least 150 experimental research licenses to orthodox medical practitioners who wished to explore the use of the Voll Machine and EAV technologies in diagnosis and therapy. This is a sign that there is slow evolutionary change occuring within the medical field, and that devices like the Voll Machine may eventually find their way into widespread use by health care professionals within the next ten to fifteen years.

From EAV to Radionics:
A Pure Frequency Model of Diagnosis & Therapy

There are a number of meridian/acupoint-based electronic systems which go beyond the Voll Machine in their sophistication. One particular system, known as the Mora device, works on the same principle as EAV but uses a different energetic linkup with the substances being tested for acupoint resonance effects. The Mora system employs special holders for remedies which are similar to the metallic shelves used by Dr. Ber to simultaneously test multiple remedies. Instead of a wire hookup between remedy and instrument, the vibrational characteristics of the remedy are electronically broadcast (via radio waves) across the room to the Mora device, where the energy enters the test circuitry. With the remedy in semi-distant energetic connection, the patient may be tested for meridian resonance phenomena via a handheld acupoint probe. A number of sophisticated acupoint treatment modes are also possible with this device, but they are beyond the scope of this text. Suffice it to say that it is possible to actually inject special frequencies of subtle energy directly into the body's meridians via special circuitry in the Mora device.

Another meridian-based instrument which goes beyond even the Mora device is the Acupath instrument. The Acupath has done away entirely with the need for the physical presence of the remedies. Inside the computerized memory programmed into the Acupath, there is an energy reference bank containing the magnetically coded vibrational signatures of hundreds of homeopathic remedies. The computer automatically carries out searches for acupoint resonance reactions among its many remedies in order to find those remedies that match the patient's unbalanced energetic system. Like the aforementioned EAV systems, the practitioner still needs to use the handheld diagnostic probe to contact the proper acupoints.

The Mora and Acupath systems demonstrate the principles of energy frequency matching between patient and remedy to a high degree. The energy frequencies of the remedies can actually be dealt with separately from the remedies themselves in such systems as the Acupath. These devices are not the first to deal with diagnosis and treatment of human illness from an energetic frequency perspective. They are actually distant cousins of a group of diagnostic systems known collectively as radionic devices.

Radionic systems have been under development and application in the United States and Europe for many decades. Various devices, often referred to as "radionic black boxes," have been used by physicians and practitioners of alternative medicine since the early 1900s. A number of early pioneers in this field, including Albert Abrams,[10] Ruth Drown, George de la Warr,[11,12] and Malcolm Rae,[13] developed and refined the basics of radionic practice and theory from its earliest beginnings.

Radionic systems are perhaps more appropriately classified as "psychotronic technologies." Unlike electronically-based systems such as the Voll Machine, radionic systems rarely make use of electricity, although many contain electrical circuitry and magnetic elements. More importantly, the successful use of radionic devices depends upon the psychic abilities of the radionic practitioner. The feedback provided by these systems is usually via an external mechanoelectrical amplifier of internal physiologic change. The physiologic changes measured by the radionic devices correlate with subtle psychoenergetic alterations that occur within the nervous system of the system operator. Radionic systems require a unique energetic sensitivity which has been referred to as "radiesthesia." Radiesthesia may be defined as a psychic sensitivity to subtle radiation of varying vibrational frequencies.

Many individuals possess this psychic ability to greater or lesser degrees. For instance, the SRI studies on remote viewing found that everyone tested had that ability in variable levels of performance.[14] Some studies of psi have found that everyone has psychic abilities to one degree or another, but that some people may actually repress this information because of incompatible belief systems. For instance, certain subjects who have been tested for ESP (extra-sensory perception) actually have statistically significant scores of psychic hits vs. misses, but in a negative direction. They scored fewer hits than should occur by random chance alone. ESP occurs at an unconscious level in all of us. Radionic systems capitalize on pathways of unconscious psychic expression within the nervous system to provide conscious data based upon extrasensory information gathering. One might say that they are ESP amplifiers. Therefore, the successful performance of radionic systems is dependent upon the consciousness of the device's operator.

The simpler prototype radionic devices usually consist of a black box with a number of tunable dials on the front, each numerically calibrated. The dials are usually attached to variable resistors or potentiometers inside the box which are also connected by wires to a circular metallic well. Within this well is placed a biological (or other) specimen from the patient— a spot of blood or a lock of hair—attached to a piece of paper labelled with his/her name. This specimen of blood or hair is referred to as the "witness."

Attached to the radionic black box is an insulated wire leading to a flat rubber surface which forms the interface between the operator and the device. While mentally tuning in to the patient in question, the radionic operator lightly strokes a finger across the rubber pad. As the practitioner does this, he or she slowly turns one of the dials on the front. The operator will register a positive response when he/she feels a sticking sensation in a finger as he/she strokes the pad. This might be viewed as a type of sympathetic resonance reaction. The resonance occurs between the energetic frequency of the patient and the subtle-energy system of the radionic operator as reflected by changes in the operator's nervous system. The dial is left tuned to the setting which induced the resonance response. The operator then moves on to a second dial, repeating the same procedure with the finger stroking until he/she has tuned all of the dials to their appropriate test settings. Each dial represents a digit in sequence which, when combined, produces a single multidigit number referred to as a "rate." The rate reflects the energetic frequency characteristics of the patient being remotely tested by the radionic device.

Based on a comparison of the patient's rate with a type of "rate reference table," the radionic practitioner is able to make a presumptive diagnosis of the patient's pathologic condition. Comparison of patient rates with the standard rate reference tables allows matching of the patient's frequency with known vibrational frequencies associated with particular illnesses. This is similar, in a way, to what happens with frequency matching in homeopathy. In homeopathy, illness frequencies are symbolically represented by individual homeopathic remedies rather than numerical rates which describe the same energy characteristics. Radionics looks toward directly measuring the patient's primary energetic frequency disturbance rather than depending upon empirical frequency matching of remedy to symptom complex.

To an orthodox physician, this description sounds very much like nonsense. Nevertheless, radionic systems have demonstrated themselves to be effective diagnostic and therapeutic tools in spite of a lack of understanding by scientific critics. Radionic devices employ two primary principles in gathering diagnostic patient information. These are the Principle of Biological Resonance and the Holographic Principle. We may come to better understand how these principles are applied in radionic systems by examining in greater detail the phenomena involved in the operation of the basic radionic device.

The key ingredient in the use of the simple radionic device is the witness. The witness is usually a biological specimen obtained from the patient in question. Frequently, the witness is a spot of the patient's blood on a piece of filter paper, or a lock of his/her hair. The blood spot contains cellular and biochemical elements removed from the body of the individual being tested. According to the holographic principle, each piece taken from the hologram contains the information of the whole. *From a vibrational and energetic standpoint, this means that a small portion removed from the whole, i.e. a drop of blood removed from the body, reflects the total energetic structure of the entire organism.* The blood cells do not have to be living to have this effect. The organic material in the blood (or hair) specimen represents an energetic sampling of the patient's dynamic frequency spectrum.

The blood spot represents more of a dynamically changing hologram than a frozen snapshot in time. Rather than capturing the energetic status of the patient at the time of venipuncture only, the blood spot witness remains in a dynamic resonant equilibrium with its source. The blood spot continues to reflect the patient's energy status over time because of energetic resonance with the person from which it came. This means that different blood spots on different days would not be needed to update diagnostic impressions of a patient's changing physiological status. This is in contradistinction to chemical testing of blood, which would require daily serial blood specimens for plotting of sequential biochemical trends.

The blood spot remains in dynamic energetic equilibrium with its source regardless of its distance from the patient. The energetic characteristics reflected in the witness will vary from moment to moment according to the energetic behavior of the patient. There is one exception to this rule which was empirically discovered by radionic practitioners. The radionic connection between patient and blood spot is rendered useless if the patient has received multiple transfusions after the blood spot was taken. Multiple frequencies injected into the patient by the transfusions appear to interfere with the resonant connection with the old blood spot. For this reason it is sometimes better to work with a lock of the patient's hair as the witness, because it continues to be a valid energetic link throughout the lifetime of the patient (regardless of transfusions).[15]

In the radionic device, the biological specimen to be used as a witness (such as the blood spot) is placed in a special metallic cylindrical well. The subtle energies of the blood specimen pass through the electrical circuitry of the radionic device via a wire beneath the witness housing. The ability of these subtle energies to flow through electrical wiring has already been demonstrated by the meridian-based technologies of the EAV systems and others which employ this phenomenon in energetic diagnosis. From the witness well to the wires, subtle energy flows into special variable potentiometers that have their dial adjustments on the front of the radionic device. By turning the dials, the resistance to subtle current flow through the potentiometer is variably impeded. From the potentiometers, the subtle currents flow to the rubber pad which is in finger contact with the radionic operator. The operator's finger strokes the rubber pad while simultaneously rotating a particular dial. When the radionic practitioner detects a sticking sensation as his/her finger lightly strokes the pad, a positive reaction is indicated and the dial is assumed to be set at the appropriate setting. The dial settings indicate the resistance level of the potentiometers which are, in turn, a reflection of the subtle energetic frequency characteristics of the patient. Each potentiometer varies progressively higher ranges of energy resistance. By repeating the process of tuning each dial in successive order, the operator arrives at a multidigit number which represents the radionic rate or frequency essence of the patient to which he/she has attuned. By comparing the rate that he/she has derived with known radionic rates of various diseases, the radionic analyst is able to diagnose the patient's illness.

Mechanisms of Action in Radionics & Radiesthesia: A Further Look into the Chakra-Nervous System Link

The consciousness of the operator plays an integral part in obtaining information from the radionic device. It is through the unconscious channels of the operator's mind that attunement is achieved with the subtle energies of the patient. The psychoenergetic link between radionic practitioner and patient is made possible by the vibrational intermediary of the witness. The radionic witness provides a subtle-energy reference which allows the higher consciousness of the radionic operator to tune in to the patient at a distance.

This psychic process of tuning in to patients occurs at the level of our higher frequency vehicles of expression. In most individuals, this energetic linkup takes place at an unconscious level. The unconscious mind acts as a passageway through which higher frequency levels of consciousness may interact with the physical body. Higher psychic impressions are translated into various forms of information expression through the various pathways of the body's neurological circuitry. If the psychic information reaches conscious awareness, it does so through the expressive mechanism of the cerebral cortex. Unconscious intuitive information may filter through the right cerebral hemisphere and then be transferred to the left hemisphere where it is analyzed and then expressed verbally. While psychic information may not always reach conscious awareness, it is still processed by the nervous system and expressed through unconscious pathways of neurological and motor activity. Radionic systems capitalize on the unconscious psycho-energetic link between the higher mind and the autonomic nervous system. Increased activity in the sympathetic division of the autonomic nervous system may reflect unconscious psychic inputs from higher frequency levels of mind.

Various studies by parapsychologists provide evidence for the common occurrence of unconscious psychic perception. Although tests to score conscious ESP may prove insignificant, simultaneous measurements of autonomic activity in telepathic receivers will significantly correlate with unconscious psi perception. Experiments by Douglas Dean at the Newark College of Engineering have revealed information about the unconscious autonomic psi link.[16] Dean measured variations in finger blood flow of telepathic receivers by plethysmography in order to obtain autonomic parameters of psychic functioning. (It is well known that sympathetic nerve activity affects blood flow through tiny arteries in the skin. The sympathetic nervous system is a portion of the autonomic nervous system.) During his study on telepathy, Dean instructed telepathic senders to concentrate on the psychic transmission of various names to telepathic receivers some distance away in the same building. Telepathic senders were given a list of target names consisting of individuals who were emotionally close to the receivers, as well as a list of dummy names chosen at random from the phone book. The senders were told to concentrate on transmitting one name at a time to the receivers at predetermined intervals. During those intervals, phethysmograph readings of telepathic receivers were studied for changes in sympathetic activity and arterial blood flow.

Although conscious awareness of telepathically transmitted names was nonexistent, there were definite and statistically significant changes in finger blood flow during periods when the names of emotionally close individual were transmitted. Significant changes in arterial blood flow through the fingers of ESP percipients reflected increased sympathetic nervous system activity at times of heightened emotional telepathic content. The increase in sympathetic activity caused constriction of blood vessels and thus a decrease in finger blood flow. *Dean's landmark experiment proved that telepathy takes place at an unconscious level. Additionally, he demonstrated that increases in sympathetic nervous system activity mirrored unconscious telepathic reception by the brain.*

Another important reflection of autonomic hyperactivity in response to psychic perception is the level of sympathetic nerve stimulation of sweat glands in the skin. A state of sympathetic hyperactivity is frequently accompanied by cool moist palms and sweaty fingers. The coolness of the skin is due to constricted superficial blood vessels. Increased activity of sympathetic nerves innervating the skin causes the skin to become moist because of autonomic stimulation of sweat glands. Radionic devices capitalize upon increased fingertip moisture as a reflection of autonomic nervous activity.

Most radionic devices utilize a special rubber membrane for feedback on the correctness of the radionic dial setting. The correct setting is signalled by a burst of increased sympathetic nervous activity when a psychic resonance reaction occurs. The feedback to the operator that this has occurred is a sticking sensation as he/she strokes a finger across the rubber membrane feedback system. The rubber membrane acts as a translational device which measures activity of fingertip sweat glands as an autonomic indicator of higher psychoenergetic inputs into the central nervous system. The rubber pad has an energy connection to the vibrational witness (i.e. blood spot) via the wires and potentiometers within the radionic device.

While the radionic operator is tuning the potentiometer dial, he/she is attempting to mentally attune his/her consciousness to the patient through the energetic link of the witness. The witness provides an energetic waveguide which allows the operator to tune in to the vibrational frequency of the patient. As he/she turns the dials of the potentiometer, the

higher mind of the radionic operator looks for a match between the energetic frequency of the patient and the frequency setting of the radionic device.
The subtle energies of the vibrational witness are variably impeded by the
resistance setting of the potentiometer. When the operator feels a resonance reaction, it is because the dial setting of the potentiometer has allowed
a maximum of frequency-specific subtle energy to move through the circuit. This energy maxima is intuitively sensed by the radionic operator as
a positive sticking reaction as he/she moves a finger across the rubber pad.
The primary psychic sensing takes place at a higher psychoenergetic level.
The increased autonomic nervous system activity of the radionic operator
is the signal that the dial setting permitting a subtle energy maxima has
been reached.

The higher mind of the radionic practitioner plays a uniquely integral
role in psychic information gathering. This is reflected by the variability of
specimens that may be used as vibrational witnesses. Although most practitioners utilize some type of biological specimen from the patient, such as
a lock of hair or a spot of blood, some radionic practitioners are able to tune
into the energies of the patient with a witness consisting only of a photograph or a piece of paper bearing the handwritten signature of the test patient. The holographic theory of "every piece containing the whole" may
only partially explain how the patient's hair or blood sample may carry information. The witness is of the same energetic frequency as the patient
from which it is derived. There is a type of energetic resonance between
the patient and witness. Photographs of patients may actually capture an
element of their vibrational essence, as evidenced by radionic practitioners'
abilities to use them as witnesses. Instead of tuning into the small representative hologram of the patient encoded within the blood or hair specimen,
it is possible that the consciousness of the radionic practitioner is able to
tune into the cosmic hologram in order to obtain psychic information
about a patient at a distance.

The process of radionic attunement may be similar to the mechanisms
underlying remote viewing, as described in Chapter 1. In remote viewing
studies, a human experimenter is sent to visit a randomly chosen geographical target site which the subject attempts to describe in detail. The
distant but familiar experimenter provides a focal point for attuning the
consciousness of the remote viewing subject to the target site selected. The
experimenter provides a type of directional psychic compass that allows
the subject to tune into the relevant portion on the vast map of the cosmic

hologram. Similarly, in radionics, the witness may provide a different type of directional psychic compass that serves as a focal point for the radionic operator's higher mind. This compass guides the operator in tuning into the relevant portion of the cosmic hologram by allowing it to hone in on the patient's unique frequency characteristics.

Another useful analogy is the concept of a psychic bloodhound. When trackers are attempting to find someone lost or missing, they will often use bloodhounds. The bloodhound will be given an article of clothing, such as a shoe, belonging to the missing person, to smell in order that it may fine-tune its olfactory senses to the scent of that person. By following the scent, the dog is able to sniff out where the missing person has been and ultimately discover his/her whereabouts. In radionics, the witness waveguide acts in a similar fashion to give the vibrational scent of the patient to the higher senses of the radionic operator. Unlike the bloodhound who must physically track the individual, the psychic capabilities of the radionic operator allow him/her to tune into the patient at any distance and be in direct vibrational attunement

While the radionic operator may not be able to consciously perceive energetic data about the patient he/she is attempting to tune into, the operator's multidimensional higher mind can. Human beings constantly receive higher frequency energetic inputs through their chakra-nadi systems. In most individuals, this perception takes place at levels outside of their conscious levels of awareness. Because the chakras possess higher frequency perceptual qualities and are intimately interconnected with the physical nervous system, pathways are provided by which the activity of the autonomic nervous system may be modulated by subtle energetic inputs. Radionic systems, such as the basic unit previously mentioned, attempt to translate the normally unconscious data of higher psychic information into consciously utilizable diagnostic data. A variety of radionic instruments have been devised which allow the practitioner to diagnose a wide range of energetic and physiologic disorders.

The radionic system is a passive device. It is entirely dependent upon the subtle energetic perceptual system of the radionic operator to provide the necessary ingredients for its successful operation. *The ability to accurately diagnose energetic dysfunction at various frequency levels is a reflection of the energetic sensitivity of the chakra perceptual systems of each individual radionic practitioner.* Therefore, the radionic systems only provide consistently accurate diagnoses if the operator has achieved some functional level of awakening and proper functioning of the major chakras. This is indeed one type of diagnostic instrument that is entirely dependent upon the experimenter effect. Therefore, the radionic devices may provide slightly different levels of information to practitioners with varying levels of experience.

Diagram 23.

THE HUMAN MULTIDIMENSIONAL ENERGY SYSTEM

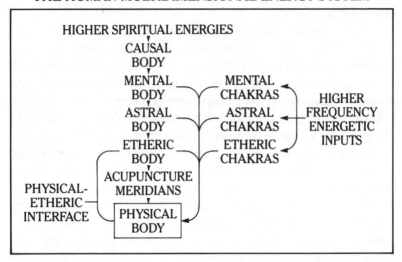

Radionic systems capitalize on the energetic links between our subtle energetic anatomy and our physical nervous system. It is known that the subtle threads of the nadi system, intimately intertwined with the physical nerves of the body, relay magnetic currents from the chakras at various energetic levels. In many radionic devices, the subtle energetic currents that affect the central nervous system are translated into conscious awareness via external indicators of increased sympathetic activity. The subtle increase in superficial moisture of the finger, due to increased sympathetic tone, causes the sticking sensation on the rubber pad which the radionic operator consciously interprets as a positive response. The sticking sensation is an external indicator of internal sympathetic activity.

As we have seen from the experiments of Dr. Dean, unconscious fluctuations in sympathetic outflow from the central nervous system may accurately reflect changes in subtle energetic input to the brain. Multiple frequencies of subtle current flow are taken into the body through various psychoenergetic channels including the chakra-nadi system (see Diagram

23). Finger stroking across the radionic rubber pad allows the conscious mind to use sympathetic nerve activity as a means of psychic feedback in tuning the radionic dials to the appropriate settings. There are alternative and equally interesting explanations for the mechanism behind the finger "stick" phenomenon, such as Tiller's model of acoustic resonance.[17] The actual mechanism is perhaps less important than the fact that the finger "stick" response does relay relevant diagnostic data to the consciousness of the radionic practioner.

The radionic dial settings connected to internal potentiometers act as a kind of bookeeping instrument, keeping quantitative records of the psychic data. Three- and four-digit frequency numbers, or rates, are psychically analyzed one digit at a time. The rates represent energetic frequencies at which the patient is resonating in health or illness. The rates describe not only the energetic condition of the patient but also the frequency of energy needed to shift the body back to a state of energetic equilibrium and homeostasis. *The rates represent relative frequency disturbances and not absolute numerical descriptors.* Radionic rates may be different for the same patient on different radionic devices. The radionic rate for pneumonia may be different from one device to another. But for a single type of radionic device the rate for pneumonia will always be the same. Tables of reference rates for health and illness have been generated and standardized for each unique radionic diagnostic tool.

The numerical rates are formed by composite numbers taken from the potentiometer dial settings, which are tuned to particular diagnostic values on the radionic device. In other words, one dial is set in increments of ten, another in increments of one hundred, etc. As we mentioned earlier, some researchers feel that the tunable resistance of the potentiometers affects the flow of subtle energetic currents passing through the circuitry to the rubber pad. Certain resistance settings allow optimal flow of particular frequencies of subtle energetic current.

While mentally tuning in to the patient, the radionic practitioner turns a single potentiometer dial and strokes a finger across the rubber membrane. One might compare this process to a safecracker listening for the tumblers of the vault mechanism to fall into place as the dial of the safe is gently turned. When the optimal resistance setting for the subtle current flow is achieved, a type of mental resonance reaction occurs. The radionic practitioner receives a conscious affirmative response to the dial setting through perception of the finger "stick" sensation. Utilizing this same process, he/she goes back again and tunes the second, third, and/or fourth potentiometer dial until each digit of the three- or four-digit frequency rate has been ascertained. Similarly our safecracker, after hearing the first tumbler fall into place, continues the process until all tumblers have been unlocked and the safe door can be opened.

Radionic systems have become quite sophisticated in their construction since the simplistic systems just described, but similar principles of operation are involved. The successful operation of radionic systems depends upon a developed radiesthetic faculty as well as skill and experience in applying this ability toward radionic diagnostics. Like any other system of medical diagnosis, technical skill and training is needed for accurate interpretation. The radionic systems are only external devices which provide a focal point of feedback and direction for the radiesthetic and healing skills of the practitioner. They translate unconscious psychic data into conscious diagnostic information. Before the development of radionic instruments, there were other translational devices which were able to decode diagnostic radiesthetic impressions.

One of the earliest applications of the radiesthetic faculty came with the use of the pendulum in medical diagnosis by such pioneers as Mermet.[18] The pendulum is operated as a device suspended from the hand, while the patient is held in the consciousness of the practitioner. While mentally asking certain yes/no questions relating to the medical status of the patient, the practitioner observes the pendulum for clockwise or counterclockwise rotation. Similar yes/no type questions are also used in obtaining information through radionic systems.

The mechanical output of the pendulum, like the radionic device, is dependent upon the unconscious nervous output induced by psychic perceptual functioning. In the instance of the radionic device, the unconscious output is conveyed through the autonomic nervous system. In the case of the pendulum, the medium of expression is tiny unconscious skeletal muscle movements. Both systems capitalize on electrical changes in the nervous system of the physical body as a means of translating unconscious psychic data into conscious diagnostic energetic information.

Diagram 24 summarizes the relationship of various radionic and radiesthetic devices to pathways of information flow through the conscious and unconscious (or autonomic) pathways of the human psychoenergetic system. It will be noted that the basic underlying process of information reception takes place at a psychic level via input through the chakra-nadi system. From there, information flows first to an unconscious level of processing in the nervous system. Outputs from this processing pathway generally occur through the autonomic nervous system and through unconsciously mediated motor activity. The conscious mind is then able to perceive and analyze the information through the various output modes of the radionic or pendulum devices. The only process which takes place at a conscious level is the attunement to the patient and the readout of the radionic device. All processes leading up to diagnostic interpretation take place at non-conscious levels of energetic functioning. Because these subtle energetic systems interface with the nervous system, it is possible to utilize indicators of unconscious nervous activity as indirect reflectors of higher psychic activity.

Diagram 24.
DIAGNOSTIC APPLICATIONS OF RADIESTHESIA:
PATHWAYS OF INFORMATION FLOW IN RADIONIC SYSTEMS

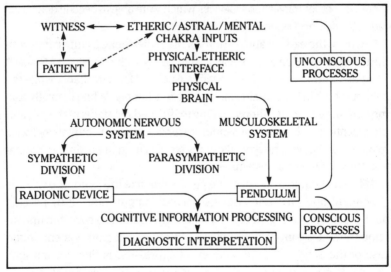

Since the information-gathering network of the practitioner includes the chakra system, it is possible to radionically diagnose ailments stemming from imbalances in the subtle bodies. Work in this direction has been largely due to research by Dr. David Tansley in England.[19] Specific chakra imbalances may be diagnosed (and treated) insofar as underactivity or overactivity of a particular psychic center is involved in the pathological processes of the patient being studied. (The issue of chakra imbalance relating to underlying physical illness will be examined in greater depth in a later chapter.)

The radionic practitioner is able to obtain this diagnostic information by achieving a mental link with the patient through the vehicle of the witness. This has been referred to by Tansley as a mental resonance link. *The vibrational witness is actually a two-way energetic focal point of attunement, in that it allows energetic information to flow from the patient to the practitioner as well as providing a subtle energetic link to the patient for distant therapy.*

After learning the energetic frequency imbalances within the patient by radionic diagnosis, *these devices allow the practitioner to transmit vibrational energy of the needed frequency characteristics back to the patient.* This type of energetic frequency matching is similar, in theory, to the diagnosis and treatment achieved by practitioners of the EAV method. Different types of radionic frequency therapies may be provided by a number of energetic modalities. Because the witness allows one to attune to a patient's vibrational frequency from anywhere in the world, one is able to establish a two-way link between the patient and the radionic practitioner. This means that it is possible to utilize various radionic systems to broadcast therapeutic frequencies of subtle energy to the patient even across great distances. Instead of giving the patient a homeopathic remedy containing a quantum dose of the needed frequency of vibration, one can directly broadcast the frequency of the homeopathic medicine to the patient using the radionic device and the vibrational witness. The Mora device, discussed earlier in the chapter, is able to transmit therapeutic homeopathic energy frequencies by utilizing similar subtle energetic principles of resonant vibrational transmission at a distance. Similarly, one can also transmit subtle energy frequencies to patients utilizing a variety of vibrational emitters, including various gems and crystals, color sources, flower essences, and even the pure, subtle magnetic frequencies of certain radionic devices themselves.

In general, radionic systems of diagnosis and treatment are harder for most conventional scientists to accept because they are predicated upon acceptance of human subtle energetic anatomy. In addition, the ability to radionically transmit healing over great distances is an idea which is not in vogue with many physicians. As we shall later see, there are a number of interesting scientific studies which substantiate the claim that healing energies may be transmitted from healers to patients over hundreds of miles. In the case of distant radionic healing, the witness provides the wave-guide necessary to direct the healing energies to the sick patient. In order to understand radionic methods of diagnosis, it is necessary to accept the fact that various types of remote viewing are possible and that sometimes these latent abilities may function at unconscious levels of perception. In addition, these clairvoyant abilities may be aided and focused by various types of psychotronic instrumentation.

Holographic theories of reality may hold the key to understanding how individuals may psychically tune in on distant sites and persons to obtain detailed information. Learning how to read the cosmic hologram may be a necessary prerequisite toward applying radionic diagnostic methods. It is likely that we all possess these abilities to varying degrees.

The attunement necessary between practitioner and device may be a necessary prerequisite of operation, not only for radionic systems, but also for EAV-type methods of diagnosis as well. *The intuitive faculties of the health care practitioner will come to play an ever-increasing role as medicine continues to explore subtle energetic approaches of diagnosis and treatment.*

Some have suggested that the EAV systems are actually a type of radionic diagnostic and treatment system, but that they are more electronically amplified than their pure radionic counterparts. Both systems involve transmission of subtle energies over wires. The EAV method works best using a direct interface with the patient's meridian system via electrical acupoint contact. The pure radionic method works without the patient having to be physically present. Radionic systems require only a vibrational representative of the patient (the witness) to tune into the same subtle energetic network.

There is clinical research which suggests that the Voll Machine is, indeed, a type of radionic or dowsing instrument. Studies have found that there may have been variations in the pressure applied by the EAV practitioner to the acupoints using the early EAV acupoint probes. More recent acupoint probes have been devised which give electronic feedback as to the pressure applied, in order to control this variable. Even when the pressure is controlled, there is still some suspicion that the Voll device may work best when the practitioner is sensitive to the energies involved, in a manner similar to the requirements for the radionic operator. The Voll device allows the practitioner to directly tap into the meridian network of the patient instead of working at a distance from a vibrational witness.

Even without the radionic connection, computerized electrodiagnostic systems such as the AMI Machine, which do not require the direct participation of the practitioner, reinforce the value of using the meridian system as a diagnostic interface.

Radionic and EAV systems commonly employ the principle of resonance to achieve their diagnostic functions and to provide effective frequency-specific energetic therapies. The radionic systems even eliminate the need for bodily ingestion of remedies, as the needed frequencies may be broadcast to the patient via the witness waveguide. Both methods provide a means of diagnosing disorders at the level of patients' subtle energetic anatomy prior to the manifestation of actual physical pathology. Radionic and electroacupuncture diagnostic systems make feasible the detection of diseases before organ damage occurs. It is clear that the widespread acceptance of both radionic and meridian-based technologies will demand a significant shift in consciousness of the medical profession toward a viewpoint that acknowledges the subtle-energy systems of human beings.

Key Points to Remember

1. The acupuncture meridian system, because of its energetic link between the physical and etheric bodies, is referred to as the physical-etheric interface.

2. Electroacupuncture diagnostic systems, such as the Voll and Motoyama devices, detect physiological and energetic imbalances in the body by measuring electrical changes in the meridian system. Because the meridian system is part of the physical-etheric interface, energy imbalances in the acupoints reflect disturbances at the etheric, as well as the cellular level.

3. Whereas the AMI Machine samples all the major meridians simultaneously, the Voll Machine is used to examine the electrical characteristics of single acupoints at a time.

4. Voll-detected imbalances at specific acupoints along a meridian may reflect physiological disturbances at different levels in the organ system supplied by that meridian.

5. The Voll Machine can also be used to diagnose specific causes of illnesses or to match specific remedies to the patient. The energetic

mechanism behind this use of the Voll system relates to a vibrational phenomenon known as the acupoint resonance reaction. When either the causative disease agent or the appropriate vibrational remedy is placed into the circuit path of the Voll Machine, this reaction produces an electrical change on the device's output meter (while the system is in electrical contact with the patient's acupuncture meridian system).

6. Using diagnostic systems like the Voll Machine to discover and treat vibrational imbalances in the body allows one to probe deeply into older layers of energetic armor. The peeling away of successive layers of this armor, which were acquired through exposure to various physiological and energetic insults, is referred to as the "onion effect."

7. Food allergies, sometimes referred to as food sensitivity reactions, are often caused by adverse reactions to phenolic chemical substances commonly found in many foods. The mechanisms by which these sensitivity reactions occur include a variety of immunological responses, and probably certain subtle energetic reactions as well. Such food sensitivities are probably responsible for more undiagnosed illness than is currently recognized.

8. The Voll Machine can be used to speed the diagnosis of various food allergies, and can also provide rapid determination of the specific homeopathic dosages of allergenic substances which can neutralize the allergic symptoms.

9. Instead of having direct contact with a patient's meridian system to gain energetic information, radionic devices utilize a biological specimen or photograph of the patient to sample their energetic makeup. Such a specimen is called a vibrational witness. The witness is an energetic focal point for the higher consciousness of the radionic practitioner to tune into.

10. Radionic devices also utilize the principle of resonance in order to get feedback about the status of the patient. The resonance reaction occurs within the autonomic (unconscious) nervous system of the radionic practitioner and is reflected by an increased activation of the sympathetic nervous system. This reaction is marked by an increased stickiness of the practitioner's finger when it is stroked across the rubber "stick pad" of the radionic device.

11. The radionic systems are devices which extend the sensitivity of the practitioner's higher energetic perceptual systems, most notably the chakra-nadi system. Therefore, the sensitivity of radionic devices is

a reflection of the psychospiritual development of their operators.

12. Radionic devices are mental scorekeepers with numbered dials which help the practitioner tune into the disease frequency of the patient. By discovering this frequency, it is possible to broadcast the appropriate and needed healing frequency back to the patient through the energetic intermediary of the vibrational witness.

13. Radionic devices and pendulums are systems which allow the sensitive health care practitioner to amplify and bring to conscious awareness psychic perceptions that usually operate at an unconscious level.

14. Because the Voll Machine operators may unconsciously vary the pressure with which they probe the acupoints, it is possible that the Voll device may also work as a kind of radionic or dowsing system.

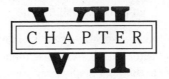

CHAPTER VII

The Evolution of Vibrational Medicine:
LEARNING TO HEAL WITH THE WISDOM OF NATURE

Throughout this text, we have examined in great detail the relationships between the physical body and the subtle light bodies which contribute to the multidimensional nature of human beings. It has become increasingly clear that it is possible to therapeutically impact upon physical and emotional illness by affecting the higher frequency structures which are in dynamic equilibrium with the physical body. Our subtle-energy bodies play a major role in maintaining our health. Energy disturbances in the etheric body precede the manifestation of abnormal patterns of cellular organization and growth. Disease becomes manifest in the physical body only after disturbances of energy flow have already become crystallized in the subtle structural patterns of the higher frequency bodies. One of the best ways to alter dysfunctional patterns in the subtle bodies is to administer therapeutic doses of frequency-specific subtle energy in the form of vibrational medicines.

When we speak of vibration, we are merely using another synonym for frequency. Different frequencies of energy reflect varying rates of vibration. We know that matter and energy are two different manifestations of the same primary energetic substance of which everything in the universe is composed, including our physical and subtle bodies. The vibratory rate of this universal energy determines the density of its expression as matter. Matter which vibrates at a very slow frequency is referred to as physical matter. That which vibrates at speeds exceeding light velocity is known as subtle matter. Subtle matter is as real as dense matter; its vibratory rate is simply faster. In order to therapeutically alter our subtle bodies, we must administer energy that vibrates at frequencies beyond the physical plane. Vibrational medicines contain such high-frequency subtle energies.

Vibrational medicines are usually essences or tinctures which are charged with a particular frequency of subtle energy. We have already examined one type of vibrational medicine in the form of homeopathy. As demonstrated by the prototypical homeopathic remedies, vibrational characteristics are usually imprinted upon the universal storage medium of nature: water. The subtle energetic patterns stored within the vibrational essence may be used to affect human beings at a variety of interactive levels.

There are a multitude of vibrational remedies which have been derived from Mother Nature. The essences of living flowers are among the most ancient of these natural healing modalities. We shall continue our discussion of the evolution of vibrational medicine with the gifts to humanity that the flowers of our planet have provided.

Learning to Heal with Flower Remedies: Dr. Bach Discovers the Hidden Gifts of Nature

One of the most respected names associated with the use of flower essences in healing is Dr. Edward Bach of England. Dr. Bach was a respected homeopathic practitioner in London during the early part of the twentieth century. Dr. Bach is credited with the discovery of the now famous Bach Flower Remedies, which are utilized by health care practitioners throughout the world. These flower essences are used in treating a variety of emotional disorders and temperaments. Like homeopathic medicines, flower essences contain minute quantities of physical substance, yet they are considered to be pure vibrational remedies. Their widespread application has opened the way for the development of flower essence healing as a unique and specialized form of subtle energetic therapy. Edward Bach was a pioneering medical thinker who discovered a link between stress, emotions, and illness decades before most contemporary physicians had begun to address the issue. From his inital insight on the emotional contributors to illness, Bach sought to find a simple and natural way to return people to a level of harmonious balance. It was this search for a cure in nature that eventually led Bach to discover the healing properties of homeopathic remedies and, ultimately, the essences of flowers.

Before becoming a homeopathic practitioner, Bach was an orthodox physician specializing in bacteriology at a major hospital in London. One of his early discoveries in this field had to do with the presence of particular types of bacteria found in the gastrointestinal tract of persons suffering from chronic ailments. He found a number of bacteria whose presence in the gastrointestinal tract was associated with persistent exacerbations of chronic illness such as arthritis and rheumatic disorders. If, in fact, the suspected bacteria were aggravating these rheumatic illnesses, then boosting the body's ability to immunologically reject these microorganisms would provide relief to such afflicted patients by diminishing their arthritic symptoms. Bach conjectured that innoculation with vaccines made from these intestinal bacteria would have the desired effect of cleansing the system of the bacterial poisons causing the chronic illness. Based on this assumption, Bach made dilute vaccines from the suspected intestinal pathogens which he had linked with exacerbations of chronic disease. When given by injection to patients with various chronic disorders, the vaccines produced significant improvements in the arthritic and other chronic symptoms.

Soon after this discovery, Bach was given a book called *The Organon of Medicine*. This was Hahnemann's famous treatise on homeopathy. Bach felt great sympathy with the ideas of homeopathic practice. His idea of giving minute doses of toxic substances to cure illness was similar to Hahnemann's homeopathic theory. Bach had empirically arrived at this conclusion strictly through trial and error. He was also interested in finding an alternative method to injecting his vaccines, as they frequently produced local tissue reactions at the injection site. Bach decided to prepare homeopathic concentrations of the illness-associated intestinal bacteria to give as sublingual dosages. He gave them to patients by the oral route, with results far more remarkable than those he had previously achieved with his injectable vaccines. In all, Bach classified seven types of bacteria associated with chronic illness, and from these he made homeopathic preparations known as Bach's Seven Nosodes (see Chapter 6 for a further discussion of bionosodes).

It was at this time that Bach made a curious discovery. He found that patients carrying each of the seven types of intestinal bacterial pathogens displayed particular personality types or temperaments. He felt that the seven bacterial types were associated with seven distinct and different personalities. On the basis of this insight, Bach began to treat patients with his nosodes. He assigned the nosodes strictly on the basis of the patients' emotional temperaments. He ignored the physical aspects of their disease and dealt only with the mental symptoms he had correlated with particular nosodes. Utilizing this method, Bach obtained positive clinical successes that exceeded his expectations.

After some refining of his techniques and analyses of personality types, Bach came to another profound insight. He concluded that individuals of the same personality group would not necessarily come down with the same diseases. Rather, confronted with any type of illness-producing agent, patients in the same personality group would react to their illnesses in a similar fashion with the same behaviors, moods, and states of mind, regardless of the disease. Therefore, it was necessary only to categorize the mental and emotional characteristics of the patient in order to find which remedy would be most applicable to curing their chronic illness. What Bach had correctly intuited was that different emotional and personality factors contribute toward a general predisposition to illness. The most significant of these factors were emotional tendencies such as fear and negative attitudes. Medical science is only now beginning to address this remarkable insight into the relationship between illness and the emotions. Bach had already reached this conclusion more that 50 years prior to current psychoneuroimmunological research.

Bach did not like giving nosodes prepared from disease-producing agents. He felt that there existed in nature various remedies of vibrational similarity which would duplicate the effects of his nosodes, as well as go beyond them in therapeutic efficacy. So he began a search for natural agents which would deal not with the pre-established pathology of illness but rather with the emotional precursors to disease. He later found these in the essences of particular flowers. Bach identified 38 essences in all. The 38th essence was a combination floral mixture known familiarly as Rescue Remedy.

Bach correctly perceived that the illness-personality link was an outgrowth of dysfunctional energetic patterns within the subtle bodies. He felt that illness was a reflection of disharmony between the physical personality and the Higher Self or soul. Reflections of this inner disharmony could be found within particular types of mental traits and attitudes which the individual displayed. This mental and energetic disharmony between the physical personality and the Higher Self was seen as outweighing the particular disease process.

Bach felt that the subtle vibrational energies of the flower essences could assist in realigning the emotional patterns of dysfunction. By increasing the alignment of the physical personality with the energies of the Higher Self, greater harmony could occur within the individual as reflected by greater peace of mind and the expression of joy. *By correcting these emotional factors, patients would be assisted in increasing their physical and mental vitality and thus be aided in resolving any physical disease.* Bach links this relationship of the physical personality to the Higher Self via a reincarnational philosophy. To quote Bach himself:

> *It cannot be too firmly realized that every Soul in incarnation is down here for the specific purpose of gaining experience and understanding, and of perfecting his personality towards those ideals laid down by the Soul. Let everyone remember that his Soul has laid down for him a particular work, and that unless he does this work, though perhaps not consciously, he will inevitably raise a conflict between his Soul and personality which of necessity reacts in the form of physical disorders...*

From time immemorial it has been known that *Providential Means have placed in nature the prevention and cure of disease, by means of divinely enriched herbs and plants and trees.* They have been given the power to heal all types of illness and suffering. In treating cases with these remedies no notice is taken of the nature of the disease. The individual is treated, and as he becomes well the disease goes, having been cast off by the increase of health. The mind, being the most delicate and sensitive part of the body, shows the onset and course of the disease much more definitely than the body, so that the outlook of mind is chosen as the guide as to which remedy or remedies is necessary...

The dawn of a new and better art of healing is upon us. A hundred years ago the Homeopathy of Hahnemann was as the first streak of morning light after a long night of darkness, and it may play a big part in the medicine of the future...

When we come to the problem of healing we can understand that this also will have to keep pace with the times and change its methods from those of gross materialism to those of a science founded upon the realities of Truth and governed by the same Divine laws which rule our very natures...

Materialism forgets that there is a factor above the physical plane which in the ordinary course of life protects or renders susceptible any particular individual with regard to disease, of whatever nature it may be. *Fear, by its depressing effect on our mentality, thus causes disharmony in our physical and magnetic bodies and paves the way for [bacterial] invasion. The real cause of disease lies in our own personality...*

[In the future], healing will pass from the domain of physical methods of treating the physical body to that of spiritual and mental healing, which, by bringing about harmony between the Soul and mind, will eradicate the very basic cause of disease, and then allow such physical means to be used as may be necessary to complete the cure of the body.[1] *(italics added)*

Bach understood the energetic relationship of the higher mind to the magnetic qualities of the higher subtle bodies. As discussed in earlier chapters, qualities of mind and emotion that are expressed through the brain and physical nervous system are a product of energetic input from the etheric, astral, and mental bodies. By the ability of the flower essences to energetically impact upon these higher bodies, their effects are ultimately able to filter down to the physical body.

Bach discovered the effects of the various flowers through observation of how they affected him. Bach himself was a psychic "sensitive." He was so sensitive that at times he had to shield and isolate himself from the bustling crowds and chaos of London, because the city life was too disruptive and draining. Living in the English countryside following an acute illness that nearly took his life, Bach took long walks in search of the healers within nature. Bach's sensitivity to subtle energies was such that he could touch the morning dew from a flower or its petal to his lips and he would experience the potential therapeutic effects of the plant. Bach was so sensitive that when he was exposed to a particular flower, he would experience all of the physical symptoms and emotional states to which the flower's essence was an antidote. The process of determining all 38 of the flower remedies was such a strain on Bach's physical and emotional nature that he died in 1936 at the relatively early age of 56.

Bach also sought a method of preparing these vibrational essences without having to pulverize the plant and potentize it in the laborious homeopathic method. (See Chapter 2 on the preparation of homeopathic remedies.) He collected the morning dew from flowers that were in sunlight, and the dewdrops from flowers that were still in shade. He examined them for differences in their ability to affect his subtle energy bodies. By comparing the two solutions, he found that the water from flowers exposed to sunlight had the most marked effect. To his delight, he found that he could place the flowers of a particular species upon the surface of a bowl of spring water for several hours in sunlight and obtain powerful vibrational tinctures. The subtle effects of sunlight were critical in charging the water with an energetic imprint of the flower's vibrational signature. This may relate to the subtle energetic qualities in sunlight which the Hindu's have referred to as "prana."

The Bach flower remedies were used to treat the emotional reactions to disease as well as the temperaments leading up to eventual cellular pathology in the body. For instance, if a patient suffered from a known fear, i.e. a phobia, he or she would be given the essence of Mimulus. Individuals suffering from a shock of any kind would be given a tincture of the Star of Bethlehem flower. Individuals exhibiting problems with constant indecision found relief in the essence made from the Scleranthus flower. Obsessional thoughts appeared to diminish when patients were treated with flower essences made from White Chestnut.

Utilizing the Bach flower remedies, many practitioners have achieved clinical success in relieving long-standing patterns of emotional distress and personality dysfunction. Unlike conventional drug therapies which impact solely at the level of physical cellular pathology, the energetic patterns contained within the flower essence work at the level of the emotional, mental, and spiritual vehicles. The subtle bodies influence the physical body by altering its susceptibility to illness from any external or internal noxious agent. What Bach was doing with his vibrational essences was working to increase the host resistance of his patients by creating internal harmony and an amplification of the higher energetic systems that connect human beings to their higher selves. Bach's flower remedies had little direct effect upon the cellular systems of the physical body. There are, however, other types of flower essences which can directly influence cellular imbalance in the physical body by their interactions with various levels of human subtle energetic anatomy.

Following Bach's death in 1936, the Dr. Edward Bach Healing Centre in England continued to prepare flower essences in the unique style discovered by their innovator. In various naturopathic schools throughout Europe and the United States, the Bach Flower Remedies were used according to the emotional and mental criteria established by Edward Bach. Various types of experimentation took place utilizing different natural flowers, but it was not until the 1970s that an entirely new series of healing flower essences was developed.

In 1979, Richard Katz established the Flower Essence Society (FES). The Society provided a framework for flower essence workers and therapists to network and exchange information on the use of essences. Additionally, they introduced a variety of new essences prepared from flowers indigenous to the United States (mainly California, where the FES is based). The FES group published data on different methods of utilizing the Bach Flower Remedies and the new essences which became known as the FES Essences.

The discoverer of the FES Essences was Richard Katz, the founder of the Flower Essence Society. Katz arrived at the selection and formulation of each particular flower through intuitive guidance, modified by experiential sharing with a small group of local practitioners. Clinical feedback to Katz indicated that the new essences worked especially well with processes of inner growth and spiritual awakening. They appeared to function as catalysts for the transmutation of specific psychoenergetic blockages such as fears about sexuality, issues of intimacy, sensitivity, and psychic and spiritual development. Much expansion of knowledge about individual essences came through intuitive or channeled guidance from a variety of psychic sources, as well as through the individual practitioner's use of the radiesthetic faculty via the pendulum.[2] Through this type of intuitive information gathering, much knowledge on the application of the essences was accumulated. Bits and pieces of flower essence knowledge trickled through the intermittently published *Flower Essence Journal,* but it was not until 1983 that an authoritative text on the therapeutic, subtle energetic aspects of flower essences was written and compiled by Gurudas, a researcher in Boulder, Colorado.

A Revolution in Healing with Flower Essences: Gurudas' Contribution toward a Synthesis of Vibrational Medicine

During the early portion of 1983, a variety of new flower essences were distributed throughout centers of esoteric healing by a company calling itself Pegasus Products, Inc. These new essences were arranged in a special display, side by side with a second group of vibrational remedies referred to as gem elixirs. Accompanying this unique display case was a single page handout listing the energetic and therapeutic uses of the gem elixirs and flower essences. Listed at the top of the handout was a reference to several books providing further detailed vibrational information. Most prominent among these references was a subtle-energy medicine textbook entitled *Flower Essences and Vibrational Healing* by Gurudas.

Several months later a book was released into bookstores which were already carrying a wide variety of published holistic medicine guides. Among its more unusual topics, the book contained scientifically detailed and technical descriptions of the subtle energetic and physical properties of 108 new flower essences. Some of these flowers were already a part of the FES Essences, but they had not previously been described in such detail. In addition, there were technical descriptions of the energy relationships between flower essences and homeopathic remedies. In this uniquely authoritative textbook of vibrational medicine, Gurudas compiled and annotated information acquired from psychic readings by Kevin Ryerson, a remarkable channel of technical psychic information who is similar to Edgar Cayce. A significant portion of the material contained within *Flower Essences and Vibrational Healing* had been acquired through a series of group psychic-research readings with Ryerson that Gurudas had attended during 1980 in San Francisco. The group had met with Ryerson to acquire channeled technical material on the clinical use of various flower essences. Among the individuals present at this unique gathering were Gurudas and Richard Katz, originator of the Flower Essence Society. In addition to these 1980 sessions, Gurudas continued to collect further psychic data on flower essences from Ryerson and to elaborate on channeled data that had already been explored in previous readings.

It should be stated here that the channeled material offers insights into what may today be considered a new healing technology, although the roots of such methods may actually be quite ancient. The earliest inroads to developing flower essences as a systematic method of healing in the twentieth century were provided by the research of Dr. Edward Bach, himself a sensitive as well as a clinician. The channeled information, as provided by Kevin Ryerson, hints at biochemical and subtle energetic mechanisms of action of flower essences, their possible applications for healing, as well as directions for further scientific research to validate the information which has been given. The effects of these new flower essences, as well as their actions, must be considered in this light as an experimental form of therapy.

Flower Essences and Vibrational Healing is a remarkable achievement in that it puts together a diverse amount of technical information on the therapeutic use of flower essences and related vibrational therapies. The historical use of flower essences is outlined in a descriptive chapter relating the discoveries and inspiration of Dr. Bach. Gurudas draws an interesting conclusion here, suggesting that Bach may have been inspired to explore the healing properties of flowers by Rudolph Steiner. Steiner, a famous metaphysician, had delivered a number of medical lectures in

England which may have been attended by Bach at the time he was still in early practice.

Additional discussion on the origins of flower essences in healing goes into great detail on their use in ancient, esoterically described civilizations such as Atlantis and Lemuria. In the first portion of the book, Gurudas describes various techniques by which flower essences may be prepared and amplified, as well as intricate mechanisms by which they affect the human energetic system. The second portion of the book deals in great detail with the properties of individual essences. There are discussions which specify the subtle energetic levels at which each essence works, and there are also lists of illnesses which each essence may best be used to treat. At the end of this section, Gurudas has organized the data in convenient tables of clinical relevance, relating the therapeutic uses of various essences and the individual energy systems with which each particular essence interacts.

Unlike any previous text on vibrational medicine, great attention is given to the subtle energetic and physiologic mechanisms by which the vibrational remedies work on the human organism. The information mentioned within this book has rarely been published or described in such detailed fashion. References to esoteric texts which substantiate the claims of the channeled material are provided wherever possible. The mechanisms by which the energies of the flowers are transferred from the water to the human system are elegantly and simply described. To quote from the text:

> In this evolutionary plan, flowers were and are the very essence and the highest concentration of the life-force in the plant. They are the crowning experience of the plants' growth. They are a combination of the etheric properties [of the plant] and are at the height of the life-force, so they are often used in the fertility portions of the plant's growth . . .
>
> The actual essence, of course, is the electromagnetic pattern of the plant form. Even as there are nutritional elements found in various plant forms that ye partake of for the physical body, so in turn are there various parameters of biomagnetic energies discharged by flowers and various plant forms. And the vitality of the life-force increases about the area of the bloom . . .
>
> [Essences prepared from the flowers are] merely an etheric imprint; nothing physical gets transferred. In this work, you are dealing strictly with the ethereal vibration of the plant, the intelligence of it. The sun upon striking the water melds into the water the life-force of the flower, and this is transferred to people when they assimilate

these vibrational essences.[3]

In addition to charging water with the vibrational imprint of flowers, Gurudas mentions the use of gem elixirs which are similarly prepared by using sunlight to energize water with the unique crystalline properties of various gems and minerals. Even more fascinating than the energetic reasoning behind the sun method of flower essence preparation is the description Gurudas provides of how the essences have their effects upon people's physical and subtle bodies. This material describing the subtle anatomy incorporates much that has already been discussed in previous chapters of this text, with new information yet to be explored. There are therapeutic interactions between the physical body and the etheric and higher frequency vehicles caused by the energetic patterns of the flower essences. Of great interest here is the description of particular crystalline or quartz-like properties of the physical body, and the role they play in forming a special subtle energetic system at the level of the physical-cellular structures. In later chapters we will examine in greater detail the healing and energetic properties of quartz and other crystals. This description of the crystalline properties of the human body will have special relevance when we talk about healing with crystals.

When a flower essence, homeopathic remedy, or gem elixir is ingested or used as a salve they follow a specific path through the physical and subtle bodies. They initially are assimilated into the circulatory system [the bloodstream]. Next, the remedy settles mid-way between the circulatory and nervous systems. An electromagnetic current is created here by the polarity of these two systems. Indeed, there is an intimate connection between these two systems in relation to the life-force and consciousness that modern science does not yet understand. The life-force works more through the blood, and consciousness works more through the brain and nervous systems. These two systems contain quartz-like properties and an electromagnetic current. The blood cells, especially the red and white blood cells, contain more quartz-like properties, and the nervous system contains more an electromagnetic current. The life-force and consciousness use these properties to enter and stimulate the physical body.

From midway between the nervous and circulatory systems the remedy usually moves directly to the meridians. From the meridians, the remedy's life-force enters the various subtle bodies, the chakras, or returns directly to the physical body to the cellular level through several portals midway between the nervous and circulatory system. Its path is determined by the type of remedy and the person's constitution.

The three main portals for the remedy's life-force to reenter the physical body are the etheric body and ethereal fluidium, the chakras, and the skin with its silica or crystalline properties. The ethereal fluidium is the part of the etheric body which surrounds the physical body, that brings the life-force into the individual cells. Hair, with its crystalline properties, is a carrier of the life-force; it is not a portal. Specific parts of the physical body are portals for the life-force of a vibrational remedy only because they are associated with different chakras or meridians. The life-force of a vibrational remedy usually gravitates toward one portal, but it may re-enter the physical body through several portals.

After passing through one of the described portals, the life-force always passes midway between the nervous and circulatory systems. Then it enters the cellular level and imbalanced areas of the physical body. This entire process takes place instantaneously, but it usually takes awhile to experience the results.[4]

According to this interpretation, the subtle energies of the flower essences work their way through the physical circulatory systems of the blood stream and nerves to reach the meridians. One of the interconnecting pathways mentioned appears to be some type of electromagnetic network of energy flow that exists between the bloodstream and nervous system. This particular energy network has been previously unknown to most esoteric physiologists. Certain researchers, such as Itzhak Bentov,[5] have noted specialized pathways of energetic resonance which link the circulatory system to the nervous system in meditation. More will be said on Bentov's model in a later chapter on meditation. From this electromagnetic pathway, the life-energies of flower essences flow to the meridians. As discussed in previous chapters, the meridians are a key mechanism of energetic interface between the higher frequency vehicles and the physical body.

From the meridians, the energies reach the chakras and the various subtle bodies. The initial upward flow of the flower-essence life-energies to progressively higher energetic levels is opposite to the usual downward flow of higher energies into the physical. It is as if energy is retracing its footsteps to progressively more subtle levels in order to be reintegrated from the appropriate higher frequency domains. It appears as though the life-force of the essences and remedies needs to be amplified and processed at special relay points such as the chakras to allow the energies to be properly utilized by the cellular systems of the physical body.

There are additional subtle-energy relay/processing stations at the cellular level that involve the crystalline network alluded to in the previous quote. The topic of crystalline structures within the human body is a subject which has not been widely approached nor understood by many of today's physicans. Bioelectronic theorists, such as Becker and Szent-Gyorgi, have tried to comprehend and therapeutically interact with the energetic amplification systems inherent in the cellular networks of the body by applying semiconductor and electronic systems theories.

Scientists have also recently begun to recognize that special types of fluid-like crystals exist, which are otherwise referred to as liquid crystals. These liquid crystals may possess some of the energetic properties of solid quartz, but unlike the naturally occurring minerals, many are of organic origin. There appears to be an entire subtle energetic network throughout the body that utilizes these biocrystalline structures. This crystalline network is involved with the assimilation and processing of the subtle energies of vibrational remedies. In the following quote from Gurudas (taken from the channeled material of Kevin Ryerson), the principle of bioenergetic resonance is again mentioned in relation to crystalline components of subtle energetic systems that form an integral part of the human body.

> *There are various quartz-like crystalline structures in the physical and subtle bodies that augment the impact of vibrational remedies.* In the physical body, these areas include: cell salts, fatty tissue, lymphs, red and white cells, and the pineal gland. *These crystalline structures are a complete system in the body but not yet properly isolated and understood by modern medicine.*
>
> *Crystalline structures work on sympathetic resonancy.* There is an attunement between crystalline properties in the physical and subtle bodies, the ethers, and many vibrational remedies, notably flower essences and gems. These properties in the body magnify the life-force of the vibrational remedies to a recognizable level to be assimilated. Indeed, *these crystalline properties are relay points for most ethereal energies to penetrate the physical body.* This allows for a balanced distribution of various energies at correct frequencies, which stimulates the discharge of toxicity to create health. In a similar fashion, vibrations of radio-wave frequency strike a crystal in a radio. The crystal resonates with the high frequency in such a way as to absorb it, passing along the audio frequencies which are perceivable by the body.
>
> *When vibrational remedies are amplified, their life-force reaches the imbalanced parts of the body faster and in a more stable state. The remedies may cleanse the aura and subtle bodies so those imbalances will no longer contribute to ill health.* If this sounds strange,

remember scientists have many times proven that subtle energies such as ultrasonics and microwaves can cause sickness. Why cannot other subtle energies produce health?[6] *(italics added)*

In reference to frequency-specific subtle energies causing the body to throw off the toxicity of illness, one is reminded of explanations in previous chapters of this textbook which have described the mechanisms by which homeopathic remedies have their therapeutic effect upon human beings. *The crystalline network of the human body assists in transducing and distributing subtle energies of homeopathic remedies and flower essences to their appropriate paths of action.*

The ultimate therapeutic action of a remedy or flower essence depends upon the energetic level at which it has the greatest effects. Homeopathic remedies would appear to have greater energy effects at the physical/molecular level, however some clinical work suggests that homeopathic remedies are also able to affect higher levels like the chakras, as well as the emotional/astral body. For instance, certain cases of manic-depressive illness and schizophrenia have benefited dramatically from treatment with homeopathic remedies. These effects may be due to correcting both the neurochemical imbalances associated with the diseases as well as the more subtle energetic illness-linked disturbances.

Flower essences appear to be especially potent in inducing changes in the chakras and subtle bodies, but certain essences also heal by working directly at the level of the physical body. Homeopathic remedies deliver frequency-specific vibrational quanta that seem to resonate more with the physical/molecular structure of the cellular body, but homeopathics can also affect the chakras and subtle bodies. Flower essences contain a higher concentration of the life-force, and possess qualities not unlike a kind of tincture of the energy of pure consciousness. Because of this subtle vibrational quality, certain flower essences may be able to effectively interact with the subtle bodies and chakras to increase their coordination with the physical body when dysfunctional patterns exist.

Homeopathic remedies usually come from denser inorganic material, while flower essences have a much higher concentration of life-force. Homeopathic remedies often vibrationally duplicate the physical disease in a person to push that imbalance out of the body. *Homeopathy integrates into the subtle bodies but still functions upon the vibrational level of the molecular structure. Homeopathy is a bridge between traditional medicine and vibrational medicine.*

In contrast, flower essences adjust the flow of consciousness and karma that create the disease state. They influence the subtle bodies and ethereal properties of the anatomy and then gradually influence the physical body. The fact that flower essence come from flowers, which are the most concentrated area of the life-force in plants, is one key reason why there is more life-force in flower essences than in other forms of vibrational medicine.[7] *(italics added)*

Karma, Consciousness, & the Crystalline Network: The Pineal Gland's Link with the Right Cerebral Hemisphere

The view expressed in the channeled material suggests that *karma plays a role in the causation of disease, and that some flower essences help the individual to better deal with these dysfunctional karmic energetic patterns.* It is a feeling shared by many esoteric thinkers that disease causation is influenced, in part, by carry-overs and unresolved traumas and conflicts originating in past lives. Certain types of hypnotic reincarnational regression techniques have supported this viewpoint. Various longstanding phobias have been permanently cured by hypnotically guided past-life recollections. When patients are able to recall traumatic events that are the source of their phobias, whether they occurred in the present life or a past one, the phobias gradually dissolve.

Even Edward Bach felt that disease was caused by a failure of the physical personality to behave in concordance with the wishes, desires, and altruistic, service-oriented motivations of the Higher Self. The higher (or causal) self has knowledge of all past lives and the patterns needed for further growth of the incarnating personality at the level of the physical plane. A lack of connection and coordination with one's Higher Self may result in feelings of separation from others, and behavior that may reflect feelings of egocentrism and alienation.

The conscious personality frequently fails to perceive the interconnectedness of all life at subtle energetic levels. Douglas Dean's study on autonomic indicators of telepathy showed that communication at higher energetic frequencies may take place constantly at an unconscious level.[8] This finding suggests that humans may be in continuous psychic communication with other individuals at higher levels of consciousness, in addition to their everyday verbal exchanges. Because this communication takes place at levels outside of ordinary waking consciousness, the conscious personality is rarely aware of its connections to the Higher Self. When we feel disconnected from our higher selves, loneliness and despair are often accentutated. At times this may lead to a sense of total isolation.

It is well known that emotional states of depression may cause stress and immunosuppression. Likewise, karmic influences may unconsciously interact with the subtle anatomy of the organism to energetically crystallize and precipitate certain specific tendencies toward illness.

These and other energetic influences may create patterns that can increasingly weaken an individual's host resistance, impair their overall vitality, and diminish their ability to repel any type of noxious influence. Certain flower essences (and gem elixirs) may be helpful in decreasing the negative karmic expressions of illness by altering dysfunctional energetic patterns which exist at the level of the subtle bodies. If left unaltered, these abnormal subtle-energy patterns may eventually move into the biomagnetic field of the physical body and create abnormal cellular changes.

An individual's ability to connect with his or her Higher Self is partly a function of specialized energy links within the crystalline network of the physical body. This crystalline network helps to coordinate the energetic structures of the higher subtle bodies with the consciousness of the physical personality. Gurudas brings out new and important information that may explain certain aspects of right-hemispheric functioning and psi abilities. Psychic abilities are mediated by special biocrystalline and energetic pathways through which the Higher Self may interact with the consciousness of the physical personality. One particular crystalline structure that is important to our psychic receptivity is the pineal gland and, more specifically, the pineal calcification: a crystal that lies in the center of the brain.

Long utilized as a structural landmark for judging x-ray parameters of symmetry within the human brain, the true function of the pineal's crystal has never been known. Some scientists have gone so far as to suggest that the more the calcification, the lesser the capacity for physiologic function left within the supposedly atrophied and aging pineal gland. Medical research in the field of chronobiology has recognized the pineal as one of the body's internal clocks. It also has hormonal control over the process of sexual maturation, and is influenced by the light cycles of day and night. The pineal gland controls our biological ascension from child to adult by inhibiting sexual maturation until the appropriate time. Interestingly, the pineal produces a hormone called melatonin which not only inhibits sexual maturation but also appears to have an additional function in regulating sleep cycles.

The pineal gland in esoteric literature has long been associated with the third eye. Our early biological ancestors actually had a rudimentary but functional third eye structure, complete with lens, as exists today within the tuatara (a lizard found in the southern hemisphere). The pineal gland is associated with the phenomenon of light from a variety of different biological and energetic perspectives. This esoteric association of the pineal with the third eye in humans stems from the pineal gland's link with the third eye (or brow) chakra. The pineal gland is linked to the chakra system by way of a special energetic circuit which has developed in human beings over the course of time. The function of this specialized energy system is uniquely involved with raising the energies of the personality toward a higher, more spiritual level of consciousness. In addition, this same energy system is responsible for awakening and balancing the major chakras in the body while releasing an individual's full creative and evolutionary potential.

In the Hindu and yogic literature, this unique energy system which activates the energy of the chakras and assists in the awakening of higher consciousness is referred to as the kundalini. The kundalini is visualized as a "coiled serpent" (the actual Sanskrit translation of the word kundalini) which lies dormant in the coccygeal region of the first major chakra. Like a coiled snake, the kundalini is ever poised to spring into action; however, in most individuals, this serpent energy sleeps quietly. When its power is unleashed in a coordinated fashion, as for example through structured meditation, the kundalini energy rises slowly up the spinal column, activating sequential chakras along the way. As the kundalini energy finally enters and activates the higher chakras (specifically the third eye and crown chakras), a sensation of light flooding the brain may be experienced by the individual, followed by a tremendous expansion of consciousness.

According to the channeled material in *Flower Essences and Vibrational Healing,* the kundalini activation process utilizes the crystalline circuitry of the body, specifically the pineal gland, as well as a special resonant energy reflex arc extending from the coccygeal region to the brain stem. Although energy flow through this pathway is primarily involved with the ascension of the kundalini, it appears that this circuit also functions on a more day-to-day basis to allow us to communicate with our Higher Self.

> *The pineal gland is a crystalline structure that receives information from the soul and subtle bodies,* particularly the astral body. The subtle bodies often act as filters for teachings from the soul and Higher Self. *From the pineal gland information travels to the right*

portion of the brain. If there is need to alert the conscious mind to this higher information, it passes through the right brain in the form of dreams. Then the left brain analyzes it to see if the information can be grasped. This often occurs with clear dreams that offer messages. From the left brain information travels through the neurological system, specifically passing through two critical reflex points—the medulla oblongata and the coccyx. *There is a constant state of resonancy along the spinal column between the medulla oblongata and the coccyx; properties of the pineal gland resonate between these two points.* Then the information travels to other parts of the body through the meridians and crystalline structures already described. *The life force of vibrational remedies activates this entire procedure.* This is a key process the soul uses to manifest karma in the physical body.[9] *(italics added)*

The crystalline circuitry herein described actually contributes to the physiological basis for the kundalini process. Additionally, this circuit permits the step-down transduction of information from the Higher Self to various levels of awareness experienced by the physical personality. It is most interesting that the right cerebral hemisphere, working in concert with the pineal, acts as a primary relay point for information moving from the Higher Self to the waking personality. It is well known that the symbolic imagery of the right hemisphere is the landscape of dreams. Many have felt that the right brain seems to express certain functions which reflect our more intuitive side.

It has been said that we live in a left-brain culture of logic, science, and language. The symbolic language of dreams represents the mode of communication of the right-brain-dominant state of sleep which occupies nearly a third of our lives. In other words, we are only left-brain dominant when we are awake; when we sleep, we switch over into our right-brain mode of information processing. We need right-brain skills to function in the metaphorical landscape of dreams.

The right/left-brain interplay of dream consciousness versus waking consciousness represents an attempt by the soul to maintain a balanced and integrated expression of interplay between the Higher Self and the physical personality. We have already established that psychic communication (via our subtle energetic anatomy) continually occurs at unconscious levels of information processing. Subtle perceptual systems such as the chakras have direct input into the right brain through pathways of the crystalline circuitry. This unique biocrystalline network allows information from the Higher Self to reach the left-brain consciousness of the personality.

The dream state represents a special time when the right brain, which is more directly connected to the Higher Self, can relay coded messages to the waking personality. An individual's ability to decode these inner messages depends upon his or her skill at unraveling the symbolism of their dreams.

The right brain is also the storehouse of each person's body image. This self-image is formed from the various positive and negative life experiences which the individual has accumulated over time. People's self-images are created from unconscious message tapes, running in their right-brain biocomputers, which tell them each about their value as a person, their physical appearance, and their sense of self-worth. Because dreams are the language of the right brain, they hold great potential as tools for understanding not only the unconscious mind, but also for deciphering the vision of inner spiritual awareness and self-knowledge.

Dreams form a pictographic/symbolic language which may represent an attempt by the right hemisphere to pass on important unconscious information to the conscious, waking, left-hemispheric personality. *Sometimes, when dreams are ignored, the right hemisphere may attempt to communicate important messages to the left-brain personality by creating symbolic disorders and diseases within the physical body.* It has been said that there is a particular metaphor to illness. Physical illness may sometimes represent our own unexpressed inner feelings and inadequacies that are crystallized in the symbolic patterns of right-hemispheric body language. The symbolic language of disease expression may also relate to particular chakras that have energy blockages which are a reflection of emotional dysfunction within the personality. When the chakras are blocked, so too are the pathways of information flow impeded in their ability to connect the Higher Self to the physical personality.

Certain flower essences (and gem elixirs) help to strengthen these natural pathways of energetic flow, thus stabilizing and integrating the personality with the Higher Self. This was one of Dr. Bach's reasons for administering his flower remedies to patients. The flower essences represented a vibrational method of correcting dysfunctional emotional patterns in the self which Bach correctly recognized as precursors to physical illness.

The Problem of Miasms:
Our Energetic Tendencies toward Illness

In addition to the ability of flower essences to modify subtle energy connections with the Higher Self, Gurudas mentions many new essences which work at the cellular level. Some of these flower essences also work at modifying certain energetic precursors to illness which are known as miasms. Miasms are energetic tendencies which predispose an individual toward manifesting particular illnesses. Most miasms are either inherited or acquired during the course of an individual's lifetime. Hahnemann, the father of modern homeopathy, felt that miasms were the root causes of all chronic diseases and a contributing factor to many acute illnesses.

Miasms represent a totally different concept in the mechanism of illness causation. Although, for example, miasms may be acquired as a result of an infectious agent, the infection itself is not the miasm. Even though the disease-causing organism may be eradicated by antibiotic therapy, subtle energetic traces of the infectious agent may persist at an unseen level. These disease-associated energy traces are incorporated into the individual's biomagnetic field and higher subtle bodies. The miasms reside there until their latent toxic potential is released into the molecular/cellular level of the body, where disruptive changes or illness may manifest. However, the delayed illness which occurs is different than the one associated with the original disease-causing agent. Miasms weaken the natural body defenses in particular areas, creating a tendency toward manifesting different types of illness at a later time. Acquired miasms may be caused by exposure to a variety of noxious agents including bacteria, viruses, toxic chemicals, and even radiation.

Hahnemann was the first homeopath to recognize the existence and influence of miasms. Among the miasms he described were those caused by exposure to the venereal-disease-related organisms of syphilis and gonorrhea. The syphilitic and sycotic (gonorrheal) miasms were felt to cause secondary manifestations of illness even after the primary infection had been cured.

Conventional research has hinted at possible medical models for miasmatic illnesses. For instance, certain viruses may not only produce illness-related symptoms, but their core DNA may incorporate itself into the chromosomes of its human host. There, the silent DNA of the virus (viral DNA) may persist and even be mistakenly replicated along with the body's own chromosomes during cell division. If the viral DNA becomes incorporated into the sex cells of the body (i.e. sperm and egg cells), then the viral DNA may theoretically be passed on to future generations. Under specific types of environmental and internal physiological stresses, the viral DNA may be activated, and the latent virus may come out of its dormant state.

There are some physicians who believe that this theory may apply to the causation of certain types of cancer. Certain tumors, such as carcinoma of the breast, have occasionally revealed the presence of viral particles when examined under the electron microscope. While this evidence does not necessarily substantiate the link between breast cancer and a viral causation, it suggests that viral particles may somehow participate in the formation of certain malignancies. The viruses that are discovered in malignant breast tissue may not be the result of infection as much as the product of a released, latent viral DNA that may have already existed in the cells of the body. In other words, the DNA coding for the expression of these viruses may be passed unknowingly from generation to generation before it becomes expressed in the individual afflicted with breast cancer. The combination of a variety of stresses—biological and environmental, as well as emotional— may work in concert with the viral DNA to create abnormal cellular changes in the body that eventually manifest as a tumor. Although the viral model suggests ways that toxic agents may adversely affect an individual and their future offspring, the primary mechanisms involved in acquired and inherited miasms are usually subtle energetic rather than molecular in nature.

Miasms usually do not involve the physical disruptive effects of the etiologic agents of disease as much as their vibrational effects upon the organism. They create energetic/physiologic influences which predispose the individual to various types of illnesses. Because they can be transmitted from generation to generation, miasms represent an energetic pathway by which events in the life of a parent can be transmitted to their offspring. Miasms provide an interesting interpretation of the statement: "the sins of the father are inherited by the son."

> *Miasms are stored in the subtle bodies, especially the etheric, emotional, mental, and, to a lesser extent, astral bodies. Some miasms are passed on to the next generation genetically by inhabiting the molecular level of the physical body, which is the genetic code. A miasm is not necessarily a disease; it is the potential for a disease.* Indeed, *miasms are a crystallized pattern of karma.* The merger of the soul's forces and ethereal properties determine when a miasm will arise in the physical body to become an active disease. This happens only when the miasm's ethereal pattern projects into the physical body from the subtle bodies. Miasms may lie dormant in the subtle bodies and aura for long periods of time. *They are organized in the subtle bodies, and gradually, through the biomagnetic fields about the physical body, miasms penetrate the molecular level, then the cellular level (individual cells), and finally the physical body...*

There are three types of miasms, including planetary, inherited, and acquired miasms. Planetary miasms are stored in the collective consciousness of the planet and in the ethers. They may penetrate the physical body, but are not stored there. Inherited miasms are stored in the cellular memory of individuals. Acquired miasms are acute or infectious diseases or petrochemical toxicity acquired during a given lifetime. After the acute phase of the illness, these acquired miasmatic traits settle into the subtle bodies and the molecular and cellular levels where they can ultimately cause other problems.[10] *(italics added)*

In Hahnemann's time it was believed that there were three inherited miasms: the psora miasm (somehow linked with psoriasis and skin disorders), the syphilitic miasm (partly caused by syphilis), and the sycotic miasm (partly caused by gonorrhea). The sycotic miasm was associated with disorders in the pelvic/sexual region, skin and digestive systems, and rheumatic afflictions of the joints. A fourth miasm relating to tuberculosis was later recognized as creating a tendency toward respiratory, digestive, and urinary problems. Many of the systems affected by miasmatic tendencies are those same organs which are potential sites of infectious spread during periods of active disease. These vibrational afflictions of various organ systems are said to continue in spite of abatement of the primary infection and "cure" of the illness by appropriate antimicrobial agents. This observation applies especially to the sycotic and tuberculous miasms.

There are, as well, acquired miasms which are due to toxic environmental influences. These miasms have relevance to the study of environmental illness and clinical ecology. They represent a subtle energetic influence which has, thus far, been undetected by the majority of health practitioners who treat occupational illnesses. The three major miasms under this category are the radiation miasm, the petrochemical miasm, and the heavy-metal miasm. To quote from Ryerson's channeled material:

The radiation miasm is associated with the massive increase in background radiation, especially since World War II. It contributes to premature aging, slower cell division, deterioration of the endocrine system, weakening of bone tissues, anemia, arthritis, hair loss, allergies, bacterial inflammations especially in the brain, deterioration of the muscular system, and cancer, especially leukemia and skin cancer. Skin disorders such as lupus, rashes, and loss of skin elasticity occur. Individuals are furthermore subject to hardening of the arteries and the full spectrum of heart diseases. Females are prone to miscarriage and excessive menstrual bleeding, while men experience sterility or a drop in the sperm count. . .

The petrochemical miasm is caused by the major increase in the petroleum and chemical products in society. Some of the problems caused by this miasm include: fluid retention, diabetes, hair loss, infertility, impotence, miscarriages, premature greying of the hair, muscle degenerative diseases, skin blemishes, and thickening of the skin's tissues. Metabolic imbalances that cause excessive storage of fatty tissue may occur. It is harder to resist stress and psychoses, especially classical schizophrenia and autism. Leukemia and cancer of the skin and lymphs also occur. Finally, it is harder to assimilate Vitamin K, circulatory disorders result, and endocrine imbalances occur. . .

At the present time, the heavy metal miasm is cross-indexed with other miasms. For instance, radioactive isotopes often latch onto heavy metals. The contents of this miasm include lead, mercury, radium, arsenic, sulphuric acid, carbon, aluminum, and fluoride. The symptom picture of this developing miasm includes allergies especially from petrochemicals, excessive hair loss, excessive fluid retention, inability to assimilate calcium, and susceptibility to viral inflammations. It is taking longer for this problem to become an inherited miasm for the planet because these minerals have existed in minute degrees in people and in the water and atmosphere for thousands of years. Consequently, a tolerance has developed. This tolerance, however, is for elements that have traditionally existed in the water. *The growing prevalence of these pollutants in the atmosphere is a key factor in this problem becoming an inherited miasm.*[11] *(italics added)*

Various types of environmental pollution from petrochemical, radiation, and heavy-metal sources are becoming more and more pervasive. By and large, the orthodox medical community is not aware of the many diseases associated with these noxious environmental agents, although they acknowledge that they do form some type of health hazard. For example, it is acknowledged that constant exposure to low-level radiation has been linked to leukemia, but the other associations of the radiation miasm have not been addressed by the majority of health care practitioners. These miasms illustrate that there are very few safe levels of radioactive, heavy metal, and petrochemical materials in our environment because, as we have seen, homeopathic doses of these substances are able to induce subtle energetic dysfunction within the human system.

Flower essences (and other vibrational remedies) provide one method of impacting upon the miasmatic tendencies toward illness. Homeopathic remedies have been used in the past for treating miasms, and will likely be useful in treating the newer miasms just outlined. The flower essences offer a slightly different approach toward releasing the potential toxicity of miasms because of their higher energetic effects. Their mechanism of action in the case of miasms is not to directly purify the subtle bodies but to integrate with the higher chakras of the body, and thus allow the consciousness of the individual to move to a level where these energies may be discharged from the bioenergetic system.

> Flower essences do not so much directly abate miasms; they merely create a clear state of consciousness that then affects the personality, the physical body, and the genetic code to entirely eliminate miasms from the physical and subtle bodies. Flower essences that notably influence the crown chakra and subtle bodies weaken all the miasms, so they can be discharged from the system.[12]

A Closer Look at Some of the Newer Flower Essences: Revolutionary Methods of Healing at the Physical & Ethereal Levels

In *Flower Essences And Vibrational Healing*, Gurudas describes 108 new flower essences which are divided into two distinct categories. The first group is characterized by essences that primarily affect the physical body. These essences are unusual in the sense that most flower essences have been used to affect the emotional body, as demonstrated by the Bach Flower Remedies. Gurudas' second group of flower essences are said to work primarily at the level of the subtle bodies, chakras, and various psychological states. The Bach remedies would fit more closely with this second group.

What is most unusual about Gurudas' book is that his descriptions of the effects of the essences upon the human body contain extremely technical biochemical and energetic information about their mechanisms of action. The data which Gurudas has accumulated and organized, derived from channeled information supplied by Kevin Ryerson, not only describes the actions of the essences but fills in gaps of knowledge in understanding the subtle workings of the physical body.

Some of the essences which are said to work at the physical level provide vibrational tools with which to therapeutically impact upon areas as diverse as potentiation of the immune system, enhancement of memory, and stimulation of neuronal reconnections in stroke victims. The explanations of how these essences work are as fascinating as the descriptions of the subtle functioning of the physiologic systems themselves.

In regards to enhancing brain functioning in patients with impaired cognitive and motor abilities, several essences appear to be helpful. The vibrational treatment of neurological disorders has great importance when one considers the limitations of current pharmacologic therapy. Allopathic physicians have a limited number of drugs to offer patients afflicted with neurological diseases. Great strides have been made in the treatment of seizure disorders and Parkinson's disease, but there are many more patients with brain disorders for whom doctors have few treatment strategies. On the other hand, there are numerous flower essences (and gem elixirs) which are said to promote neurological regeneration and assist in rebalancing at both the cellular and subtle energetic levels. It would be useful if Ryerson's channeled information were applied toward experimental validation utilizing such essences to study their effectiveness in stimulating nerve regrowth and repair in existing animal models of neurological dysfunction. One useful flower essence which may enhance neurological function is derived from the white flowers of the Yerba Mate tree, a small evergreen indigenous to Paraguay and Southern Brazil. To quote from the channeled material:

> Yerba Mate increases tissue regeneration of brain cells, yet this is only the subtle aspect. It actually facilitates remapping cell patterns for unused portions of the brain; for instance, if there is damage to the left-hand portion of the brain, the right brain compensates for this. This essence, moreover, increases memory, visualization, and development of the attention span . . .
>
> It is applicable in the full spectrum of mental disease, particularly when psychochemical imbalances cause mental illnesses. It also affects the pituitary gland, which influences the personality far beyond that which western science now understands. In addition, it alleviates the psora miasm. This essence influences the ethereal fluidium, enhancing its role of surrounding and nourishing the cells with the life-force.[13]

Another essence which may also be helpful to patients with impaired cognitive abilities is made from the flowers of the Mugwort, a plant found in Europe and the eastern United States. The Mugwort plant has been used as a medicinal herb since ancient times for treating gout, digestive problems, skin diseases and nerve disorders. While the essences prepared from the flowers of many plants have special therapeutic properties, their effects may often differ from the herbal properties of the roots and stems. In the case of Mugwort, however, many of the herb's therapeutic effects upon nerve tissue are also shared by the flower essence.

Mugwort's most beneficial effect is its ability to reintegrate the synapses and enhance communication between the individual neurons in the brain. For instance, a person with left-brain damage from any cause, especially using creative visualization with this essence, could rechannel the energy from certain neurons, so the damaged portions of the brain could again be used. Brain damage involving the syphilitic miasm can also be treated with this essence. It increases one's IQ, and it helps a person enter the alpha state.

It is a general tonic for all the subtle bodies, meridians, nadis, and chakras. Mugwort helps assimilation of the B vitamins, and on the cellular level, it enhances the properties of RNA.[14]

Another unique essence which might be useful in treating neurological disorders is prepared from the Macartney Rose, a flower native to central and western China. The explanation given in Gurudas' text for its effectiveness is quite interesting if viewed from the perspective of neuronal electrophysiology. Macartney Rose essence apparently can be used to alter the electrical charge carried by neurons. As discussed in Chapter 5, the electrical charge and membrane potential of cells helps to modulate the activity of individual neurons. One can see that the potential benefits of flower essence (and gem elixir) therapy in treating neurological disease may be very significant. It is imperative that clinical studies on animal and human models be conducted to investigate the therapeutic claims contained in Ryerson's material.

Flower essences which are said to have regenerative effects upon the nervous system could assist doctors in treating stroke victims. Currently, all that can be done with individuals suffering from cerebrovascular accidents (strokes) is to prescribe intensive physical therapy, speech therapy, and lifestyle modification. Medical intervention attempts to control the risk factors which may precipitate further strokes, but nothing is actually done to enhance recovery aside from basic retraining of the nervous system. Many elderly patients with decreased brain functioning are unable to regain lost abilities, and may remain semi-paralyzed and bedridden. It appears that specific flower essences (and gem elixirs) might help these seemingly hopeless patients recover neurological function and autonomy. The Macartney Rose essence, for example, may prove helpful in working with various forms of neurological disorders when used in combination with other essences such as Yerba Mate and Mugwort.

This essence increases telepathic abilities. It balances the right and left brain, in part, by increasing the sensitivity of the neurons.

This increased telepathic ability also creates a greater sense of self in comprehending one's total being. Macartney Rose eases epilepsy, alleviates various forms of schizophrenia such as autism, and balances motor neurological tissues.

On the cellular level, Macartney Rose increases the distribution of the RNA and stimulates tissue regeneration of the neurological tissues, particularly in the brain. In addition, it increases the ability of the cellular structure to hold an electrical charge. This has implications in tissue regeneration because electrical charges within cells activate cellular memory. The astral and mental bodies are brought into greater alignment, which also increases telepathy.[15]

A unique point brought up in this quote concerning the actions of Macartney Rose was that telepathic ability was enhanced by this essence. It is interesting to note that this increased telepathic capacity is due to changes produced by the flower essence at both the cellular and subtle levels. At the neuronal level, telepathy may be enhanced by increasing the sensitivity of individual nerve cells to stimuli. At the subtle level, telepathic interactions are augmented because the astral and mental bodies are brought into greater alignment.

Telepathy is a form of subtle communication which occurs between individuals. Telepathy is suggested to occur when thought energies are transmitted from one individual to another. The telepathic effect is somewhat analogous to a kind of energy field resonance between the brains and chakra systems of the telepathic sender and receiver. Thoughts are transmitted not so much in words, but in general content. The brain of the telepathic receiver translates received thought patterns according to symbols, pictures, words, and feelings that are common to the mental vocabularies of both sender and receiver. The telepathic phenomenon is a reflection of energetic resonance between the mind fields of sender and receiver. In other words, thought waves are received and then, by induction, seem to resonate with particular memory circuits of pictures, words, and feelings which the brain uses to interpret the received thought. When telepathy takes place between two individuals, they will frequently arrive at the same thought simultaneously. This is a by-product of resonance induction between mind fields. Often, in conscious telepathy, neither individual can distinguish who first came up with the idea.

More commonly, telepathy occurs between two individuals at a level of higher consciousness. Signal transduction of higher energies occurs through the chakra-nadi and meridian interfaces that link the subtle bodies to the physical nervous system. For telepathic perception to occur at a conscious level, there must be balanced organization of not only the physical brain but also of the subtle energetic systems which feed higher frequency information into the nervous system.

The point to be made here is that flower essences (and gem elixirs) may be helpful in assisting with various types of psychic development. The essences that would be most beneficial in this regard are those that work primarily at ethereal levels of human subtle anatomy. Certain essences, such as California Poppy, may assist an individual to become more balanced and psychically attuned. This essence might assist one in becoming more aware of information originating from past lives, especially those lives that may have bearing on current situations and health problems. The inflow of information from past lives is mediated through the solar plexus chakra and its subtle connections to the astral body. One's ability to access various types of higher energetic information, especially that originating in past lifetimes, depends upon proper alignment and functioning of the chakras and the subtle bodies. The California Poppy essence seems to help our subtle anatomy to achieve this balance and alignment.

> The need for psychic and spiritual balance is a major indication for prescribing this essence. A sense of inner balance is maintained during psychic awakening. Past life information and psychic information in general are released and properly integrated. Much of this information is released through dreams. Used over a six-month period, people would start seeing auras and nature spirits.
>
> The essence creates these effects because it aligns the mental, causal, and spiritual bodies with the astral body to release past life and psychic information in a coordinated pattern. The integration point of this psychic information is the solar plexus region because past life information residing in the astral body enters the physical body through the solar plexus. The other three bodies assist in this process.
>
> It moderately invigorates the pineal and pituitary glands, but this is more the etheric portion of the glands. On the cellular level, it oxygenates the circulatory system. Morever, it facilitates the ingestion of vitamin A. Since the psychic qualities in the eyes are strengthened, telepathic and clairvoyant vision is stimulated. The eyes are the physical vehicle involved in clairvoyantly seeing auras and nature spirits.[16]

The issue of aligning the subtle bodies and chakras in order to attain meaningful insight is a pervasive one throughout Gurudas' book. It becomes quite clear by the end of the book that the personality and its physical body are unable to reach harmony and inner balance unless true alignment of the spiritual with the physical vehicle occurs. Although the subtle energetic alignment must involve spiritual work by the individual to achieve this integration, the flower essences (and gem elixirs) offer vibrational assistance which may augment and accelerate this natural process of enlightenment.

Another essence which appears to be complementary in respect to the ethereal integrating effects of California Poppy is the essence prepared from the flowers of the plant known as Angelica. This flower is native to Europe and Asia, and has been used to treat certain forms of nervous tension. Angelica is a good example of a flower essence which might be used in conjunction with various forms of psychotherapy, biofeedback, and meditation. It is said to help the individual to connect in a more meaningful way to information flowing from the Higher Self. In this way, meaningful personal insight may be gained at an accelerated pace via the use of essences such as Angelica in conjunction with various psychotherapeutic integrative techniques.

> This is an excellent remedy to use with meditation and many forms of psychotherapy. This essence actualizes clearer insight into the cause and nature of problems, but it does not create a solution. For instance, it helps an alcoholic understand the nature of his or her problem, but other remedies would usually be needed to ease the problem...
>
> When pondering a problem, Angelica provides intellectual or rational information to resolve the issue, but it does not actually solve the problem. This takes place because higher information manifests in the individual. This higher information manifests because Angelica integrates and aligns all the chakras, nadis, meridians, and subtle bodies, but it does this without actually strengthening or changing these forces...
>
> Angelica augments the nervous system, particularly by connecting the sympathetic and autonomic nervous systems. Many neurological disturbances such as epilepsy can be treated with Angelica. Furthermore, it enhances the effectiveness of the mind to extend and actually control all portions of the physical body. Thus, this is a fine essence to use in biofeedback, hypnosis, and hypnotherapy.[17]

Ryerson's channeled information suggests that various flower essences may augment many of the currently existing forms of medical and psychological therapies. For instance, the use of visualization to augment the immune response of cancer patients is well known to practitioners of holistic

medicine. Various types of flower essences might be used to assist psychological growth techniques which are already being applied as adjunctive
therapies. Flower essences may even aid the body in tolerating the effects
of anti-cancer treatments. In regards to working with cancer patients, the
essence prepared from the flowers of the Spruce tree (an evergreen native
to the Rocky Mountains) seems to offer the ability to detoxify the body and
prevent the side effects of chemotherapy and radiation.

> Spruce is good to use during a detoxification program; for in-
> stance, when people have been exposed to various pollutants such
> as asbestos. This is also an excellent remedy to take when undergo-
> ing chemotherapy or radiation therapy. It detoxifies the body to pre-
> vent side effects developing. But once disease is manifest in the
> physical body, other essences should be used. . .
> Spruce should be considered when there is a general disorien-
> tation or lack of direction in a person. This tends to happen when the
> etheric and physical bodies are not properly connected. This essence
> bonds the etheric body closer to the physical body by enhancing the
> ethereal fluidium. This is important because a loose knitting between
> the etheric and physical bodies often leads to diseases such as cancer,
> even though the outer subtle bodies may be aligned. You might call
> this imbalance a precancerous state on the level of the subtle bodies.
> Therefore, when there is a high level of toxicity present this is an ex-
> cellent remedy which may prevent cancer from developing.[18]

It has become increasingly clear that a multidisciplinary approach to
achieving health and inner balance is the only technique that will have
lasting effectiveness. Flower essences offer us a unique vibrational tool
which can help mobilize the unseen subtle energetic factors of health and
illness in the direction of greater balance and homeostasis. These essences
set the stage for positive patterns of growth and alignment. But flower
essences (and gem elixirs) must work in conjunction with natural cellular
and subtle energetic systems to allow the body, mind, and spirit to reachieve
proper orientation and balance along the most natural routes.

Although only a small number of flower essences have been discussed
here, the remaining essences mentioned in Gurudas' book seem to offer
significant advances in treating a variety of illnesses many of which have
no effective medical or surgical therapies at this time. Ryerson's channeled
information offers us a greater understanding of the subtle energetic interplay between consciousness and human illness. With continued research
over the next 20 to 30 years, many of the new flower essences introduced
by Gurudas have the potential to revolutionize the art of healing and our

understanding of humans as spiritual beings.

Gem Elixirs & Chromotherapy:
Further Explorations into Healing with Vibration

The basic property of water as a universal storage medium of vibrational energy allows other types of therapeutic essences to be prepared utilizing the sun method. Already alluded to in the earlier material are the gem elixirs. These are prepared by placing one or several gems of a particular crystalline nature into pure spring or distilled water, leaving the combination in direct sunlight for several hours during the early morning sun. The solar energies are most potent in their pranic forces in the early hours of the day. As with the flowers, certain etheric properties from the gems become transferred to the water, which becomes charged with their particular vibrational characteristics.

Following the publication of Gurudas' first book, two further volumes dedicated to the uses of crystals and gem elixirs were released. These two texts, *Gem Elixirs and Vibrational Healing, Volumes I and II,* are similarly compiled from information channeled by Kevin Ryerson and Jon Fox. Both books offer detailed descriptions of the historical origins and vibrational properties of many gem elixirs, as well as a variety of charts compiling their potential uses for different ailments and energetic imbalances. In addition, there is a section describing case histories and therapeutic successes in the use of gem elixirs and flower essences for various disorders, based upon feedback Gurudas has received from practitioners utilizing his vibrational preparations.

There are unique energetic differences between flower essences and gem elixirs in regard to their therapeutic benefits in healing illness.

Gemstones function between flower essences and homeopathic remedies. When a physical gemstone is ingested after being crushed, it is closer to homeopathy and notably influences the physical body with medicinal, nutritional, and antibiotic properties. When a gem is prepared into an elixir, however, using the sun in a method similar to preparing flower essences, that remedy functions slightly closer to flower essences and is more ethereal in its properties.

With either method of preparation gems influence specific organs in the physical body, while homeopathic remedies have a wider impact on the entire physical body. Gems carry the pattern of a crystalline structure, which focuses the physical body's mineral and crystalline structures on the biomolecular level; therefore gems work more closely with the biomolecular structure to integrate the life force into the body. Finally, gems function between the other two systems of vibrational medicine because they have a stronger impact on the ethereal fluidium. Flower essences come from the living vehicle that holds the pattern of consciousness, while gems amplify consciousness.[19]

Diagram 25 is a general guideline to the energetic differences between various vibrational modalities in their abilities to affect the many bioenergetic levels of human functioning.

Diagram 25.
LEVELS OF ACTION OF VIBRATIONAL ESSENCES

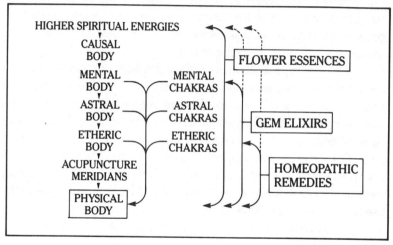

In the above chart, the solid darker lines and arrows indicate the spectrum of areas where each vibrational remedy has its strongest effect. As indicated, various flower essences may strongly influence all levels of the multidimensional human system, from the physical/biomolecular levels on up to the higher subtle and soul levels. The dotted lines and arrows in the chart indicate significant action of individual remedies and elixirs at higher energetic levels where there may be a lesser degree of strength of action. For instance, most commonly used homeopathic remedies operate strongly at the level of the physical/molecular and biomagnetic fields of the body. However, many homeopathic remedies can affect higher levels like the chakras and subtle bodies, but less often and less effectively than the other modalities. Also, certain gem elixirs (and homeopathics) are capable of affecting the causal and higher spiritual bodies. Therefore, the distinction between levels of energetic action affected by homeopathics, gem elixirs, and flower essences is less clear-cut than the chart might imply.

The chart gives a general idea of the energetic levels at which various commonly used vibrational essences and remedies may have their effects. Individual homeopathic remedies and gem elixirs may be capable of stronger effects at the higher subtle levels than the chart would suggest at first glance, and so this must be kept in mind. It is perhaps unfair to compare such vibrational remedies in their efficacy at the various levels because each different modality is capable of rather dramatic healing influences on a wide variety of psychospiritual and physical illnesses. The analysis of energetic level of influence is more a general systems approach to vibrational healing and is presented more for its teaching value than for its applicability to each individual essence or remedy.

Gem elixirs as a form of vibrational therapy are able to amplify the energies already moving through the subtle structures of higher dimensional anatomy. Gem elixirs help to balance the physical body with the subtle bodies in a way that is closer to the flower essences, but they do not contain the energy of the life-force to the same extent as do flower essences. Gem elixirs operate on the principle of sympathetic vibrational resonance. Gemstones and crystals have a unique molecular arrangement of geometrical symmetry. The geometrical symmetry of crystalline structure also has unique, frequency-specific vibrational properties which are transferred to water during etheric imprinting via the sun method of gem elixir preparation. The molecular regularity of crystalline structures offers a stabilizing energetic influence to cellular and biomolecular systems within the physical body. Certain gemstones have a special harmonic resonance with particular points of human physical anatomy. Healing through the use of gem elixirs takes place when crystalline patterns stored in the elixir are resonantly transferred to unstable biomolecular structures within the diseased physical body. As vibrational energy is transferred to specific molecular systems within the body, stabilization of biochemical processes causes increased cellular organization, organ repair, and a general shift toward physical health.

Gem elixirs also affect the psychospiritual dynamics of individuals. When they work at this level, they influence the subtle structures of consciousness more than the molecular chemistry of the physical body. Gem elixirs can have powerful effects upon the meridians, chakras, and subtle bodies. By modifying the subtle elements that contribute to conscious awareness, they may promote illumination that can eventually lead to behavioral modification. By themselves, they do not influence behavior so much as the consciousness upon which behavior is based. As illumination is assisted by taking gem elixirs, the individual can better focus upon inner problems or decision-making.

Although gem elixirs work more closely to the physical body than many flower essences, they can still work on various levels of consciousness. Gem elixirs, like flower essences, are tinctures of liquid consciousness containing evolutionary patterns of the life-force itself. When gem elixirs are ingested, they become an evolutionary force that may stimulate inspiration and eventual change in the consciousness of the individual. The elixirs are not the causative force behind change, but they can be the inspiration behind such causal forces. Unlike flower essences, however, gem elixirs may work strictly at the biomolecular level of the physical body without directly influencing the psychospiritual dynamics of the individual.

Ryerson's material suggests that gem elixirs are also slightly different in their effects upon the acupuncture meridians of the body. When flower essences are used, they tend to affect specific meridians in the body. Gem elixirs, however, tend to influence all the meridians of the body. When gem elixirs affect specific meridians, their energetic influence tends to spread to the other meridians through the terminal or command acupoints located in the fingers and toes. This is a phenomenon that does not occur with flower essences. This effect may be partly due to the more powerful vibratory effect of gemstones.

Another interesting vibrational remedy, which can be prepared without the use of either flowers or gems, is color tinctures. Distilled water may be placed in direct sunlight in either a bottle of colored glass or one which has been wrapped with colored plastic. During exposure to the pranic forces of sunlight, the water becomes charged with the energetic frequency of the particular color filter used. The use of color in healing is unique in that the pure energies of light are used therapeutically in a variety of forms. The essence prepared from the color treatment can be given orally to treat a variety of disorders. Color therapy, or chromotherapy, has many forms and applications. The use of color tinctures (or hydrochromatic therapy) is a less known form of color therapy, but it demonstrates the principle by which water may be imprinted with a variety of vibrational characteristics for the purposes of healing.

Color therapy is not new to the twentieth century. This unique art was

Diagram 26.
SUBTLE ENERGETIC EFFECTS OF COLOR

COLOR	CHAKRA	ENERGIES	DISEASES AFFECTED
VIOLET	Crown Chakra	Higher Mind	Nervous & Mental Disorders
INDIGO	Third-Eye Chakra	Vision	Disorders of the Eye
BLUE	Throat Chakra	Self-Expression	Thyroid & Laryngeal Diseases
GREEN	Heart Chakra	Inner Harmony	Heart Disease & Hypertension
YELLOW	Solar Plexus Chakra	Intellectual Stimulation	Disorders of Stomach, Pancreas & Liver
ORANGE	Spleen Chakra	Assimilation Circulation	Disorders of Lungs & Kidneys
RED	Root Chakra	Vitality Creativity	Blood Disorders Anemias

applied in ancient times in the healing temples of light and color at Heliopolos in Egypt, as well as in early Greece, China, and India. Of modern researchers, Edwin Babbitt[20] and Dinshah Ghadiali[21] are among the most prominent pioneers mentioned in the color therapy literature. Many esoteric color theorists feel that the colors of light in the visible spectrum are lower octaves of higher vibrational energies that contribute to the auric field and subtle bodies. Esoteric sources refer to these higher octaves as the seven major rays which influence the personality nature and growth of the soul. These seven rays are of celestial origin. Their characteristics are beyond the scope of this textbook, but specific references provided at the end of the chapter may be sought for further details.

Each major visible color has particular qualities that are linked to the chakra with which it resonates. An understanding of the nature of the chakras and their higher energetic links to body physiology helps one to understand the reasons for using particular colors to heal specific illnesses. For instance red, being of the lowest frequency energy, resonates with the first or root chakra in the coccygeal region. Because the root chakra regulates the vitality of the physical body, disorders such as anemia, which are associated with severe fatigue, can sometimes be treated by exposing the body to light in the red spectrum. Ingestion of water charged with the frequencies of the color red may be used instead of direct therapy with red light rays.

Certain color therapists feel that the lower two chakras, the root and splenic chakra, mirror the energetic relationships between the physical and etheric bodies. The root chakra resonates with the lower frequency physical energies, while the splenic chakra processes energy of an etheric frequency. While red stimulates the root chakra and physical vitality, the orange ray energizes the splenic chakra and strengthens the etheric body. Because the etheric and physical body are so interrelated, these two lower chakras are sometimes dealt with as a single unit.

The splenic chakra also acts as a type of intermediary between the etheric and astral energies. Orange light affecting the splenic chakra may also therefore modify an individual's emotional nature. Because it stimulates the splenic chakra, an important center which directs prana flow throughout the body, the use of the orange ray may also affect the processes of assimilation, circulation, and distribution of pranic energy. At the physical level, diseases of the lungs have been treated by the use of the orange ray. Breathing is a process of energy assimilation through the lungs. Both life-giving oxygen and vitalizing prana are absorbed into the pulmonary system and distributed throughout the body via the bloodstream. Because the orange ray seems able to augment pranic energy assimilation, disorders of the lungs and airways which interfere with this process (i.e. asthma, emphysema, and bronchitis) might benefit from orange light therapy.

The yellow ray stimulates the solar plexus chakra, which is linked at the physical level to the major digestive nerve plexus in the same region. The so-called solar plexus nerve ganglion is actually considered to be a type of visceral brain. This "lower mind" of the body is felt to regulate, at a physical level, the digestive processes through the gastrointestinal system. The solar plexus chakra is tied in to the higher astral and lower mental forces. Thus, the lower mind is considered to be the objective, material mind which is affected by various emotional influences. The yellow rays are assumed to have a stimulating effect upon our rational, thinking, and intellectual nature. In the auric field, yellow is usually associated with the color of intellect and the use of the mind in concrete, scholarly ways. Because many individuals with various stress-related disorders, such as ulcers, tend to be mentally focused and sometimes emotionally repressed, the yellow ray can be helpful in treating various types of stomach problems and indigestion.

The green ray resonates most vibrantly with the heart chakra. At a higher energetic level, the heart chakra processes energies associated with the higher mental body as well as with the higher emotional energies such as love and compassion. The green ray is a vibration of harmony and balance and is naturally radiated by the verdant foliage of nature. The green ray also exercises some control over distribution of the blood supply through its effects upon the heart. Many heart diseases have their root in the emotional nature or astral body. Strong emotion is an exacerbating factor in many types of angina pains. Because of its balancing effects upon the heart and its soothing influences upon the sympathetic nervous system, the green ray could prove useful in treating heart disease and hypertension.

The upper three chakras are closely connected with the spiritual nature of human beings. They mediate the integration of higher spiritual forces into the physical personality, while the lower three chakras regulate more of an individual's physical nature. The heart chakra stands as a midpoint between the two worlds of spirit and matter. For spiritual energy to ascend up the kundalini pathway from the root chakra to the crown center, each chakra along the path of energy ascent must be unblocked. Thus, it is no coincidence that an ability to freely express love and harmony through an open heart chakra appears to be an important personality trait for the full blossoming of one's psychic and spiritual gifts of perception.

The throat chakra is the first of the spiritual triad of higher centers, and it resonates most vibrantly with the blue ray. The throat chakra is the center of communication and self-expression. At the psychic level, this chakra is associated with clairaudience, or the ability to hear things at a subtle energetic level. The throat chakra is also the center of religious devotion and the mystical instinct, partly because of its association with the energies of the causal body. This center is sometimes referred to as the center of will or power. Since personal power is often a reflection of freely verbalized inner feelings as well as an exertion of one's will upon others through the use of the voice, the association seems most appropriate. Disorders treated by the blue ray revolve around diseases in the throat area that interfere with the will and the verbal expression of thoughts and ideas. Laryngitis, sore throats, and goiters may improve significantly after treatment with subtle energies of the blue ray.

The energies of the brow or third-eye chakra are so named because of this center's association with the psychic gift of clairvoyance. This chakra presides over the higher spiritual phenomena of the soul. The opening and proper functioning of the third-eye chakra is usually seen in those who are highly developed at the intuitive level. The color indigo resonates most forcefully with this center. Indigo appears to control physical and higher aspects of vision as well as olfaction (smell) and physical hearing. Various types of eye diseases, like cataracts, may be treated by the subtle energies of the indigo ray. Indigo may also be helpful in treating disorders of hearing and loss of smell.

Lastly, the violet ray is associated with the crown chakra. The crown chakra is considered by many to be the sanctuary of the spirit, or the gateway to the highest spiritual influences that can affect human beings. The main areas which the violet ray seems to influence are the physical brain and the spiritual nature of the higher mind. Leonardo da Vinci maintained that the power of meditation could be enhanced tenfold if carried out under the influence of violet rays passing through the stained glass windows of a quiet church.[22] Violet is felt to provide nourishment of a subtle energetic nature to those neurons in the cerebral cortex that contribute toward a greater understanding of our divine nature. Because the violet ray has positive therapeutic effects upon various mental and nervous disorders, it may be effective in relieving headaches, neuroses, and even certain forms of schizophrenia and dementia.

There are intricate systems and approaches to color healing which are utilized by various practitioners. The general outline of the effects of color therapy which has been presented here is of a highly simplified nature. The selective use of color vibrations to treat human illness is a complex and intricate healing art. Colors may be applied alone or in special therapeutic combinations which tend to enhance the potential of color healing through synergistic effects. The forms by which the frequencies of color may be transmitted to patients are numerous. These methods include direct lighting from electric lamps (or natural sunlight) which has passed through various types of color screens and filters, as well as hydrochromatic therapy, which utilizes color-solarized water.

Other forms of therapy include color breathing. A physical-etheric method of color breathing involves deeply inhaling air that has been pranically charged with the energies of a particular color. A more common method of color breathing involves visualizing oneself breathing in a particular color during the inspiratory phase of respiration. Following inspiration, the visualized color is mentally directed to areas of illness, blockage, and dysfunction, or to those bodily systems which are in need of vitalization. There are many variations on this particular technique of color breathing which allow visualized colors to be used for altering the level of one's consciousness and for cleansing the chakras, as well as for achieving particular types of healing. Color breathing at the mental level involves directing energies that work with the mental and astral bodies and chakras.

In general, visualization of the color, gem, or flower being vibrationally applied (through tinctures, essences, etc.) can powerfully augment the effectiveness of the treatment. Mental affirmations—inwardly spoken statements that reaffirm the desired physical or emotional change—can also be helpful in amplifying the efficacy of the various vibrational therapies. Many of the older Bach flower therapists gave their patients specific affirmations to use with the prescribed combination of flower remedies. The more the individual becomes actively involved with the therapy (either vibrational or allopathic), as in the use of visualization and affirmations, the greater the chances are for a successful healing outcome to occur.

The Healing Power of Sunlight & Water: New Revelations in Understanding the Vibrational Gifts of Nature

The significance of healing with tinctures of color, gem elixirs, and flower essences is that the physical body may be therapeutically affected in profound ways by the most simple ingredients found in nature. The plants and flowers of the field are most abundant upon the planet we inhabit. The strata of the earth contains numerous gems and minerals which hold undreamt-of subtle energetic healing potentials. The unifying forces—sun and water—that allow these energetic sources of natural healing to influence the human organism, are the most abundant resources on the planet which we inhabit.

By combining the subtle energetic storage properties of water with the pranic-charging capabilities of sunlight, early researchers of vibrational medicine created a simple yet powerful method of extracting key healing frequencies from nature. The physiological effects produced by such ethereal medicines are difficult to detect by most medical systems. Their effects, as their name implies, are so subtle in quality that current methods of medical monitoring are inadequate for recording the hard proof demanded by a skeptical scientific community. It is only with the acceptance of electro-acupuncture, and radionic, Kirlian, and other etheric-based technologies, that the subtle energetic effectiveness of particular vibrational medicines can be measured and substantiated.

As discussed in an earlier chapter, technologies such as the Voll Machine utilize the network of acupuncture points to create a diagnostic interface with the meridians of the physical body. The meridian system is part of an energetic grid which moves the life-force energies from the etheric into the physical body via a special mechanism known as the physical-etheric inte: - face. The energies of the subtle bodies are intimately connected to the physical body through this unique interface. Because of this natural energetic linkup, EAV monitoring of the acupuncture points can provide an accurate indication of specific needs for flower essences and vibrational remedies.

A number of EAV practitioners have researched the application of the Voll Machine for prescribing flower essences as well as homeopathic remedies. One pioneer in this field of endeavor is Dr. Abram Ber, mentioned in Chapter 6. Dr. Ber has successfully experimented with the use of the Voll Machine in prescribing Bach Flower Remedies. Dr. Ber has also investigated the Voll Machine's ability to determine patients' energetic needs for some of Gurudas' new flower essences. Ber empirically found a strong correlation between the flower essences which produced acupoint resonance reactions in asthmatic patients and the particular essences listed as useful in treating asthma in the book *Flower Essences and Vibrational Healing.*

Utilizing the EAV method, Ber studied a young boy that had been referred to him for pituitary growth failure and dwarfism. Previous medical attempts to alter the boy's height had been unsuccessful. Dr. Ber gave the boy a combination remedy prepared from multiple flower essences which had produced positive reactions on the Voll Machine. As it turned out, these were also the essences listed in *Flower Essences and Vibrational Healing* which were recommended for the treatment of growth failure. After a two-month period of using the combination flower-essence mixture, the boy achieved a remarkable growth spurt of approximately two inches. Although this is an anecdotal case history, it tends to substantiate the potential usefulness of flower essences for treatment, as well as the utility of using Voll and other EAV based technologies for both medical diagnosis and the pinpointing of appropriate therapies. Meridian-based technologies offer a unique diagnostic potential for discovering vibrational medicines that may offer effective therapy to patients whose diseases might otherwise be deemed untreatable. To quote from Ryerson's channeling:

> There shall be large advancements made in this particular field
> when instruments, that are approximately in current levels of develop-
> ment and shall be of more popular level and knowledge in the public

consciousness in approximately three to five years, for measuring the existence of the ethereal anatomies, come into focus and play. For these shall eventually be the instruments that are used to evolve and isolate through scientific method and practice the impact of various forms of vibrational therapies, including flower essences, homeopathic remedies, and gem elixirs upon the subtle anatomies. When these become an accepted isolated science, it is then that these ethereal properties will reach the greatest level of appreciation.

Some of these instruments are, in part, in use, such as those which measure the activities of brain waves, those which measure the capacities of neurological points relative to acupuncture, galvanic skin response, and above all those that measure the pulsation of biomagnetic energy from cellular division. These machines allow for measuring the physiological responses of the body physical when the essences are prescribed. They will likewise allow for the scrutinization in laboratory tests the potency of the essences and their fields of effect in same.

As is given, the subject material on flower essences is as staggering in its implications, particularly if they were to become the complete medicine. The content and nature of using them as medicine in these days would reintegrate man's focus upon his link vibrationally with nature through a particular area of study, concentrating on healing. Eventually, the entire emphasis must become reintegrated with the entirety of these energies.[23]

A deeper understanding of how these abundant tools of vibrational healing can have beneficial effects upon emotional and physical disease is predicated on a working knowledge of human subtle energetic anatomy. The chakras, the nadis, the meridians, and the subtle bodies are inseparable parts of our extended anatomy. These subtle structures allow us to interface with the multidimensional universe which we are an integral part of. The subtle bodies serve specific functions that influence how the personality of the individual expresses itself upon the physical plane. The subtle forces help to determine the vitality, purpose, and creative expression of human beings as they work to understand their lives upon the Earth/ School of Life into which they have chosen to incarnate.

When the connections between the Higher Self and the physical personality become interrupted or blocked, egocentrism, alienation, and feelings of separation occur. The flower essences, gem elixirs, color tinctures, and homeopathic remedies work at the level of the biomolecular structure of the physical body as well as the subtle bodies, meridians, and chakras to increase the coordination and harmony between the physical self and its higher energetic influences. If used properly, these natural vibrational remedies may alter the course of illness at the physical, emotional, mental, and spiritual levels of experience, and facilitate a more comprehensive and lasting healing of the human mind/body/spirit complex. As the physicians/healers of our culture begin to acknowledge the spectrum of subtle energies that influence the human form, there will be an abundance of information produced on new ways of healing which will ultimately uplift the spirit of humankind.

Key Points to Remember

1. Vibrational medicines, such as flower essences, gem elixirs, and homeopathic remedies, are derived from various biological and mineral sources. These unique medicines utilize the energetic storage properties of water to transfer a frequency-specific, information-bearing quantum of subtle energy to the patient in order to effect healing at various levels of human functioning.

2. Dr. Edward Bach was a pioneer in the development of flower essences—the so-called Bach Flower Remedies. These remedies are used primarily to balance the mental and emotional energies of the individual which, if unbalanced, can predispose to, as well as exacerbate, the various physical manifestations of illness. Bach was a sensitive, and used his intuitive abilities to define the various healing qualities of the Bach remedies.

3. More recent research has focused upon sources of intuitively derived information to examine and explore the uses of many other flower essences for healing. Certain sources of channeled information suggest that flower essences may be helpful in healing both at the physical level as well as at the subtle levels of human functioning.

4. Because flowers contain the very essence and life-force of the plant from which they are derived, tinctures and essences prepared by the sun method actually transfer an aspect of this life-force to the remedy.

5. When vibrational remedies, such as flower essences, are taken internally, their energies are amplified and assimilated with the assistance of a unique biocrystalline energy system within the physical body. This crystalline system has certain qualities similar to quartz,

which allow a resonant transfer of the remedies' energies into the physical body in order to reach the subtle bodies.

6. Through its link with the pineal gland, this biocrystalline network helps to coordinate information transfer from the higher dimensional aspects of consciousness (i.e, the astral, mental, and causal levels) to the physical personality by way of the right cerebral hemisphere. This higher information appears in the form of dreams and symbolic imagery during meditation, which can be analyzed by the left brain for meaning. Flower essences can help strengthen this inner connection, and thus help reconnect the personality to the Higher Self.

7. Certain flower essences are said to work primarily at the cellular level, while other essences affect the more subtle levels of functioning, i.e. the chakras and nadis, meridians, and subtle bodies.

8. Miasms represent a unique energetic state which, in itself, is not an illness, but predisposes the individual to illness. The most common miasms are acquired through exposure to various bacteria, viruses, and toxic agents. They can also be inherited along familial lines. Miasms can be treated and neutralized using specific homeopathic remedies, as well as particular flower essences and gem elixirs.

9. In addition to making flower essences via the sun method, water can be charged with the subtle energies of crystals, or with the pure vibrations of colored light in order to provide another source of energetic healing. These therapeutic modalities are referred to as gem elixirs and color tinctures, respectively.

10. The color energies have their effects primarily because certain color frequencies resonate strongly with particular chakras. Through resonant energy exchange, the color frequencies energize and rebalance chakras which may be abnormal or blocked as a reflection of the disease process. By balancing the dysfunctional chakra, the proper flow of subtle energies are re-established to the diseased organ system.

11. Electroacupuncture systems, such as the Voll Machine, may be useful in matching the subtle frequencies of the various vibrational essences with specific disease states and energetic imbalances. Through research and experimental validation using such devices, flower essences and other vibrational remedies will eventually gain acceptance as useful healing modalities.

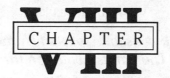

CHAPTER

The Phenomenon of Psychic Healing:

EXPLORING THE EVIDENCE FOR AN UNDISCOVERED HUMAN POTENTIAL

In the last several chapters we have examined various systems of subtle energy healing. Most of these methods involve the therapeutic application of different frequencies of vibrational energies that occur within nature. For example, the healing qualities of flower essences, gem elixirs, color tinctures, and homeopathic remedies are used to treat illness by supplying a frequency of vibration that is needed by the human energy system. It is also possible to transmit energies of a healing nature to individuals in need without having to depend upon external sources of vibrational energies. The multi-dimensional human energy field is a unique transmitter and receiver of vibrational energies.

Various esoteric sources have long suggested that human beings are capable of healing one another by utilizing the special energy potentials which are brought into each lifetime. This healing ability has had many names through the centuries, including laying-on-of-hands healing, psychic healing, spiritual healing, and Therapeutic Touch. Only in the last several decades has modern technology and the consciousness of enlightened scientists evolved to the point where laboratory confirmation of subtle energetic healing has been made possible. Although certain aspects of these laboratory findings have been touched upon in earlier chapters, we will now re-examine these studies in a fuller perspective as we examine the history of our growing understanding of psychic healing.

Psychic Healing as an Aspect of Human Potential: An Historical Look at Its Evolution through the Ages

The use of laying-on-of-hands to heal human illness dates back thousands of years in human history. Evidence for its use in ancient Egypt is found in the Ebers Papyrus dated at about 1552 B.C. This document describes the use of laying-on-of-hands healing for medical treatment. Four centuries before the birth of Christ, the Greeks used Therapeutic Touch therapy in their Asklepian temples for healing the sick. The writings of Aristophanes detail the use of laying-on-of-hands in Athens to restore a blind man's sight and return fertility to a barren woman.[1]

The Bible has many references to the laying-on-of-hands for both medical and spiritual applications. It is well known that many of the miraculous healings of Jesus were done by the laying-on-of-hands. Jesus said, "These things that I do, so can ye do and more." Laying-on-of-hands healing was considered part of the work of the early Christian ministry as much as preaching and administering the sacraments. In the early Christian church, laying-on-of-hands was combined with the sacramental use of holy water and oil.

Over the following hundreds of years, the healing ministry of the Church began to gradually decline. In Europe the healing ministry was carried on as the royal touch. Kings of several European countries were purportedly successful in curing diseases such as tuberculosis (scrofula) by laying-on-of-hands. In England, this method of healing began with Edward the Confessor, lasted for seven centuries, and ended with the reign of the skeptical William IV. Many of the early attempts at laying-on-of-hands healing seemed to be predicated upon a belief either in the powers of Jesus, or the king, or a particular healer. There were other contemporary medical theorists who felt that special vital forces and influences in nature were the mediators of these healing effects.

A number of early researchers into the mechanisms of healing theorized on the likely magnetic nature of the energies involved. One of the earliest proponents of a magnetic vital force of nature was the controversial physician Theophrastus Bombastus von Hohenheim, otherwise known as Paracelsus (1493-1541). In addition to his discoveries of new drug therapies, Paracelsus founded the sympathetic system of medicine, according to which the stars and other bodies (especially magnets) influenced humans by means of a subtle emanation or fluid that pervaded all space. His theory was an attempt to explain the apparent link between human beings and the stars and other heavenly bodies. Paracelsus' sympathetic system may be viewed as an early astrological insight into the influences of the planets and stars on human illness and behavior.

The proposed link between humans and the heavens above was through a subtle pervasive fluid, perhaps an early construct of the "ether," which existed throughout the universe. He attributed *magnetic* qualities to this subtle substance and felt that it possessed unique qualities of healing. He also concluded that if this force was possessed or wielded by someone, then that person could arrest or heal diseases in others. Paracelsus stated that *the vital force was not enclosed inside an individual but radiated within and around him or her like a luminous sphere which could be made to act at a distance.*[2] Considering the accuracy of his description of the energies surrounding people, one wonders whether or not Paracelsus could clairvoyantly observe the human auric field.

In the century following Paracelsus' death, the magnetic tradition was carried on by Robert Fludd, a physician and a mystic. Fludd was considered to be one of the most prominent alchemical theorists of the early seventeenth century. He emphasized *the role of the sun in health as a source of light and life. The sun was considered the purveyor of life beams required for all living creatures on earth.* Fludd felt that this supercelestial and invisible force in some way manifested in all living things and that *it entered the body through the breath.*[3] One is reminded of the Indian concept of *prana*, the subtle energy within sunlight which is assimilated through the process of breathing. Many esotericists feel that by mentally directing the visualized stream of inhaled prana, healers may focus this etheric energy through their hands and into the patient. Fludd also believed that the human being possessed the qualities of a magnet.

In 1778 a radical healer stepped forward to say that he could achieve remarkable therapeutic success without the need for patients' faith in the healing powers of Jesus or himself. Franz Anton Mesmer claimed that the healing results which he obtained came through the enlightened use of a universal energy which he called fluidum.[4] (There is an interesting similarity between the terminology of Mesmer's fluidum and the ethereal fluidium mentioned in Ryerson's channeled material, i.e. the substance of the etheric body.) Mesmer claimed that fluidum was a subtle physical fluid that filled the universe, and was the connecting medium between people and other living things, and between living organisms, the earth, and the heavenly bodies. (This theory is quite similar to Paracelsus' astrological concept of sympathetic medicine.) Mesmer suggested that all things in nature possessed a particular power which manifested itself through special actions upon other bodies. He felt that all physical bodies, animals, plants, and even stones were impregnated with this magical fluid.

During his early medical research in Vienna, Mesmer discovered that placing a magnet over areas of the body afflicted with disease would often effect a cure. Experiments with patients who had nervous disorders often produced unusual motor effects. Mesmer noted that successful magnetic treatments frequently induced pronounced muscle spasms and jerks. He came to believe that the magnets he used for therapy were mainly conductors of an ethereal fluid which issued forth from his own body to create subtle healing effects in patients. *He considered this vital force or fluid to be of a magnetic nature, referring to it as "animal magnetism"* (to distinguish it from mineral or ferromagnetism).

Through his research, Mesmer came to believe that this subtle energetic fluid was somehow associated with the nervous system, especially when his treatments would often cause involuntary muscle spasms and tremors. He hypothesized that the nerve and body fluids conveyed the fluidum to all areas of the body, where it animated and revitalized those parts. Mesmer's concept of fluidum is reminiscent of the ancient Chinese theory of ch'i energy which flows through the meridians, feeding the vital force to the nerves and tissues of the body.

Mesmer realized that the life-sustaining and regulating actions of the magnetic fluidum were integral to the basic processes of homeostasis and health. When the individual was in a state of health, he or she was considered to be in harmony with these most basic laws of nature, as expressed by a proper interplay of the vital magnetic forces. If disharmony occurred between the physical body and these subtle forces of nature, sickness was the end result. Mesmer later realized that the best source of this universal force was the human body itself. He felt that the most active points of energetic flow were from the palms of the hands. By placing the practitioner's hands on patients for direct healing, energy was allowed a direct route to flow from healer to patient. Because of Mesmer's influence during this revolutionary period in French history, the technique of laying-on-of-hands, otherwise known as "magnetic passes," became quite popular.

Unfortunately, many scientific observers at the time considered Mesmerism to be merely an act of hypnosis and suggestion. (To this day, many scientists still refer to hypnosis as "mesmerism," thus the origin of the term "mesmerized.") In 1784, the king of France appointed a commission of inquiry into the validity of Mesmer's experiments in healing. Among the commission were members of the Academy of Sciences, the Academy of Medicine, the Royal Society, as well as the American statesman-scientist Benjamin Franklin. The experiments which they devised were constructed to test the presence or absence of the magnetic fluidum which Mesmer claimed was the healing force behind his therapeutic successes. Unfortunately, none of the tests devised by the commission were concerned with the measurement of fluidum's medical effects. The conclusion of this prestigious commission was that fluidum did not exist. Although they did not deny Mesmer's therapeutic successes with patients, they felt that the medical effects which Mesmer produced were due to sensitive excitement, imagination, and imitation (of other patients). Interestingly, a committee of the Medical Section of the Academie des Sciences examined animal magnetism again in 1831 and accepted Mesmer's viewpoint. However, despite this validation, Mesmer's work never achieved widespread recognition.

As more recent laboratory investigations into the physiological effects of laying-on-of-hands have confirmed the magnetic nature of these subtle healing energies, researchers have demonstrated that Mesmer's understanding of the magnetic nature of the subtle energies of the human body was centuries ahead of his contemporaries. As will be shown, direct measurement of these energies by conventional tools of electromagnetic detection are as difficult today as during Mesmer's time.

Mesmer also discovered that water could be charged with this subtle magnetic force and that the stored energy from bottles of healer-treated water could be transmitted to sick patients by way of metallic iron rods which the patients would hold in their hands. The storage device which was used to relay healing energy from the charged water to patients was known as the "bacquet." Although today many consider Mesmer to have been a great hypnotist, there are few who really understand the pioneering nature of his research into the subtle magnetic energies of healing.

Modern Investigations into Psychic Healing: Scientists Examine the Biological Effects of Healers

Over the last several decades scientific investigation into the medical effects of laying-on-of-hands healing has shed new light on Mesmer's findings. In addition to confirming the actual exchange of energy between healer and patient which Mesmer and others suggested, researchers have demonstrated an interesting similarity between the biological effects of healers and high-intensity magnetic fields. The energetic fields of healers, although magnetic in character, also demonstrate other unique properties which have only recently begun to reveal themselves to scientific inquiry.

One of the most extensive studies into the energetic qualities of laying-on-of-hands healing was conducted during the 1960s by Dr. Bernard Grad of McGill University in Montreal.[5] Dr. Grad recognized the potential therapeutic power of so-called spiritual healers and psychic healers. He knew that many physicians who tried to explain the legitimate therapeutic effects of these healers often relied on the potent power of belief. This belief is sometimes known as the placebo effect. Grad suspected that in addition to the placebo effect of the patient's faith, there were other psychoenergetic factors which were operating but were more difficult to separate and study. Grad tried to devise an experiment which could distinguish between the psychological effects of the patient's belief from true energetic effects of the healer's hands upon cellular physiology. He wished to apply the scientific method to try and learn whether there were actually subtle forces at work aside from the patient's faith in a particular healer. In order to isolate the effects of belief from his experiments, Grad chose to work with non-human models of illness by substituting animals and plants as healing subjects.

The animals Grad selected to work with were mice. From a financial perspective, mice were easy to house and feed, and took up little room in his laboratory. Dr. Grad chose the formation of thyroid goiters as a model of illness that could be affected by a healer's energies. He was influenced by the fact that one of the healers he was studying had particular success in treating this disorder. (This issue has significance to researching healing energies, as it has been noted that certain healers seem to have better success rates with particular illnesses.) Grad chose to work with a healer by the name of Oscar Estebany, a Hungarian colonel with a reputation for curative powers in his healing touch. He referred to Estebany as Mr. E in his experimental studies.

In order to produce states of illness in the mice, Grad placed them on special "goitrogenic diets." These diets consisted of food that was deficient in iodine, a necessary nutrient for proper thyroid functioning. The water administered to the mice was laced with thiouracil, a known thyroid hormone blocking agent. The combination of iodine deficiency plus thiouracil was more than enough to create conditions of thyroid goiters in the experimental mice. The mice on the goitrogenic diets were then separated into healer-treated and non-healer-treated groups.

The first group of mice (which were not exposed to healing hands) served as a control group. To control for factors such as thermal effects from the heat of the healer's hands and the behavioral effects of humans holding the mice, several other control subgroups were also added. The first control subgroup received no treatment at all. The second control subgroup of mice was placed in cages that were wrapped by electrothermal tape to simulate the heat of human hands. A third control subgroup of mice was held by individuals who were non-healers. While holding the mice, they attempted to do laying-on-of-hands healing. Additionally, all mice were initially handled by lab personnel to accustom them to being held as well as to distinguish calm from very nervous mice. Anxious mice were found to be poor laboratory subjects for healing experiments, and they were excluded from the pool of test mice following the "gentling" procedure.

The mice in the treatment group were placed inside a special container that would allow the healer to treat a number of mice at the same time. The mice were put into small individual compartments in a specially constructed container of galvanized iron mesh similar to an ice cube tray. The container was large enough that nine mice could be held by the healer simultaneously. In this way, the mice in the small wire containers would be held for fifteen minutes at a time by a healer, and then returned to their cages.

The experiment lasted forty days. At the end, all mice were examined to determine the number in each group which had significantly large thyroid goiters. While all animals showed an increase in thyroid size over the testing period of forty days, it was demonstrated that *mice in the healer-treated group had a significantly slower rate of goiter development.* Grad performed an interesting variation on this experiment which examined the possibility of removing the healer's hands entirely. Instead of having the healer work with the mice directly, the healer performed laying-on-of-hands healing on pieces of cotton and wool in hopes of charging them with the healing energy. The charged cotton and wool pieces were placed on the cage floors of mice on goitrogenic diets. The charged material was left with the mice for an hour in the morning and an hour in the afternoon. Similar but untreated pieces of cotton and wool were placed in the cages of control mice on the same diet. Mice in both groups were found to be sitting on piles of the cotton and wool cuttings at the end of the treatment periods.

Grad performed statistical analysis on the two groups, comparing thyroid size between mice. *Grad found that even when the healer's hands had no direct contact with the mice, animals who had been exposed to the healer-charged cuttings showed a slower rate of goiter formation.* Both of Grad's experiments suggest that a healer may have measureable energy effects in retarding the formation of goiters. This positive finding was consistent with Mr. Estebany's reputation as a healer with an ability to alleviate thyroid goiters in humans. A more fascinating conclusion from these experiments was that the energies of a healer could be absorbed into a common organic storage medium, such as cotton, and transmitted to the sick patients (i.e. the mice with the goiters). These findings will have later significance when we talk about the use of Therapeutic Touch by the nursing profession.

Grad was intrigued by his success in demonstrating the healer's ability to prevent the development of thyroid goiters. What his study had shown was that psychic healing could counteract the goitrogenic effects of iodine deficiency and thiouracil. *The healing energy had not actually caused an existing condition of illness to disappear. It had prevented the appearance of the anticipated thyroid disorder.* In order to observe the effects of healing energies on accelerating a natural process of recovery from illness, Grad selected an animal recovering from surgery. The physiologic process which Grad wished to study was the phenomenon of wound healing. He wondered whether the healers could be effective in accelerating the rate of healing and closure of a specially created surgical wound.

In the experiment, mice were anesthetized and their backs shaven, after which equivalent coin-sized areas of skin were surgically removed from each animal. In order to follow the gradual shrinking in wound size over time, the wound outlines were traced onto a transparent piece of plastic with a grease pencil. Following this procedure, the outlines were copied onto pieces of paper which were then weighed on sensitive balance scales. The weight of the traced paper piece was directly proportional to the size of the wound on the back of each mouse. This original method allowed Grad to make quantitative daily measurements of the size of the wounds over time.

Forty-eight mice were subjected to the surgical wounding procedure and then separated into three groups of sixteen each. The first group was a control group to which no special treatment was given. The second group of mice was held between the healer's hands in a special wire cage (similar to the container used in the goiter experiment). This metallic container prevented direct physical contact between the healer and the mice during periods of psychic healing. The third group of mice was handled in a manner similar to the second group except that the wire cage was exposed to heat similar to the temperature of human hands. This group was added to simulate the thermal effects of the healer's hands on wound healing. In all three groups of mice, the wounds were measured in the manner described over a period of thirty days. At the end of the experimental period, the three groups of mice were examined for statistically significant differences in the final size of their nearly healed wounds.

The final tally showed that wounds on the mice in the healer-treated group had either healed completely or were very tiny and nearly healed. Wounds in the other groups showed various stages of healing. Although gross visual inspection of the two groups revealed striking differences in the size of their wounds, statistical analysis confirmed what appeared to be obvious. *Mice in the healer-treated group had a significantly faster rate of wound healing.*

Grad's studies of the effects of psychic healing on wound healing in mice were later replicated under strict double-blind conditions by Dr. Remi Cadoret and G. I. Paul at the University of Manitoba.[6] In addition to using larger groups of mice (300 instead of 48), another control was added whereby mice were treated by persons not claiming healing ability. Cadoret and Paul's results were similar to Grad's in that mice treated by healers demonstrated significantly faster rates of wound healing.

Grad's early studies with mice suggested that healers did, indeed, possess some type of bioenergetic influence that affected the cellular expression of disease states. This influence was above and beyond anything that might be attributed to the effects of suggestion and faith. Although the placebo effect may be operative in humans at times, it would have been difficult to suggest that mice in the healer-treated group improved because they believed in the healer. The studies with mice had been useful, but long periods of time were needed to observe significant physiologic changes in the animals. Because the time necessary to observe a healer's effect on mice was usually three to five weeks, Grad sought another biological model which could produce more rapid results. Based on this time criterion, Grad eventually shifted to a plant model for studying the energetic effects of healers. He decided to use barley seeds as the experimental subjects. To make the seeds ill, they were initially treated with a one-percent salt solution (salt being a known inhibitor of plant growth). This saline treatment was followed by several days of drying, after which the seeds were watered with tap water at suitable intervals.

Grad separated the seedlings into two groups. The first group was watered with untreated saline, then dried, and watered with tap water in the described procedure. The second group of seeds was treated differently in that the saline used had been held by a psychic healer for a period of fifteen minutes. (Mr. Estebany was again used as the healer.) In early studies, the healers held flasks of saline that were open to the air. Some critics argued that the saline could be exposed to some physical agent from the healer such as sweat or exhaled carbon dioxide. To tighten the controls, Grad later modified the procedure by having the healer treat the saline in a flask sealed with a ground glass stopper.

Elaborate double-blind conditions were used which prevented the experimenters from knowing which were the treated and untreated saline solutions. Technicians soaked the seeds in saline that was arbitrarily numbered 1 or 2, so that only Grad knew which was the treated seed group. Following watering with healer-treated or untreated saline, the seedlings were put into numbered seed pots containing soil. The pots were then placed in a specially heated incubation chamber for 48 hours at 38-40 degrees centigrade. Following this incubation procedure, the pots were removed and randomly arranged in rows in an appropriate location. They were watered with equal amounts of untreated tap water until the end of the experimental observation period. At the end of twelve to fifteen days, the experiment was terminated, and the treated and untreated seeds were compared for percentage germination rate, plant height, and later for chlorophyll content.

Following statistical analysis, *it was shown that seeds exposed to healer-treated saline were more abundant in yield and larger in plant size than the untreated group. The healer-treated plants also showed a higher chlorophyll content than the untreated plants.* These experimental results have since been replicated in Grad's lab with the same healer, and in other laboratories utilizing different psychic healers. It seemed obvious to Grad that some type of healing energy had been transmitted from the healer's hands through the glass flask into the salt water solution, as evidenced by the effect of treated saline on plant growth. *The fact that water could be charged with healing energy and transmitted to living organisms is significant in light of Mesmer's claim that his bacquet could be useful in treating patients by exposing them to the stored energies of healer-treated water.*

Grad carried out an interesting variation on this experimental theme of charging water with psychic energy. He gave an individual with a "green thumb," and a psychotically depressed patient, water to hold and charge in a manner similar to that utilized with the healers. Sealed bottles of water treated by the individual with the green thumb caused an *increased* growth rate in plants, whereas *water treated by the severely depressed patient resulted in a retarded rate of plant growth,* (as compared with controls). Grad had clearly demonstrated that some type of healing energetic influence could be transmitted through glass to the water. The healing energy which was stored in the water was then passed on to the seeds in a manner similar to his early experiments which showed that healer-charged cotton could transmit a healing influence to the mice with goiters. This energy, whatever its character, seemed to have both positive and negative polarity in its physiological effects. Healers and individuals with green thumbs appeared to possess energy of a positive, nurturing character, while severely depressed individuals seemed to give off negative energy which had inhibitory effects upon plant growth.

Energetic Similarities Between Healers & Magnetic Fields: Science Takes a Closer Look at Animal Magnetism

The fact that ordinary water could absorb healing energy made Grad wonder whether or not the water had been changed in any way by its exposure to the healer's energy field. Grad later performed quantitative scientific analysis on the water to see if the healers had caused any measureable changes in the physical properties of the water. Utilizing infrared absorption spectrometry, Grad discovered that the bond angle of the water molecule had undergone a subtle but detectable shift. Because the healer-induced changes in the normal bond angle had caused a slight alteration in the way the water molecules were able to align themselves in solution, hydrogen bonding was found to be indirectly affected.

Hydrogen bonding is a unique phenomenon associated with water (H_2O). Hydrogen bonding occurs when the slightly negative oxygen atom of one water molecule is attracted to the slightly positive hydrogen atom of another water molecule. This weak attraction between water molecules is responsible for the way water climbs the root systems of plants (through capillary action). The delicate membrane-like effect created by hydrogen bonding at the surface of water allows water striders and similar insects to actually walk on water. The surface tension of water is directly affected by slight changes in hydrogen bonding such as those induced by exposure to healers' energy fields. By their ability to diminish the hydrogen bonding ability of water, Grad found that healers were able to cause a slight but measureable decrease in surface tension.

Dr. Robert Miller of Atlanta, Georgia, is a research chemist who has studied the biological effects of healers. Miller has been able to experimentally confirm Dr. Grad's discovery of the healer's ability to disrupt hydrogen bonding in water. Miller also found a significant similarity between the energetic effects of magnetic fields and the field-effects noted with psychic healers.[7] Utilizing a Du Nouy-type tensiometer, Dr. Miller attempted to measure the surface tension of water which had been exposed to healers' energies or magnetic fields. Treatment of water by several healers produced significant reductions in surface tension. *Miller discovered that water which had been exposed to magnetic fields also showed significant reductions in surface tension similar to that observed with psychic healers.* He studied the relative stability of energized water to see how long the surface bonding would remain disrupted after treatment.

Experiments which were designed to test the stability of the energized water demonstrated that healer or magnet-treated water would gradually release its excess energy to the environment over a 24-hour period, at which time the surface tension became normal. This gradual release of energy was speeded up to become a rapid discharge if someone used a metallic rod to touch the magnetically-charged water. Miller also found that pouring the healer or magnet-treated water into a stainless steel beaker caused within minutes a sudden dissipation of stored energy into the environment, with a quick return to normal surface tension. The metal appeared to act as a type of energy sink that provided a pathway of flow for the magnetic healing energy. Dr. Miller and Dr. Grad's work suggested that water could be charged with magnetic and healing energies, and that metals and organic substances provided intermediate pathways of flow for this unique energy to direct it where it might be needed.

Miller discovered that metallic stirring rods placed in contact with the energized water would provide a route for the healing energy to flow in a specific direction. This discovery helps confirm the rationale behind the bacquet that Mesmer used for treating patients nearly 200 years ago. The bacquet was formed by several bottles of magnetically treated water which were connected to sick patients via metallic rods leading from the bottles. Individuals in the first circular row around the bacquet were often connected to a second row of patients via fabric cords around their waists. Grad's observation that cotton and wool could act as natural organic capacitors, which could store and later transmit healing energy to mice, gives additional rationale to Mesmer's idea of connecting patients in a unique healing circuit by utilizing fabric cords.

In later studies, Dr. Miller found a number of other interesting similarities between magnet-treated and healer-treated water. He created a unique experiment which used the natural process of crystallization to reveal subtle energetic changes in the water. Miller knew that adding copper sulfate to water to create a supersaturated solution would ultimately allow the natural growth of crystalline patterns if the solution was allowed to sit undisturbed. With untreated water, the copper sulfate would ordinarily crystallize out of solution as a jade green monoclinic crystal. However, if the copper sulfate solution was pre-treated by exposure to a healer's hands, the crystals formed were always turquoise-blue in color and of a coarser grain. Miller duplicated the experiment with the copper salt solutions, but this time substituted a magnetic field for a healer's field. He placed a solution of supersaturated copper sulfate in a magnetic field of 4500 gauss for fifteen minutes. *When the crystals eventually formed, Miller noted that they were of the turquoise-blue variety noted in the healer-treated solutions instead of the usual jade-green.* Here again we see *a qualitative similarity between the effects of healers' hands and magnetic fields.*

Miller carried out another experiment to measure further physiologic similarities between the effects of magnet-treated and healer-treated water. As in Grad's earlier studies, Miller chose to examine the rate of seedling germination after exposure to healer-treated water. Miller looked at the growth-stimulating effects of normal tap water in comparison to magnet-treated and healer-treated water. He selected three groups of seeds, each composed of 25 rye grass seeds. One group of seeds was watered with ordinary tap water. The second group was watered with tap water that had been exposed to a magnetic field. The third group of rye seeds was watered with healer-treated tap water. At the end of four days, he looked to see how many of the 25 rye seeds in each group had sprouted. Dr. Miller found that seeds which had been watered with regular tap water had an eight-percent germination rate, whereas *seeds watered with healer-treated water showed a 36-percent germination rate—or a fourfold increase in the number of new sprouts.* Even more surprising was Miller's discovery that *seeds which had been watered with magnet-treated water showed more than an eightfold increase (68-percent rate) of seedling germination.*

In addition to measuring germination rates, the plants were examined for differences in growth rates as indicated by the final height of the plants after eight days. Although the seeds watered with healer-treated water were only slightly higher than those in the tap water control group, the seeds watered with magnet-treated water produced plants that were approximately 28.6-percent taller at the end of the same time period. What Dr. Grad and Dr. Miller had discovered in their respective laboratories was the unique qualitative similarity between the energies of healers and of magnets: an observation which had been noted by Franz Anton Mesmer nearly 200 years ago. The results of Dr. Miller's and Dr. Grad's studies provided new experimental evidence for the magnetic nature of the energies of healers, as Mesmer had previously speculated. They also found evidence for the possible mechanisms behind Mesmer's bacquet, which could heal a number of patients at the same time by distributing the subtle energies among many individuals through the use of a special healing circuit. Like Grad, Mesmer had discovered that bottles of water could be charged with the energies of healers like a battery, similar to the use of the Leyden jar to store electricity in the early days of experimentation. Because of this subtle energy's tendency to flow from areas of high to low potential in a fashion similar to electricity, some healers, such as Ambrose Worrall, have referred to it as paraelectricity.

When Grad's work was published, there were many scientists who speculated on the possible mechanisms by which healers might have accelerated plant growth and wound healing. One theory which seemed plausible was that healers accomplished their acceleration of the normal growth and healing processes of living organisms by speeding up the activities of the cellular enzymes which normally carried out these functions.

At the same time period that Grad's work became public, a number of studies were published which demonstrated the ability of high-intensity magnetic fields to accelerate enzyme kinetics. Among the researchers in this area was Dr. Justa Smith, a nun and biochemist working at the Human Dimensions Institute at Rosary Hill College in New York.[8] Dr. Smith had confirmed other researchers' published findings that strong magnetic fields were able to accelerate the reaction rate of various enzymes, depending on the length of time that the enzymes were magnetically treated. Dr. Smith's work in magnetic fields and enzymes had been the subject of her recently completed doctoral thesis. Soon after completing her work, she came across Dr. Grad's study on the biological effects of healers. Dr. Smith speculated that the healer's potential to accelerate natural enzyme activity would be the most plausible explanation for increased growth and healing. Because enzymes are the cellular workhorses that perform all the metabolic functions in the physical body, it was a natural assumption that accelerating their activities could result in enhanced healing of wounds and speeded growth. As her laboratory was already geared to measure enzyme kinetics, this hypothesis could be easily tested. Smith's previous observations on the biological effects of high-intensity magnetic fields also tied in well with Miller's newly discovered data, which revealed striking similarities between healers' fields and magnetic fields.

Dr. Smith set up an experiment where she could compare the effects of healers' hands with magnetic fields as to their ability to increase enzyme reaction rates. She obtained the assistance of Mr. Estebany, one of the healers that Grad had used in his studies on the laying-on-of-hands. Dr. Smith had Mr. Estebany hold a test tube containing a solution of the digestive enzyme trypsin while thinking about doing a laying-on-of-hands healing. The trypsin utilized in this experiment was a pure crystalline form with standardized activity, purchased from a biochemical firm. She would take periodic small samples of the treated enzyme over the time the healer did his work. Each sample was then tested in a spectrophotometer, which registered the level of activity of the enzyme in its ability to catalyze a chemical reaction. *What Dr. Smith found was that Mr. Estebany was able to increase the enzyme reaction rate over time, and that the longer the healer held the test tube of enzymes, the more rapid the reaction rate. Similar effects on enzymes had been noted with high-intensity magnetic fields,* as was demonstrated in her previous study.

The similarity between the abilities of the healer's energies and the magnetic fields to accelerate the activity of enzymes prompted Dr. Smith to investigate the possibility that healers might radiate some type of magnetic energy to achieve their healing results. To test this hypothesis, she used sensitive magnetic recording devices around the healer's hands during attempts at healing. She was rather dismayed to find that no magnetic fields could be detected around the healer's hands. In order to obtain the effects on enzymes that were noted, the healer would have had to produce a magnetic field of significant intensity. The strength of the magnetic fields utilized in her earlier study were about 13,000 gauss, which is approximately 26,000 times the intensity of the earth's magnetic field.

Dr. Smith decided to carry out further variations on the enzyme experiment to see if there were differences between the healer's energy field and the magnetic field. She also utilized several other healers in her study of enzyme changes to see if they produced similar energetic results. She tested each healer's energetic effect on different enzymes, utilizing the same type of experimental protocol as she had used with the trypsin. In one experiment, she substituted an enzyme which synthesized the chemical NAD (nicotinamide adenine dinucleotide, an important member of the mitochondrial electron transport chain).[9] She discovered that healers would uniformly cause a decrease in the activity of this enzyme. Experiments with other enzymes showed consistent increases in activity with some enzymes, and decreases in activity of other enzymes following exposure to the energy of healer's hands.

Although initially perplexing, this seemingly conflicting data was later shown to make biological sense when viewed from the perspective of cellular physiology. *The type of change in enzyme activity noted after exposure to healers was always in a direction of greater health of the cells, and thus the organism.* For instance, let us examine the case of NAD-synthetase, one enzyme noted to be decreased in activity by healers. NAD, the chemical produced by this enzyme, is a chemical intermediate in the electron transport chain of the mitochondrion, the tiny powerhouse in each of our cells. Chemical reactions which take place in the mitochondria are responsible for extracting the greatest amount of energy from the food we eat. Chemical energy from food is partially released in the form of electrons that flow through the battery-like structure of the mitochondria. It is at the mitochondrial level that life-giving oxygen has its greatest function: to accept the electrons of the energy-producing electron transport chain.

NAD is the precursor of NADH, a charged energy intermediate that the mitochondrion uses to make ATP, which is the energy currency of the cell. (ATP is the cellular equivalent of energy dollars used to pay the enzyme workers of the cell to stay on their respective production-line jobs.) The higher the amount of NADH that is present, the greater the available energy (and ATP) to the cell for healing and proper metabolic functioning. After NADH gives up its energy to make ATP, it is broken down to NAD, a chemical intermediate which has had its energy potential reduced. There is always a balance known as the NAD/NADH ratio between the amount of NAD and NADH in the cell. The greater the amount of NAD that is present relative to NADH, the less energy the cell has available to do metabolic work. Dr. Smith discovered that healers would decrease the activity of the enzyme that converts high-energy NADH to low-energy NAD. Therefore, the enzyme which Dr. Smith found that healers had reduced in activity was one which normally robs the cell of needed energy. Thus, a decrease in NAD conversion by the healer's suppression of NAD-synthetase would have an overall positive energetic effect upon cellular metabolism.

This type of cellular metabolic reasoning helped to put into perspective the direction of enzymatic change which the healers produced. *Whatever the enzyme used, the healers always caused changes in activity which would result in a push toward greater health and energy balance of the sick organism.* Thus, Dr. Smith's speculation about healers' effects on growth and wound healing via enzymatic change was experimentally validated. This healing energy appeared to have an almost innate intelligence in the way it could therapeutically distinguish between the different test tubes of enzymes. To the eyes of the healers, the test tubes appeared to contain only clear solutions. They were not trying to induce a change in enzyme activity in any particular direction. They were only thinking about healing. This demonstrates a significant qualitative difference between healing energies and magnetic fields. *The magnetic fields could only produce a nonspecific increase in the activity of enzymes.* On the other hand, *the energy fields of healers could cause variable changes in different enzymes. The direction of change was always consistent with greater health of the cell and organism.*

Healing Energies & Negative Entropy: The Drive toward Increasing Order & Cellular Organization

Dr. Smith carried out a further enzyme experiment which was to eventually show an even greater similarity between the energies of a healer and the magnetic fields. This experiment was designed partly from suggestions provided by Dr. Grad, whom Dr. Smith had consulted. Grad said that in his experiments on measuring healing energies, he had never asked a healer to heal a well person. Since Dr. Smith was testing whole enzymes, why not try to damage the enzymes first? Acting on Grad's suggestion, she tested the ability of healers to affect enzymes which had been damaged so that they no longer had full functional activity.

She placed test tubes of trypsin in ultraviolet (UV) light, a frequency of energy which is known to disrupt the normal structure of proteins, so that their active site of reaction was destroyed. Following this UV treatment, the trypsin was given to the healer (Mr. Estebany) to treat in the usual manner. Baseline measurements of the enzyme activity revealed that the UV light had significantly decreased its activity due to structural disruption. Following treatment by Mr. Estebany, Dr. Smith was surprised to find that the damaged enzymes recovered enzymatic activity and that their activity continued to rise linearly over time with continued exposure to the healing energies. *The activity remained at the new level following healing, suggesting that the healer had repaired the damaged enzymes.* Interestingly, high-intensity magnetic fields had similar effects in repairing and accelerating enzyme activity. This was an entirely new dimension of measured energetic effect. Enzymes which had been physically disrupted by UV light were found to undergo structural reorganization following exposure to the healer's energy field. In physics terms, this biological enzymatic system had undergone a decrease in entropy.

As mentioned in Chapter 4, entropy is a term which describes the state of disorder of a system. The greater the disorder, the higher the entropy; the more ordered the system, the lower the entropy. Crystals, because of their mathematically precise, highly ordered lattice structures, are held to represent the lowest entropic states possible. Most processes in the physical universe are believed to head toward increasing positive entropy; that is, given time, everything tends to fall apart. The unique exception to this thermodynamic rule is the behavior of biological systems. Living organisms utilize energy to create increasing levels of order within their physiological systems. However, when this self-organizing energy or life-force leaves the system (i.e., the body dies), then its component parts return to dust and disorder.

As discussed in previous chapters, the life-force seems to possess negative entropic characteristics. This energy moves biological systems toward increasing levels of cellular order and self-organization. The most dramatic demonstration of this principle of life is seen in its opposite form: death. Dust, decay, and disorder follow the separation of this inhabiting life-force from the impermanent physical body.

In reality, it is the organizing principle of the etheric body which maintains and sustains the growth of the physical body. At death, the etheric vehicle dissolves and returns to the free energy of the environment. Because the physical shell is so intertwined with the etheric template, either form cannot exist independently for any period of time. (This is one of the reasons

Kirlian photographers have so much trouble in capturing the Phantom Leaf Effect. The etheric structure of the amputated portion tends to dissipate quickly without the stabilizing influence of its physical counterpart.)

Throughout its holographic energy-interference pattern, the etheric body has encoded structural information about the spatial organization of the physical-cellular structures. The unique energies of the etheric template possess magnetic characteristics, as has been indicated by the aforementioned experiments comparing magnetic fields with healers' energy fields. These particular magnetic characteristics demonstrated by the energy fields of psychic healers fit quite nicely with Dr. Tiller's predictions of the behavior of etheric or negative space/time energies.

As discussed in Chapter 4, the Tiller-Einstein Model attempts to mathematically describe the behavior of energy/matter at velocities beyond the speed of light in order to establish a reality base for subtle energies and subtle bodies which are beyond ordinary human perception. The domain of physical matter, which is so familiar to us, is the world of positive space/time (+S/T). The domain of energies beyond the speed of light are referred to as the world of negative space/time ($-S/T$). The first level of energies which move faster than light velocity are the etheric frequencies of matter and energy. Beyond this level is the astral domain. Although there are frequencies of existence beyond the astral level, i.e., the mental and the causal, this model is unable to describe domains beyond the astral at its present level of development.

According to the Tiller-Einstein Model, +S/T matter and energy are primarily electrical in nature (i.e., matter is composed of particles such as the electron and proton, which are electrically charged.) Positive space/time is the realm of electromagnetic radiation (EM). On the other side is $-S/T$ energy, which is distinguished by its primary magnetic nature, and energy which is described as magnetoelectric radiation (ME).[10] Because it moves faster than light, ME radiation does not interact with conventional EM detectors. Besides its magnetic nature, $-S/T$ energy has another unique characteristic (among many): *the tendency toward negative entropy.* In the Tiller-Einstein Model, etheric energy is seen to possess magnetic characteristics and is associated with a negatively entropic drive. That is, *the energies of the etheric body have qualities which move cellular systems toward states of higher order and organization.* The removal of this negative-entropic tendency following the dissipation of the etheric vehicle at death is the reason that the body decays after dying. Once the organizing influence of the etheric body has dissipated, the body follows a positively entropic downward spiral of cellular breakdown and dissolution. *These magnetic/negatively-entropic qualities of etheric energy and matter are also the same attributes found to be associated with the fields of psychic healers.* Healers appear to have an abundance of this same organizing etheric energy, and are somehow able to resonantly transfer some of it to their patients.

Because healer-associated fields are likely to be a function of $-S/T$ energies, they demonstrate similarities to magnetic fields in their qualitative effects on water, yet are almost undetectable with conventional EM recording equipment. However, new measuring systems have evolved since the time of Dr. Smith's experiments which have helped confirm the magnetic nature of healers' energy fields. Dr. Smith was originally unable to detect any magnetic fields around healers' hands using sensitive gaussmeters. However, recent experiments by Dr. John Zimmerman[11] with highly sensitive SQUID (Superconducting Quantum Interference Device) detectors (as mentioned in Chapter 4), which can measure infinitesimally weak magnetic fields, have found increased magnetic field emission from the hands of psychic healers during healing. Although the increases in magnetic field strength coming from healers' hands were a hundred times higher than normal body activity, these healer-associated magnetic fields were far weaker than the magnetic fields used to accelerate enzymes in Dr. Smith's experiments. Yet these same, barely detectable healer-fields had powerful effects upon biological systems which could only be produced by treament with the high-intensity magnetic fields.

This very elusive nature of the etheric fields is such that scientists today still have difficulty in measuring their presence, as did Benjamin Franklin in Mesmer's day. It is only through observation of their secondary effects on biological (enzymes), physical (crystallization), and electronic systems (electrographic scanners) that science is beginning to amass evidential data on the validity of etheric energies. One indirect indication of the presence of the healing/etheric field is through its effect on increasing order within a system, i.e., its negative entropic drive.

A number of researchers have come to understand this negatively entropic property of healing energy. Dr. Justa Smith's research suggested that healers have the ability to selectively affect different enzyme systems in a direction toward greater organization and energy balance. By speeding up different enzymatic reactions, healers assist the body to heal itself. (This is also one of the great unrecognized principles of medicine. Doctors are only successful healers to the degree that they are able to use drugs, surgery, nutrition, and various other means to assist the patients' innate healing mechanisms to repair their own sick bodies.) Healers provide a needed energetic boost to push the patient's total energetic system back into home-ostasis. This healing energetic boost has special negatively-entropic, self-organizational properties that assist the cells in creating order from disorder along selectively defined routes of cellular expression.

An experiment was recently devised to test this negatively entropic property of the energy of healers. In Oregon, a multidisciplinary team met with Olga Worrall, a spiritual healer who had participated in Dr. Smith's studies of healers, magnetic fields, and enzymes.[12] They wanted to test the hypothesis that healers enhance an organism's own ability to increase order. They speculated that a healer might also affect the self-organizing properties of a special chemical reaction known as the Belousov-Zhabo-tinskii (B-Z) reaction. In the B-Z reaction, a chemical solution shifts between two states, which are indicated by unfolding, scroll-like spiral waves in a shallow petri dish solution. If dyes are added to the solution, one observes an oscillation of colors from red to blue to red. This reaction is a special case of what is known as a "dissipative structure." (Ilya Prigogine won the 1977 Nobel prize for his Theory Of Dissipative Structures,[13] an innovative mathematical model which explains how systems like the B-Z reaction evolve to higher levels of order by using novel connections produced by entropy or disorder.)

Since the B-Z reaction is considered a self-organizing chemical system, the research team wondered if the healer could affect its entropic status. Worrall was asked to try to affect a B-Z reaction. Following treatment by her healing hands, the solution produced waves at twice the speed of a control solution. In another experiment, the red-blue-red oscillation in two beakers of solution became synchronized after Worrall's treatments. The conclu-sion of the research team was that the healer's field was able to create greater levels of order in a nonorganic system along the lines of negative entropic behavior. These results are consistent with the other studies like Dr. Smith's which showed that healers (such as Olga Worrall) could cause UV-damaged enzymes to reintegrate to their normal structure and function. Enhanced growth in plants and faster wound healing in mice are other examples of the healers' effect on increasing the organization and order within cellular systems.

The diverse range of experimental data on the biological effects of healing is supportive of the hypothesis that a real energetic influence is exerted by healers on sick organisms. The biological systems examined in the previous experiments were all non-human in nature. Animal, plant, and enzyme systems were utilized in hopes of removing any influence of suggestion or belief on the part of the test subject. Having validated the existence of a real therapeutic energy exchange between healers and non-human subjects, one is left to wonder about what actually occurs between healers and human patients.

If one accepts the fact that healers are able to induce measureable effects in living organisms, then one must ask important questions about the nature of healers in general. Are healers merely an elite group of humans in our society who possess a rare gift at birth? Or is healing an innate human potential which, like any other skill, might be enhanced by learning? If so, how does one go about teaching healing to others? Could healing be taught to individuals in the health-care professions to amplify their academically derived medical skills with natural energetic methods of therapeutic interaction? These questions have only recently begun to find meaningful answers. The growing impact of such issues reflects an undercurrent of subtle change in the evolving health-care field. The story of how psychic healing began to work its way into the teaching curriculums of the medical and nursing professions is a fascinating one.

Dr. Krieger Looks at Healers & Hemoglobin: The Evolution of Therapeutic Touch

Following the publication of Dr. Bernard Grad's experiments on the biological effects of psychic healing, various researchers began to think about the leads which had been provided for future directions of inquiry. Among those intrigued by Dr. Grad's findings was Dr. Dolores Krieger, now professor of nursing at New York University. Krieger was particularly fascinated by Grad's observation that plants watered with healer-treated water showed an increase in the amount of chlorophyll present in their leaves.[14]

Chlorophyll in plants is a pigment molecule which is biochemically similar to hemoglobin in humans. They both contain porphyrin rings surrounding a metal atom. In the case of chlorophyll, the central metal is a magnesium atom. In hemoglobin, iron forms the central metallic atom. Krieger reasoned that since plant chlorophyll is structurally similar to hemoglobin in humans, then humans exposed to the energies of healers might show an increase in blood hemoglobin, just as healer-treated plants had demonstrated rises in chlorophyll content. Krieger felt that hemoglobin levels in the blood would be a good biochemical parameter to measure because of its integral role in many life-sustaining processes.

Heme, the central metal-containing ring in the hemoglobin molecule, has three major functions. In its hemoglobin role, the most important and well-recognized function of the heme component is the transportation of life-giving oxygen from the lungs to the bodily tissues. Secondly, heme has a place in the cytochrome chain within the mitochondria of the cells, and serves as a carrier molecule in the electron transport chain. Through its mitochondrial function, the heme group allows electrons to create new metabolic energy intermediates (ATP) in a process that ultimately involves the oxygen brought by its better known counterpart (hemoglobin). Thirdly, heme participates in the cytochrome oxidase pathway of the liver and other tissues, where various potentially toxic chemicals and metabolites are degraded and removed from the body. Because the heme molecule is so integral to proper health and functioning of the organism, and because hemoglobin levels were easy to directly measure, Krieger chose hemoglobin as a biochemical indicator of healing energy influences in humans.

Krieger wished to examine and confirm the effects of healers on humans in an analytical method which would separate the influence of belief. The experimental work of Grad and Smith had convinced her that true energy effects occur between patient and healer, even when the patient is only a sick plant or a wounded mouse or even a damaged enzyme. She wished to extrapolate the known information from studies of healing in non-human systems toward creating an experiment which would confirm the healing energy influence in humans. In 1971, shortly after his work with Dr. Grad, Mr. Estebany (the healer used in Grad's studies) was asked to participate in just such an experiment. The research was being conducted by a medical doctor (Otelia Bengssten, M.D.) and a clairvoyant (Dora Kunz) who were studying the healing process. Krieger joined the group as a fellow researcher, offering her skills as a health-care professional.

The study was conducted on a farm in the foothills of the Berkshire Mountains in New York, utilizing as subjects a large group of medically referred patients with various illnesses.[15] There were nineteen sick people in the experimental group and nine similarly sick individuals in the control group. The age and sex distribution of the patients was comparable for both groups. The experimental group had direct laying-on-of-hands treatment by Mr. Estebany, while the control group did not. In addition to the healing touch of Mr. Estebany, patients in the experimental group were given rolls of cotton batting that had been "magnetically charged" by Mr. Estebany (as had been done in the experiment by Dr. Grad with the goiterous mice). (One year following the study, some of the patients that were given these charged rolls reported that they could still feel an energy flow from the cotton). Krieger measured hemoglobin levels in both groups of patients before and after a series of healing treatments to the experimental group. *She found a significant increase in hemoglobin values in the healer-treated group compared to the control group, as predicted by her initial hypothesis.*

Krieger's study was repeated in 1973 with a larger group of patients and even stricter controls to answer criticisms directed toward the design of her previous study.[16] She used 46 sick patients in the experimental group and 33 ill patients in her control group. Again she obtained similar data, with sick patients demonstrating significant elevations of hemoglobin levels following laying-on-of-hands healing by Mr. Estebany. The tendency for healing energy to increase hemoglobin has been found to be so strong that cancer patients who have undergone laying-on-of-hands healing have occasionally shown rises in hemoglobin levels in spite of treatment with bone marrow-suppressive agents which predictably induce anemias.

Krieger was fascinated by the implications of her research findings. By measuring changes in hemoglobin levels, she was able to obtain biochemical confirmation of her hypothesis that healers induce bioenergetic changes in the patients they treated. In both of her studies using Mr. Estebany, elevations in blood hemoglobin were found to reliably indicate true bioenergetic and physiologic changes induced by the application of healing energies. In addition to changes in hemoglobin levels, Krieger was amazed by the first-person reports of improvement or complete disappearance of symptoms in a majority of the patients who had experienced the healing touch of Mr. Estebany. The diagnoses of these patients covered all known systems of the body. They had pancreatitis, brain tumor, emphysema, multiple endocrine disorders, rheumatoid arthritis, congestive heart failure, and other diseases. Nearly all had experienced significant improvement in their illnesses following healing by Mr. Estebany. It was clear that hemoglobin rises were reflective of some type of bioenergetic change induced by healer-healee interactions, but these changes were by no means the only changes that had occurred.

Because measurement of hemoglobin is easily accomplished in most clinical laboratory settings, *Krieger now had a reliable biochemical yard-stick by which she could analyze healing energy interactions.* Now that she had validated the true energetic nature of laying-on-of-hands healing, she was left to ponder a great question she had not yet been able to answer. Was it necessary for a healer to be born with this healing gift, or might it possibly be learned through some special instructional process? She was particularly interested in whether or not she, as a nursing practitioner, might learn this unique healing art. She asked Mr. Estebany if he thought that others might learn to heal as he could. It was Mr. Estebany's opinion that people could not be taught to heal others; rather, they had to be born with the gift. However, Dora Kunz, the clairvoyant who had participated in Krieger's first study, felt differently about the subject.

Kunz began a workshop to instruct others in the art of healing, which she opened to all those who had a desire to demonstrate this ability. Enthusiastically, Dr. Krieger became one of her early students. One of Kunz' remarkable abilities was her gift to clairvoyantly perceive the subtle energetic interactions between people as well as to observe and diagnose the energy blockages in a person's chakras and auric field.[17] Using her clairvoyant powers of observation, she had been studying the process of healing and the subtle interactions that take place between healer and healee. Through her remarkable intuitive abilities and her esoteric knowledge of the healing arts (Kunz was also former president of the Theosophical Society), she was an effective instructor to Krieger, who learned to use her hands to help and heal others in need.

Following her healing education with Kunz, Krieger intuitively felt that this tool should be taught to health-care professionals. She began to develop a curriculum for fellow nurses to instruct them in the art of laying-on-of-hands healing. She gathered information from different disciplines, both Eastern and Western, to try to explain to other practitioners the rationale behind the therapeutic interactions induced by the healing touch. Because the term psychic healing was fraught with negative associations for many health-care professionals, Krieger endeavored to create a new, less-threatening term by which the healing process might be called. She settled upon Therapeutic Touch as her new nomenclature for healing. It was accurately descriptive, yet innocuous enough to avoid prejudgement by the inquisitive yet skeptical minds of the nurses who would attend her class. The first class on Therapeutic Touch was taught at a master's level to nurses at New York University, where Krieger was on staff. Krieger's class in healing was offered under the title: "Frontiers in Nursing: The Actualization of Potential for Therapeutic Field Interaction."

During her investigation into the mechanisms behind healing, Krieger had discovered the Hindu and yogic concept of "prana". She had learned that prana was a vital form of energy taken in from the environment which was carried by a subtle energetic component of sunlight. This subtle energy, which is taken into the body via the process of breathing, was felt to be in abundance in the body of the healer. The healthy individual was thought to have an overabundance of prana. Conversely, a sick individual demonstrated a relative prana deficit. Prana in this instance might be viewed as a subtle energy equivalent of physical vitality. In the process of laying-on-of-hands healing, the healer acts in a fashion similar to a jumper cable. The healer's energetic system represents a charged battery (at high potential) which is used to energize (or jump start) the subtle energetic system of a sick individual who is at low potential. This flow of healing energy from high to low potential appears to be similar to the flow of electricity, which behaves in a similar manner. Because of this superficial similarity to electricity, some healers, as mentioned previously, have referred to healing energy as paraelectricity.

Nurses who had taken Krieger's course slowly became proficient in doing laying-on-of-hands healing. Krieger herself found that the more she worked with it, the more effective a healer she became. Healing seemed to be a kind of subtle energetic gymnastic exercise. The more time and work an individual would put into it, the better at healing they became. This relatively small group of nurses whom Krieger had trained began to practice their healing on some of their hospital patients. Although some felt they were a bit strange, patients did appear to get better faster when Therapeutic Touch was added to their regimen of therapy. The nurses printed a bunch of T-shirts emblazoned with the words "Krieger's Krazies" to denote their alliance to the cause of healing. They also worked their healing ministrations on anyone who would be willing to "try an experiment." This would occasionally include sick and wounded stray dogs and cats with whom certain nurses achieved remarkable healing results.

After observing some of the results obtained by her healer-nurse trainees, Krieger became firmly convinced that non-psychic individuals could be taught to do healing. *She concluded that Therapeutic Touch was a natural human potential which could be demonstrated by individuals who had a fairly healthy body (and thus an overabundance of prana) as*

well as a strong intent to help or heal ill persons. In addition to these qualities, the potential healer had to be educable because, although Therapeutic
Touch might seem like a simple act, she found that in reality it was quite
complex to do in a conscious manner.

Krieger was sure that her nurse-healers could create similar healing-
associated physiological changes in patients to those Mr. Estebany had
demonstrated in her earlier studies. By showing that nurses could replicate
the healer-induced rise in hemoglobin noted in her previous research, she
could prove that laying-on-of-hands healing could indeed be taught and
verified by laboratory testing. To measure the healing energies of her nursing
students, Krieger designed a research protocol which would examine the
abilities of these fledgling healers to induce physiological changes in patients.

Krieger's study utilized registered nurses who were under her direction in hospitals and other health facilities in the metropolitan New York
area. In its final form, the study included 32 registered nurses and 64 patients
in a design similar to her two previous research projects with Mr. Estebany.
Instead of born healers, as in Mr. Estebany's case, Krieger used nurse-
healers who had been recently trained in her "Frontiers in Nursing" course.
Sixty-four sick patients were divided into two groups of 32 each: an experimental group, and a control group. The control group had regular
medical and nursing care under the direction of sixteen "non-healer"
nurses. The experimental group of patients had similar care, except that
sixteen Krieger-trained nurses performed Therapeutic Touch in addition
to their regular medical care. Hemoglobin levels were measured in both
groups of patients before and after the time period during which healing
was performed.

The two groups were compared for differences in hemoglobin values
between the beginning and the end of the experiment. In the control group,
there was no significant change in hemoglobin levels. *However, in the
nurse-healer treated group there were statistically significant increases in
hemoglobin.* Her statistical analysis showed that the odds against the results
obtained being due to chance were less than one in a thousand. Krieger
had demonstrated that trained nurse-healers could induce significant increases in the hemoglobin levels of patients treated by Therapeutic Touch
as compared with their control group counterparts.[18]

In 1979, Krieger wrote a book entitled *The Therapeutic Touch: How to
Use Your Hands to Help or to Heal.* The book was based on the experiences
and feedback of many nurses who had taken her course at NYU. In the

book, Krieger states that as of 1979, almost 350 professional nurses had taken "Frontiers In Nursing" as part of their curriculum for either the M.A. or Ph.D. degree. In addition, she had taught another 4,000 professionals in the health field via continuing education programs at various univei sities in the United States and Canada. A number of Krieger's nursing students have gone on to teach Therapeutic Touch to health-care practitioners and lay people throughout the country.

Many unique applications have come from the use of this healing art in the hospital setting. In one "premie unit" in New York, nurses began to use Therapeutic Touch on premature infants as part of their medical care. The medical staff began to note such tremendous strides in infant progress and weight gain that they sheepishly asked the nurses what they were doing that was different from the usual regimen. Eventually, all the doctors and nurses in the neonatal unit were taught to use Therapeutic Touch on the infants, including many inquisitive parents who wished to give their children every possible chance for a healthy survival. In another hospital in New York, doctors and nurses in the Emergency Room began to use Therapeutic Touch to ease and quiet many of their patients coming in with psychedelic drug overdoses. Utilization of this technique has met with interesting success, as demonstrated by patients' reduced need for sedation. There are indications of the medical community's increasing interest in Therapeutic Touch, as evidenced by recent funding for studies within this area by government-funded health agencies such as the National Institutes of Health (NIH).

Through the pioneering efforts of Dr. Krieger, psychic healing has begun to earn a place in the armamentarium of tools employed by health-care practitioners in their fight against illness and disease. A number of medical and osteopathic schools have begun to consider adding Therapeutic Touch to their curriculums of medical education. So-called "magnetic healing" has come a long way since the time of Mesmer. However, there is a diverse spectrum of phenomena that are embraced by the term psychic healing. There were some healers, such as Olga Worrall, who referred to their work as spiritual healing as opposed to psychic healing. It is possible that there are actually subtle differences in healing that distinguish these two approaches. In order to understand the different varieties of healing experiences possible, it will be necessary to examine these phenomena from the level of human subtle energetic anatomy.

From Magnetic Passes to Spiritual Healing:
A Multidimensional Model of Healing Energies

As discussed earlier in this chapter, the energies involved in laying-on-of-hands healing bear a unique resemblance to magnetic fields. Laboratory studies designed to measure the characteristics of these healing energies demonstrate interesting similarities to magnetism, including special negative entropic qualities. The healing approach employed by Mr. Estebany and practitioners of Therapeutic Touch usually involves direct contact with the sick patient or healee. Occasionally, this type of healing may employ the use of an intermediary such as water or an organic material (such as cotton) capable of absorbing and transferring healing energies to the patient. There are, however, certain methods of so-called distant healing which may transmit healing energies over great distances separating patient and healer.

As mentioned previously, Dr. Robert Miller has done extensive studies on the similarities between magnetic fields and healing energies. Much of his work was performed with the assistance of spiritual healers Olga and Ambrose Worrall. Subtle energies emanating from the Worralls' hands had been shown to decrease the surface tension of water, alter copper chloride crystallization properties, and increase the growth rates of plants via the intermediary of healer-charged water. Such effects had also been noted with the use of powerful magnetic fields. Of even greater significance than these previous studies was an experiment Miller conducted with the Worralls to measure the effects of distant healing. Because of their unusual nature, the findings from this segment of Miller's research have far-reaching implications for our understanding of the energetic dimensions of the healing process.

Although the Worralls did laying-on-of-hands healing on occasion, their usual modus operandi was to mentally hold patients in their thoughts and prayers while entering a healing state of consciousness. Dr. Lawrence LeShan, a psychologist studying psychic healing, has referred to this state of consciousness as the "clairvoyant reality." In this domain, all perceived boundaries of separation between people dissolve. Feelings of separation are often replaced by a deep inner sense of connectedness with all life and its divine nature.[19] Miller had already confirmed that healers like the Worralls were able to directly impart growth-promoting energies to plants via the intermediary of charged water. He now wondered if this other type of distant mental healing could also affect the growth rate of plants.

Miller built a special electromechanical transducer (first used by Dr. H. Kleuter of the U.S Dept. of Agriculture) to measure the hourly growth rate of rye grass. The device had a tiny lever which was attached to the growing tip of the plant to be measured. As the plant grew, the lever was lifted. The resulting signal change was recorded on a slowly moving graphic paper strip. The device had been previously shown to be accurate in recording plant growth rates to a thousandth of an inch per hour. Miller asked the Worralls if they would participate in a special experiment whereby they would hold the rye seedlings in their thoughts at their usual 9 P.M. prayer time. The unusual part of the experiment was that the Worralls were to be working from their Baltimore home *600 miles away* from Miller's laboratory in Atlanta, Georgia.

Prior to the experiment, the rye seedlings were attached to the tranducer and their growth rate measured for a period of several hours to assure that plant growth proceeded at a constant rate. The strip recorder showed a continuous slope, indicating a stable growth rate of 6.25 thousands of an inch per hour. Miller locked his laboratory so that no external physical variables could interfere with the healing experiment. At exactly 9 P.M., corresponding to the Worralls prayer time, the tracing from the plants began to deviate upward.[20] *By morning, the strip recorder revealed that the growth rate of the rye seedlings had risen to 52.5 thousands of an inch per hour, which was an increase of 840 percent!* The growth rate then steadily decreased, but never returned to the level of the original baseline. When asked how they had accomplished this healing feat, the Worralls replied that during their prayer time, *they had visualized the plants filled with light and energy.*

Miller was fascinated with the experimental outcome and endeavored to find another method of indirectly measuring the energetic influence of the healer. Miller utilized a special cloud chamber which was used to measure the vapor trails of tiny energetic subatomic particles. The cloud chamber contained a cooled vapor of liquid alcohol which permitted the observer to see a visual smoke trail formed by ionized molecules as a charged particle passed through. Miller asked Mrs. Worrall to place her hands around the cloud chamber and try to influence the vapor within. While placing her hands around the chamber without actually touching the surface, she concentrated on healing as she would with a patient. Experimental observers noted a wave pattern developing in the mist which was parallel to the position of her hands. When Worrall shifted her hands 90 degrees, the waves also shifted to a position at right angles from their former location. Similar cloud-chamber phenomena have since been produced by Ingo Swann and two other psychics.

Miller later repeated the experiment with Mrs. Worrall concentrating on visualizing her hands around the cloud chamber from her home in Baltimore. All motion in the cloud chamber was videotaped. *At the time that Worrall visualized placing her hands around the cloud chamber, similar wave motion appeared in the mist as had been observed when her hands were physically near the cloud chamber.* Worrall then visualized herself rotating her hands to a different position, at which time the wave motion in the chamber also rotated as had occurred when Worrall had been present in the laboratory. The wave motion in the cloud chamber persisted for another eight minutes following the conclusion of the experimental period. *Again, as in the seedling experiment, Worrall had been able to influence the cloud chamber at a distance of nearly 600 miles.*[21]

The results of Miller's cloud-chamber and rye seedling experiments offer new information about the dimensions of the process of healing. Although earlier experimentation on the energetic effects of healing required the physical presence of the healer in the laboratory, Miller now demonstrated that the phenomenon could be measured with the healer hundreds of miles away. This suggests that there are a wide spectrum of multidimensional energy influences being observed in different experimental settings.

The ability of Mrs. Worrall to cause energy changes at a distance of 600 miles is strong evidence for a non-electromagnetic energy influence. It is known that electromagnetic energy decreases in intensity proportional to the square of the distance from the source of energy. In physics vernacular, this is known as the inverse square law. This law is applicable to both electromagnetic, electrostatic, and gravitational forces. However, we have a repeatable experimental effect which cannot be explained away using conventional electromagnetic theory. In the Tiller-Einstein Model of negative space/time energies (i.e., ME or magnetoelectric energy), we have an energy which operates at speeds beyond that of light velocity. Tiller's model places the etheric spectrum of energies as moving at velocities between the speed of light and 10^{10} times the speed of light. Astral energies (another variation of magnetoelectric energy) are theorized to operate between 10^{10} and 10^{20} times the speed of light. As one approaches such incredible velocities of ME energy transmission, movement through the universe becomes nearly instantaneous. This could easily explain how Mrs. Worrall's energy influence could create simultaneous distant effects at a distance of 600 miles. One might literally say that the time for magnetoelectric energy to move from the mind of the healer to the experimental setup (or patient) is limited only by the speed of thought. Indeed, such energies are reflections of the higher vibrational characteristics of consciousness at the etheric, astral, and higher dimensional levels.

Depending upon the vibrational frequency from which a particular healer operates, we can see that there are a variety of energy levels at which healing can occur. On the one hand, we have a phenomenon which might be referred to as *magnetic healing*. It is perhaps akin to the therapeutic ministrations first studied by Mesmer over 200 years ago. This type of healing appears to require direct contact of the hands between the patient and the healer, or the intermediary of some energetic storage medium such as water or cotton. (Krieger's nurses on occasion will give energized rolls of cotton wadding to sick patients to hold, as Estebany had done in the original research study.) Alternatively, there is a different therapeutic method which has been referred to as *spiritual healing*. The practitioners of this art usually attune through meditation to the "forces of the divine," and attempt to mentally project energy to the sick individual as well as heal by the direct laying-on-of-hands.

Healers employing both methods often refer to themselves as "vehicles" or "channels" of a higher source of energy. Most feel that this energy has its origins at a divine level. The healer acts as a type of waveguide to direct these higher energies into the mind/body of the sick individual. In both types of healing, an energetic boost is delivered to the subtle energetic and physiological systems of the sick individual, which assists in the resolution of the disease process and in a return to homeostasis.

It has been shown that the energies relayed by laying-on-of-hands healing have definite and measureable effects upon enzymes and other physical systems of the body. The negatively entropic properties of the healer's energies can cause denatured, inactivated protein molecules to reintegrate and realign themselves to a state of functional activity. Following the process of molecular healing, one further notes healers' abilities to selectively affect enzyme kinetics. Depending on whether the treated enzyme is one that adds to the energy reserve of the cell or depletes its metabolic resources, the healer is able to speed or slow the reaction rate. The direction of enzymatic change produced by healers seems to always be in accordance with the natural cellular intelligence of the body.

Healer's energies are qualitatively similar to powerful magnetic fields and also possess negative entropic properties. Both of these characteristics fit well with the postulated properties of etheric energies. It would make sense that some healers might have their primary healing effects by supplying particular frequencies of etheric (and higher) energies to patients' etheric bodies We know that the etheric body is a holographic energetic template. It is a type of spatial waveguide that assists the molecular/cellular systems of the body to achieve proper organization, orchestration, and energetic balance. If the etheric template is healthy and orderly, the body resides in a state of health. When the etheric body is distorted and its organized patterns become disrupted by a wide variety of influences, the physical body slowly follows suit by manifesting illness. The organization of the etheric template controls the orderly cellular behavior of the body's systems. When the influence of the etheric body has totally ceased, as in death, the component molecular parts return to the chaotic disorder of inorganic matter.

Our etheric templates are the waveguides that control the flow of life energies into the body. Patterns of illness occur at the energetic level before they become manifest at the cellular level. Dysfunctional subtle energetic changes in the etheric body may precede physical/cellular changes of

Diagram 27.
A MULTIDIMENSIONAL MODEL OF HEALING

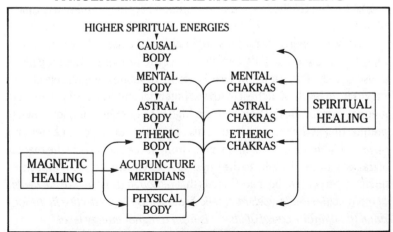

overt disease by weeks to months. Therefore, it would be useful to restructure the etheric template toward a more healthful, beneficial pattern to effect a healing of established physical illness. It is possible to influence even higher components of our subtle anatomy in order to effect healing at the physical level. To see how this would operate, we need to look back at the higher vibrational systems that feed energy into the physical body.

It is likely that *magnetic healing takes place mostly at the level of the etheric and physical bodies.* There is direct energy transfer from healer to patient, often through the intermediary of the hands. There are actually minor chakras in the palms of the hands which act as centers of energy flow into and out of the body. However, *spiritual healing is able to interact with not only the physical/etheric levels but with higher levels as well.*

Since the time of Edward Bach (the originator of the Bach Flower Remedies), physicians have begun to realize that the mind and emotions play a significant role in the origins and exacerbations of many (if not all) illnesses. The emotions work at a subtle energetic level through the influence of the astral body, which feeds into the etheric body. It has become increasingly clear that depression and other emotional disorders can cause a suppression of the body's natural defenses against illness. This state of immuno-incompetence can later become translated into physical illness through an increased susceptibility to viral and bacterial agents as well as through internal sources of disease like cancer cells. Distortions originating at the level of the astral body take time to work their way down through the etheric to the physical levels. This is why it may be weeks or months before changes in the emotional/astral constitution become manifest as physical illness.

Likewise, energy distortions originating at the mental level from aberrations in the mental body can also affect the proper functioning of the physical body. There is a downward cascade of subtle energetic effects that moves from levels of highest to lowest potential and frequency. There is a gradual signal transduction of these higher frequency energies down to manifesting at the physical level. This process occurs through a stepping down of higher vibrational frequencies from the causal level to the mental, astral, etheric, and finally to the physical level via the physical/etheric interface. The point to be made here is that *although disease may be healed at a physical/etheric level, magnetic healing may be ineffective in the long run if the ultimate cause of illness is from a higher energy level.*

An example of the lack of long-term benefit from magnetic types of healing can be seen with certain healings done by the "psychic surgeons" of the Phillipines. In some cases, cancer patients have travelled to these healers in search of cures and have returned with objective laboratory and clinical evidence of complete remission. However, some of these individuals have later returned to the same psychic surgeon several years later with a new tumor in a different organ system. Although a case may be made that the recurrent tumor was merely a metastatic lesion which was microscopic at the time of the original healing, there is a suggestion that the emotional/mental patterns of these patients which may have originally contributed to tumor formation were never addressed by the magnetic healer who worked primarily at the physical/etheric level.

In contradistinction to magnetic healing, *spiritual healing attempts to work at the level of the higher subtle bodies and chakras* to effect a healing from the most primary level of disease origins. *The spiritual healer works as a power source of multiple-frequency outputs to allow energy shifts at several levels simultaneously.* It is theorized that there may be a transient energy link between the chakras of the healer and the patient. This chakra-to-chakra link may allow for a direct resonant transfer of multiple subtle frequencies, which can shift the multidimensional energy structure of the patient back toward a perfect balance of mind, body, and spirit. *While most magnetic healers work strictly at the level of the body, spiritual healers usually work with the many levels of mind and spirit as well.* The nature of this higher dimensional energy is that it transcends all limitations of space and time by virtue of the fact that levels from the etheric and higher energies are in the domain of negative space/time. As such, the energies working at these levels move in a dimension which is outside of the usual references of ordinary (or positive) space/time to which the conscious mind is limited in its perception. However, the frequencies at which spiritual healing takes place often extend to the same levels at which the Higher Self exists and operates.

A demonstration of the transcendental nature of these higher frequency energies can be found in Dr. Miller's experiments with Olga and Ambrose Worrall. The Worralls were able to create measureable increases in the growth rate of rye seedlings at a distance of over 600 miles while working at a level of higher dimensional consciousness. The fact that the laboratory and the healer were separated by great distances at the positive space/time level is irrelevant because the energies that were operating were working at the negative space/time level, which we have seen is an entirely different reference system. The cloud-chamber experiment where Mrs. Worrall was able to create standing wave patterns in Atlanta from her home in Baltimore is another demonstration of the higher dimensional nature of these energies.

It is possible that Mrs. Worrall may have been operating at the astral and higher levels, because the astral body is able to move great distances almost instantaneously by focusing thoughts on a particular place. This is the nature of the astral domain: matter is much more plastic than at the physical level. (See Chapter 4 for a more complete description of behavior at the astral levels.) If, in fact, she were working from the level of her astral body, she would be able to communicate and work directly on the astral form of her patient. Drs. Elmer Green and Norman Shealy experimentally tested Mrs. Worrall's distant healing and her ability to affect the biological rhythms of her patients at a distance. Mrs. Worrall sat in a room down the hall from her patient while both were attached to EEG, EKG, GSR, and other physiological monitoring devices. While Mrs. Worrall visualized herself working astrally on the patient's throat area, the patient would actually report that he or she could feel a sensation of warmth and tingling in that bodily region. Even more remarkable was the researchers' observation that there was a sychronization of brainwave activity and other bioelectric rhythms between healer and patient during the healing process.

In England, researcher Maxwell Cade has reported similar biorhythm entrainment between healers and patients. Utilizing a special device known as the Mind Mirror, a computerized EEG power spectra analyzer, Cade also discovered a unique complex brainwave pattern found only in advanced healers, that became prominent in the brainwaves of patients during the healing process.[22] Cade measured these unique healing-induced brainwave synchrony patterns between patient and healer during times when the healer was both in direct contact as well as at a distance from the patient. This observation that healers can achieve biological rhythm entrainment with direct laying-on-of-hands and with healing at a distance, confirms the higher dimensional nature of the energies involved in healing as well as the energy resonance hypothesis of healing. Olga Worrall and others have repeatedly demonstrated that distance poses no great challenge to the advanced spiritual healer when attempting to send healing energies to patients. Such spiritual healers operate primarily at the negative space/time levels of people's higher dimensional components which feed, organize, and support the molecular/cellular structures of the physical body.

It is important to remember that illness can originate at many levels of our multidimensional anatomy and not just at the level of the physical body. Although there are many external agents of disease—bacteria, viruses, environmental toxins, and carcinogens—they are less likely to affect the body of an individual who is in good physical and mental health. The key concept of host resistance tells us that illness is a combination of factors both external and internal. The internal factors are more important than doctors currently recognize. These internal factors are not merely physico-chemical factors (although vitamins and proper nutrition can obviously assist the body in resisting the influence of carcinogens) but also higher energetic factors involving the realms of spiritual consciousness.

At the spiritual levels of human consciousness, there exists a level of perfection and energetic balance which cannot be affected by distortions of mind and emotion. At these highest levels, the soul is working to positively influence the energies integrating with the physical form. According to the reincarnational philosophy, our bodies are only a temporary vehicle of expression upon the physical plane. Our physical personalities are a manifestation of the soul in chemical clothes. This level of understanding is an aspect of humanity that most doctors have not yet discovered, but it is hopefully a dimension that the spiritual physicians of the future will address.

> Frankly, it is amazing that any physician or psychologist can fail to appreciate that there is an ensouling consciousness which uses the matter of thought, emotion, and dense substance to create the various bodies of manifestation. The very performance of their duties should lead them to try to discern the Idea and inner purpose which is ensouling the forms they treat, so that they can better help this Idea manifest. To put this in pragmatic terms, the physical or emotional body of a person might be sick, but the inner being and inner Idea is quite healthy and seeking to heal the substance, pattern, and function of these sick bodies. That should be a basic premise of medical science. It is a FUNDAMENTAL law of life and its manifestation . . .
>
> *Some of the ideas about the magnetic aspects of physical and emotional sickness will be the focus for some real breakthroughs in medicine, and perhaps inspire similar breakthroughs in other scientific disciplines.* In many ways, it is medicine and psychology which will have to lead the rest of the scientific community to a discovery of the ensouling consciousness and its relation to matter, because they deal more directly with the subtle levels of matter.[23] *(italics added)*

As we have seen throughout this chapter, there is increasing evidence to suggest that the ability to heal is an innate human potential. The levels at which healing may take place can vary from a purely physical healing at the physical/etheric level, to the spiritual levels where the Higher Self is already attempting to integrate with the physical body and personality. Science is beginning to evolve toward a place where New Age technologies may confirm what biblical prophets dating back to Jesus have told us all along. As Jesus said, "These things I do, so can you do and more."

Dr. Krieger found that the ability to do healing was an expression of a deep inner desire by the individual to help or heal another. It is pure compassion, an expression of love at the highest level. The experience of connectedness between patient and healer through unconditional love is a level which must be reached and addressed by more in the so-called "healing professions" for greater healing to occur. If more health-care professionals can begin to acknowledge and activate their innate healing potentials, the nature of our cultural healing institutions will begin to radically shift. As the New Age approaches and more scientists and theologicans begin to readdress the painful schism between the material and spiritual dimensions of human existence, our civilization will begin to move forward toward a greater understanding of health and illness from a truly multidimensional perspective.

Key Points to Remember

1. Laying-on-of-hands healing has been practiced throughout the world for thousands of years. In the late 1700s, Franz Mesmer theorized that a subtle life-energy of a magnetic nature was exchanged between healer and patient during laying-on-of-hands. Mesmer also discovered that water could effectively store this subtle force for transfer to sick patients in need of healing.

2. In the 1960s, Dr. Bernard Grad essentially replicated Mesmer's findings that healing energy from laying-on-of-hands could be transferred to water. Grad, however, went further to show that this subtle energy could actually stimulate the growth rate of plants, the rate of wound healing in mice, and the prevention of goiter development in susceptible animals. Grad's results with healers and accelerated wound healing were later replicated in another laboratory.

3. Dr. Robert Miller went on to show a striking energetic similarity between healer-treated and magnet-treated water, supporting Mesmer's contention that healing energy was of a magnetic nature. Miller showed that changes in water tension and hydrogen bonding, as well as alterations in crystallization patterns in copper sulfate, were similar for healer-treated and magnet-treated water.

4. Dr. Justa Smith found that, again, magnetic fields produced qualitative effects similar to healers' energies, in that both could accelerate the action of enzymes in solution.

5. Dr. Smith found that different enzymes would be affected differentially by healing energies, but that the direction of change always paralleled greater cellular health.

6. Dr. Smith found that healers could also repair damaged enzymes. This demonstrated the principle that healing energy was negatively entropic in nature, meaning that it caused systems to become more ordered. Further research with different healers showed that healing energy could produce other negative entropic effects on nonliving chemical systems.

7. In the healing experiments by Dr. Smith, she used sensitive magnetic detectors to measure magnetic fields coming from the healer, however none were ever detected. More recent work with new, ultrasensitive SQUID (Superconducting Quantum Interference Device) magnetic detectors found small but measureable increases in magnetic field emission from healers' hands during healing. Thus, laying-on-of-hands healing energies are indeed magnetic in nature, are qualitatively similar to intense magnetic fields in some of their effects upon biological systems, but are exceedingly difficult to detect with conventional measuring devices.

8. The characteristics of healers' energies are that they are negatively entropic and are also qualitatively similar to magnetic fields, but that they are poorly measured by conventional EM detectors. These characteristics are identical to the qualities of magnetoelectric or negative space/time energies as predicted in the Tiller-Einstein Model of positive-negative space/time.

9. Dr. Dolores Krieger's research demonstrated that healer's energies could increase hemoglobin levels in patients similar to the way that they increased chlorophyll content in healer-treated plants. This was one of the first parameters to be established which could allow quanti-

tative biochemical measurements in humans to detect the effects of healing energy.

10. Dr. Krieger went further to show that people could be trained to do healing. Her nurse-healers were able to increase hemoglobin levels in patients similar to the naturally gifted healers, demonstrating that healing was an innate human potential and that it could be a learned skill.

11. Experiments by Dr. Miller with healers Olga and Ambrose Worrall showed that healing energies could affect living and nonliving systems at a distance of 600 miles.

12. The varieties of healing energies occur along a spectrum of phenomena. Laying-on-of-hands healing may be more accurately described as "magnetic healing." It's effects tend to be more at the physical-etheric levels of rebalancing, and it is performed with the healer's hands in close proximity to the patient. Conversely, "spiritual healing" works not only at the physical and etheric levels, but also helps to rebalance the astral, mental, and higher energetic levels of dysfunction as well. In addition, spiritual healing may be performed either in the presence of the patient or at great distances which may separate the patient and healer.

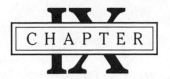

CHAPTER IX

Crystals & the
Human Subtle Energetic System:
THE REDISCOVERY
OF AN ANCIENT HEALING ART

Throughout successive chapters of this book, we have endeavored to paint a realistic portrait of humans as multidimensional beings. Each human being is an organized interweaving of many bodies of differing vibrational frequencies. Through our interconnection to the chakras and our higher frequency bodies of light, we are able to assimilate energy and information from the highest levels of being. Energy and information originating at the soul level undergoes progressive transformation and translation until it becomes manifest as a conscious personality which must exist in the molecular/cellular vehicle at the level of the physical plane. Due to the limited nature of the physical brain at its present level of linear expression, we become locked into the perspective of a seemingly fixed space/time frame. Thus, the multidimensional universe is beyond our undeveloped insight.

To most individuals, the higher dimensional energies are in the realm of invisibility. To a fortunate few with clairvoyant perception, the beauty of these invisible realms can be perceived with great ease. The only thing that seems to limit human potential is its definition of itself. As technology makes visible what was previously seen only by clairvoyants, *the invisible becomes visible.* We are slowly coming to a point in the evolution of our technology where the realms of the invisible are being made visible with increasing frequency. The growing knowledge of the use of crystals to transmute and transform electromagnetic energy has played an increasingly important role in the evolution of these new technologies. The use of crystalline technologies for the development of electronic systems has resulted in great strides in the way scientists are able to perceive the universe around us. Because of the role of silicon technology in intergrated circuitry and the development of computer systems, we have been provided with new tools that can amplify our powers of memory and information storage. Crystals are beginning to provide human beings with the power to manipulate and transform knowledge itself in many new ways.

Crystals have played important roles in many scientific discoveries which have begun to revolutionize the way we think about the structure of consciousness and the universe itself. For instance, a ruby crystal was a key component in the first laser developed by Bell Laboratory scientists in the early 1960s. As discussed in the first chapter, the model of the laser and the holograms it can be used to produce have given birth to the holographic model. Energy interference patterns as typified by holography have been adapted by Karl Pribram and other neuroscientists to explain certain aspects of memory storage within the brain. Additionally, the holographic model provides us with a new way of appreciating the multidimensional universe.

Recent research into the integration of laser and holographic technology for information storage has revealed new ways of utilizing crystals. More than ten years ago, Philips Research Labs of Hamburg, Germany, recorded a demonstration holographic movie in a crystal of lithium niobate. Since that time, new work with other niobate-related crystals at Oak Ridge National Laboratories in Tennessee has revealed the possibility of storing thousands of three-dimensional images in single crystals. By rotating the crystal slightly, a new storage opportunity is created. Applications based on this work point toward a time when tremendous amounts of data may be holographically stored in a specially tailored crystal. It has been said that the potential for archival storage is tremendous, as niobate crystals could be used to store all of the Social Security information for the United States as well as entire technical or literary libraries.[1]

Aside from the theoretical implications of lasers and holography, the practical development of lasers for use in medicine and surgery, as well as laserpuncture, have made a reality of healing with frequency-specific energies. Laser-related advances in communications have provided a new means of transmitting large quantities of information over great distances via fiber-optic cables. Crystals such as gallium arsenide have provided the tools to create tiny solid-state lasers no bigger than a match head, as well as devices for displaying information via light-emitting diodes (LEDs).

Another type of crystal which science has only recently begun to explore is the "liquid crystal." Experimentation with liquid-crystal technologies has resulted in inexpensive temperature-biofeedback devices, numerical displays, and even miniaturized color television sets. The harnessing of the regular oscillations of electrically stimulated quartz crystals, combined with the technology of liquid-crystal displays (LCDs), has made accurate and inexpensive timepieces commonplace. In addition, as our understanding of artificially created liquid crystals has grown, so have biologists come to recognize that many of the cellular membranes and structures within the human body are liquid crystals as well.

It has only been within the span of the last century that the knowledge of electromagnetism has given humanity the ability to explore potential healing applications and other beneficial gifts of the crystals and gems which grow naturally within the earth. By studying the process of crystallization, scientists have learned to artificially grow crystals of great purity with special energetic characteristics. Certain artificially grown crystals, such as the silicon used to create solar cells, have enabled us to harness the energies of sunlight to power many of our technological marvels both on Earth and in outer space.

From utilizing crystals for communication, information storage, solar power, and laser applications in industry and medicine, we are slowly discovering that the gems and minerals of the Earth hold undreamt-of potentials for serving humankind. Modern thinkers are very narrow-minded, however, in believing that our present culture is the first to develop such crystalline technologies. In general, scientists have tended to believe that the more ancient in time a civilization, the more primitive its technology must have been. One need not go further than the sophisticated astronomical calendar of the Mayans, the electrical battery discovered from ancient Baghdad, and the navigational computer found on an undersea shipwreck, to realize the egocentricity of today's minds. There are legends of an ancient civilization, Atlantis, which utilized crystalline technologies to a degree that surpassed even present-day scientific applications. It is important to closely examine these so-called legends because the information contained within such myths has accurately foretold the development of many of today's great technologic achievements with crystals. Also, we can often understand an ancient device, image, language, or archaeological ruin only when our present technology attains a similar result.

An Esoteric History of Crystalline Technologies: The Roots of Silicon Valley in the Lost Continent of Atlantis

There are few who know the ancient mythologies of the Earth who have not heard of the ancient continent of Atlantis. There are many stories told about the greatness of this now extinct civilization, and there were 6,000 books about Atlantis in existence by the 1970s. In the past, these stories have been viewed with extreme skepticism. However, there is now a growing body of information which seems to support the existence of this land mass in the Atlantic Ocean and its untimely demise beneath the tidal waves that brought about its destruction.

Even if it is viewed only as a parable, the legend of Atlantis is important because it tells the story of a people whose technologies and self-importance grew to a point where self-destruction became a prophecy fulfilled. We cannot afford to scoff at such tales, for like the Atlanteans at the peak of their civilization, we are ever poised upon the brink of atomic destruction and nuclear winter. There are some who say that America is the new Atlantis. In order to understand why this statement may have a ring of truth to it and to compare the possible parallels between ancient Atlantis and modern-day America, we shall have to examine some of the legends surrounding this once great culture.

It is said that Atlantis was a great continent which existed in that body of water now known as the Atlantic Ocean. Although modern archaeologists have tended to view human civilization as a fairly recent development, the old legends suggest that Atlantis flourished during a period dating from at least 150,000 B.C. until approximately 10,000 B.C., when it was supposed to have sunk during a flood of biblical proportions. The esoteric literature tells us that Atlantis was not destroyed in a single flood but that there were two, earlier, man-made cataclysms that reduced the land mass to a series of smaller continents before its eventual and complete annihilation in 10,000 B.C.

Although the Atlantean civilization was said to have existed over a period of more than 100,000 years, its people began as a purely agricultural society. Over thousands of years, the population evolved to more advanced levels of society and culture. During its last 30,000 or more years, the technology and sciences of Atlantis evolved to a high degree of sophistication. At its peak, sometimes referred to as the Golden Age of Atlantis, the Atlanteans had grown to become a race of highly developed individuals who were skilled in all manners of architecture, engineering, astronomy, agriculture, and especially the healing arts.

The advanced technologies of Atlantis were quite different than present-day achievements. Whereas today science has learned to exploit the latent energies of coal and petroleum products to create heat, light, and electricity to power our everyday conveniences of living, the Atlanteans had developed a technology based upon the higher dimensional energies of consciousness and the life-force.

The Atlanteans could control what one calls the "life force." As today one extracts the energy of heat from coal and transforms it into motive power for our means of locomotion, the Atlanteans knew how to put the germinal energy of organisms into the service of their technology. One can form an idea of this from the following. Think of a kernel of seed-grain. In this an energy lies dormant. This energy causes the stalk to sprout from the kernel. Nature can awaken this energy which reposes in the seed. Modern man cannot do it at will. He must bury the seed in the ground and leave the awakening to the forces of nature. The Atlantean could do something else. He knew how one can change the energy of a pile of grain into technical power, just as modern man can change the heat energy of a pile of coal into such power.

Plants were cultivated in the Atlantean period not merely for use as foodstuffs but also in order to make the energies dormant in them available to commerce and industry. Just as we have mechanisms for transforming the energy dormant in coal into energy of motion in our locomotives, so the Atlanteans had mechanisms in which they, so to speak, burned plant seeds, and in which the life-force was transformed into technically utilizable power.[2]

As alluded to in the chapter on flower essences, it is suggested that the art of healing with the vibrational essences of flowers and gems had its origin with the Atlantean culture. Numerous flower essences and other similar remedies were developed to treat illnesses that arose for the first time in Atlantis. It is said that many of the stress-related disorders commonly seen in technologically advanced societies had their origins in Atlantis. The roots of early homeopathic and vibrational medicines may be more ancient than any of today's holistic practitioners realize.

Flower essences began to be used as a system of medicine in Atlantis for herein is where diseases like those orthodox physicians study had their origins. Then the blooms were put on water so the flowers could be as exposed to the pranic forces of the rising sun. Because the Atlanteans were not properly in tune with nature many diseases developed for the first time on the planet.

Man in Atlantean days divided into three specific senses of social attitudes and studies of the origins and predominance of society. There were those who were *purely spiritual*, those of the *priesthood*, integrated between science or the material and the spiritual, and those who were *purely materialistic* and studied only the material and the various patterns of the material seeking the origins of life, having forgotten their own foundations. These are the foundations that led to the necessary homeopathic systems of science, the divisions into allopathic medicines, and of those who practiced more on the spiritual path. Those who travelled the spiritual path apart from the homeopathic and allopathic medicines were those who were purely spiritual and used more the accord of flower essences. Those of the priesthood were homeopathic for they travelled the patterns between the spiritual and the material. Those of the material accord were allopathic.[3]

It is interesting to note that in ancient times the materialistic or allopathic approach may have been practiced by those in the minority viewpoint. The Atlanteans appear to have been oriented toward the use of vibrational medicines more than drug therapies, although a distinct allopathic faction existed then as now. It is almost as if human culture has followed a reverse pattern of medical development since the fall of Atlantis, with materialistic allopathy being the cultural norm at the present and the homeopaths forming a rival minority. In addition to the use of homeopathic remedies and flower essences, the Atlanteans were famous for their knowledge of the healing powers of crystals.

In addition to the Atlanteans' knowlege of utilizing the life-force to do work through various devices, much of the sophisticated Atlantean technology was based upon the energetic applications of crystals, specifically the quartz crystal. It is said that the Atlanteans possessed various modes of transportation that included flying vehicles. The flying ships, as many other devices, were usually powered by a distant energy source known as the great crystals. These crystals, sometimes referred to as the firestones, were constructed of specially faceted quartz crystals which were capable of transmuting the sun's energy into utilizable power. This crystalline energy could be broadcast to a distant geographical location and used to power various devices including the flying ships.

It is not difficult to believe that crystals could be used to capture and transform the rays of the sun. Today, silicon solar cells are commonly found in calculators, watches, and power-generating stations around the world. The concept of broadcasting utilizable energy to a distant location is an idea which was successfully developed earlier in the twentieth century by the electrical wizard, Nikola Tesla. The Atlanteans had discovered how to tap into the energetic properties of crystals to a high degree. They could grow crystals of specific qualities and sizes for particular uses. Many of the technological wonders of the Atlantean era were powered by smaller crystals utilizing similar energetic principles used to create the great crystals.

One of the Atlanteans' key discoveries was the tremendous power inherent in sunlight. Crystals helped them tap into particular energetic applications of sunlight such as the powering of aircraft and communication systems. The creation of flower essences and gem elixirs enabled the Atlanteans to fuse the vibrations of nature with the subtle energetic properties of sunlight. They knew the pranic forces carried by sunlight which were of subtle energetic significance to all living cells. They also knew about the therapeutic use of colors produced by sunlight passing through crystalline prisms, as well as the healing properties of the higher octave color rays.

> Over the course of many civilizations the Atlanteans rose to a high state of technological achievement. They tapped into and used the energy of the Sun for the creation and sustenance of their society. Man today ignores this, the greatest factor in his life and takes the Sun's powers for granted. He knows little of the real gifts of the Sun, but the Atlanteans recognized its true power and used it. They used it not only for transportation, for building, for healing, but for every aspect of their spiritual life as well. They used it for worship. The Atlanteans recognized that because there is an aspect of the Godhead in each cell of matter, which is energized by the Sun, all matter is controlled by the Sun. They discovered the relationship between the energizing factor of the Sun and life on this Earth.[4]

Whereas modern-day applications of quartz crystals involve circuits which carry electrical energy, it is suspected that the Atlanteans exploited what would today be considered the more subtle energetic applications of crystals, i.e., the transformation and utilization of negative space/time energies. In addition to the use of crystals for powering everyday conveniences of living (lighting, communication systems, transportation, etc.), the Atlanteans had extensively explored the application of crystalline energies for healing devices. Various types of artificially grown crystals were used in what we would today refer to as laser surgery. A number of crystalline devices were also utilized in the diagnosis as well as treatment of diseases.

In instances of disease or illness the Atlanteans recognized that the source of the disease lay not in the physical but in a higher body. Therefore they always cured the higher body, not the physical. If a person was ill he was taken to a place of healing, a temple, and placed in a healing room. This room was constructed of a certain type of stone, of crystal, and was so shaped and angled that the power of the Sun was diffused into beams of different colored cosmic light and energy. The person was then placed in the middle of the room, depending upon the nature of his illness, so the correct rays of light, and therefore color, were directed onto him.

Also, of course, the priests of that time, being evolved souls with a high degree of consciousness, could look at the akashic record of the person who was ill, for illness is not necessarily only of one's present life, but can stretch back through many previous lives. They could cure, or attempt to cure, the true cause of the dis-ease in that person.[5]

Atlantis remained a powerful culture for many thousands of years. However, during its earlier technological stages, the energies broadcast from the great crystals are said to have been tuned too high. Due to this artificial energetic imbalance, Atlantis was rocked by major earthquakes which resulted in the loss of much technology and the separation of the continent into several smaller, island-like land masses. In addition to accidental disasters due to the misuse of technology (with respect to the planetary energetic environment), other destructive periods of Atlantean history were caused by wars involving the perverted use of crystalline and atomic weapons.

The reason for the eventual destruction of Atlantis had to do with the development of two ideologically divided groups in Atlantean culture. One faction of the Atlanteans, which were historically the first to evolve, were the more spiritually directed individuals. They believed in the unity of all life in its relationship to a single, all-encompassing creator or God-force. They lived according to this philosophy, which was expressed most simply as "the Law of One." Those that followed the Law of One were altruistic and selfless. They sought to uplift the spiritual and physical conditions of those around them and always endeavored to maintain a balance with the cosmic and planetary forces of nature as an expression of the one God. In opposition to this group were those who have been referred to as the Sons of Belial. These individuals were very materialistic and self-oriented. They tended to be more concerned with the sensual pleasures of life and with power. They misused the technologies discovered by the followers of the Law of One, appropriating them for destructive and materialistic purposes.

Due to the influence of the Sons of Belial, many of the religious temples of Atlantis eventually became degraded to temples of sin, in which spiritual laws were applied to the satisfaction of the physical appetites. The Atlanteans were also more psychic than today's population. But the misuse of such ability by the followers of Belial brought strife in many quarters. Conflicts arose over who would receive special privileges and who would be the ruling class. The Atlantean knowledge of the application of the life-force in genetic engineering was misused to create a mutant race of disfigured, yet physically strong, ignorant workers sometimes referred to as "the Things." A type of caste system grew up whereby the Things became abused as slave laborers that carried out most of the lowly tasks felt to be beneath the ruling classes.

Over time, party lines became sharply drawn between the two opposing factions. Although those of the Law of One were ostensibly in power, the Sons of Belial gradually cut large inroads into their authority and power. In the end, civil war erupted. The sun crystals became cruelly adapted as a means of coercion, torture, and punishment. They became known among the common people as the "terrible crystals." By 10,700 B.C., a new low in morality and human dignity had been reached by the Sons of Belial in their disrespect for all lives but their own. It seemed apparent that the materialistic faction's misuse of the crystalline and other technologies would eventually cause another major disaster as had shattered the continent of Atlantis in ages past.

> Why then did Atlantis fall? Atlantis fell for the same reason that all other civilizations have fallen: Man's erroneousness. Although the people of Atlantis had reached a high point of evolution, although they had tapped into cosmic powers and, because of the era in which they lived, they developed their psychic abilities way beyond your comprehension, they did not motivate themselves correctly. They used their knowledge of the Cosmos, their point of evolution, not to fulfill the will of their Creator, and His divine Plan but to fulfill their own ideas of creation. They used their knowledge for personal satisfaction and gain, to obtain power, to amass wealth, to control other beings, to further their own plans, no matter what the cost. The powers which the Atlanteans were given, and which in the initial stages they had used for construction, were eventually used for destruction, and so the downfall of Atlantis, with its eventual subsidence beneath the waves, began.[6]

Those who followed the teachings of the one God realized, through their naturally clairvoyant powers, that the destruction of Atlantis, with the final breakup of the remaining land masses, would slowly be upon them. They knew that the misuse of the powerful crystals would eventually have profound effects upon the environment, as had happened in a previous man-made cataclysm which nearly destroyed their civilzation. Those who followed the teachings of the Law of One prepared for the disaster by organizing groups of individuals who would leave Atlantis via three major migratory routes. Some would go to Egypt, a country with which contact had previously been made. Others would go to the area now known as Peru in South America, and to the area of land now called the Yucatan Peninsula. With them they would carry many of the record crystals and aspects of their technology which could be preserved for humanity's future. In addition, survivors would bring to these distant lands the traditions and beliefs of the Law of One. These record crystals are said to still safely exist in special pyramidal chambers in Egypt, South America, and the Yucatan Peninsula.

In approximately 9,600 B.C., the final cataclysm occurred which carried Atlantis beneath the waters of the ocean. Some sources have suggested that the reason for the flood was due to a shift in the earth's axis, which caused the polar icecap to become closer to the sun. In addition to the major quake and earth-shifting activity this would have caused, the melting of the arctic ice would have resulted in significant flooding and rearrangement of the borders of the countries of the world.

There is information today which seems to support the idea of an immense flood occurring in 9,600 B.C., the year Atlantis was supposed to have sunk beneath the waves. Much of what the scientific community knows about the destruction of Atlantis is derived from the writings of Plato. Plato lived in Greece in approximately 400 B.C. He learned of Atlantis from the writings of his ancestor, Solon, the great law-giver of Athens who had lived two-hundred years previously (about 600 B.C.). Solon had acquired his knowledge of Atlantis from conversations with priests whom he had encountered on a visit to Egypt. The Egyptian priests told Solon that the deluge which destroyed Atlantis took place in approximately 9,600 B.C. If the legends of Atlantean migration to parts of Egypt were correct, then it would lend credence to the accuracy of the Egyptian priests' story.

Modern research in the area of ancient climatic and weather conditions (paleoclimatology) has lent support to the timing of Atlantis' inundation at exactly the time told to Solon by the Egyptian priests.[7] In September 1975, University of Miami scientists reported in the journal *Science* that there had indeed been widespread flooding about that time. Cesare Emiliani, a paleoclimatologist, and his colleagues based their conclusion on sediment cores taken from the Gulf of Mexico. These cores contained fossil shells that, when originally formed, had incorporated isotopes of oxygen that were traceable either to sea water or to fresh water as is found in arctic ice. Their calculations showed that the salinity of the Gulf, as deduced from fossils in their core samples, had declined by about 20 percent when that layer of sediment was laid down. By carbon-14 dating of the shells, they determined that the layer had been deposited around 9,600 B.C., the date of the destruction of Atlantis!

This information led credence to the theory that the fresh-water-containing arctic icecap had been melted by some type of warming effect. The warming, which may have resulted from a variety of factors, including a possible axis shift of the earth, caused the ice sheet to suddenly surge southward and spread into what is now the northern United States. Here the ice melted rapidly. Fresh water from the melting glaciers surged down the Mississipi to the Gulf of Mexico and decreased the salinity of the Gulf. At the same time, fresh water from melting arctic ice poured into Hudson Bay and the North Atlantic, thus raising sea levels dramatically and giving rise to flooding of low-lying coastal areas such as Atlantis.

Although thought by many to be pure myth, the legend of Atlantis is important to modern civilization and the study of vibrational medicine because the Atlantean culture contained the earliest seeds of today's movement toward holism in healing. From a reincarnational perspective, it is said that those who were in the ranks of the Atlantean homeopathic and flower-essence movement and those who scoffed at the allopathic materialists (then the minority thinkers) have now reincarnated as today's (majority) proponents of drug therapy and surgery. This might, indeed, be a humorous irony if only this were known by the parties who today still vie for prominence and power. It would also be a unique demonstration of the principle of reincarnation, which allows a soul many lives to experience all sides of an issue and many approaches to life.

The tale of Atlantis is also important because it warns of the misuse of technology for purposes of personal power and self-aggrandizement. The nation of America stands as a growing power in the world today both in technical and ideological achievement. Many of the ideas originating in

Atlantis have again come to pass (perhaps by the reincarnating Atlanteans themselves) in such fields as communication, solar energy, and laser development. We are only now reaching the point where the true energetic potentials of crystals are being tapped, and modern scientists have only seen the tip of the iceberg. Like the gift of atomic energy, the tools of technology may be used for either healing or destruction. It was with great trepidation that Albert Einstein and other scientists gave their powerful knowledge to the world because they knew of the inherent dangers as well as the possible benefits of the energy that would be unleashed.

The story of Atlantis serves as an appropriate introduction to what may be considered the realm of science fiction: the art of healing with crystals. The Atlanteans had discovered many of the principles of directing crystalline energies for the purpose of healing. They had developed a sophisticated technology which was based upon the manipulation of subtle energies. The Atlanteans understood that these energies worked at the same levels as our higher dimensional bodies of light. They knew of the true link between the physical and subtle bodies, and their healing arts were based upon a recognition of this relationship.

Within the next twenty years, the myth that was the civilization of Atlantis may become archaeological fact. We may be on the verge of discovering the holographically encoded record crystals of Atlantis, which were to have been positioned in places of safety by the Atlantean priesthood. It is interesting that our technology is only now evolving to the point where we may be able to decode the stored knowledge of the so-called Atlantean library crystals. The New Age that America and the planet itself is moving into may be a cyclic mirror image of the latter part of the Golden Age of Atlantis. We are currently faced with similar divisions in thinking between the material/industrialists and the holistic/spiritualists. We seem to be moving toward a future which may bring either global nuclear destruction or a New Age movement of peace. It is hoped that humanity may learn a lesson from its past mistakes and utilize the insights of previous civilizations that did not profit from their erroneous thinking. Hopefully, we are headed in a direction that may be the future time the Atlanteans hoped would eventually occur in human evolution, where the tools of their advanced civilization might again be shared with individuals spiritually advanced enough to use them properly.

In a related note, there was a recent archeological excavation in Egypt near the Sphinx and the Great Pyramid, conducted by the Edgar Cayce

Foundation, a team from Stanford University, and the Egyptian government. The excavation site, chosen on the basis of psychic information derived from the Cayce readings, has led to the discovery of a buried roof of Aswan granite which may be part of a tunnel leading to the Pyramid of Records, where it is said that an Atlantean time capsule containing record crystals and other devices awaits discovery. If they are discovered in such places as the Pyramid of Records in Egypt, much of human history will have to be rewritten. It is from this point, a perspective seemingly between fantasy and reality, that we will explore current explorations into the use of crystals for healing disease.

Healing with Quartz Crystals: The Rediscovery of Ancient Tools for the Transformation of Illness

Quartz crystals have found their way into many of the electronic devices common to our present-day culture. As mentioned earlier, they are the central components of many of today's timepieces. The reason that quartz crystals are useful in telling time is that when they are stimulated with electricity, their oscillations are so regular and precise that they form a handy reference by which bits of time may be measured and displayed. This property of quartz crystals is a reflection of what is known as the "piezoelectric effect." When quartz crystals are subjected to mechanical pressure, they produce a measureable electrical voltage. Conversely, when an electrical current is applied to a crystal, it will induce mechanical movement. Most electronic devices utilize a slice or plate of quartz. Each plate of quartz has a particular natural resonant frequency which is dependent upon its thickness and size. If an alternating current is passed through the crystal plate, the charges oscillate back and forth at the resonant frequency of the crystal.

This phenomenon is the basis for crystal oscillator components used in many electronic systems to generate and maintain very precise energy frequencies. Another demonstration of the piezoelectric effect is seen when the crystal at the tip of the phonograph needle transduces mechanical vibration from patterns in the record grooves into electrical oscillation. This electrical oscillation is then translated by the electronics of the record player into music and words.

Quartz crystals are actually composed of silicon dioxide (SiO_2). While quartz crystals form the components of many electronic systems, it is the crystals of elemental silicon which have been used as primary components of computer and solar technologies. Scientists have learned to grow special silicon crystals which are infused with precise amounts of other elements during their formative stage. These added elements produce variants of silicon crystals that demonstrate specific degrees of electrical conductivity, optical activity, thermal conductivity, etc. This process is known as "doping," and has allowed scientists to create crystals with specialized properties of energy transduction.

While scientists have chosen to explore the electronic properties of silicon crystals, it is quartz crystals which bear the greatest potential in the manipulation of subtle energies. All crystalline structures are formed of mathematically precise and orderly lattice arrays of atoms. In addition to the variety of grid-like lattice structures, some researchers feel that there are also spiral arrangements interwoven into the crystal structure. Crystals represent the lowest state of entropy possible because they have the most orderly structure in nature.

The crystalline structure will respond in unique and precise ways to a wide spectrum of energies including heat, light, pressure, sound, electricity, gamma rays, microwaves, bioelectricity, and even the energies of consciousness (i.e., thought waves or thoughtforms). In response to these varying energetic inputs, the molecular structure of the crystal will undergo particular modes of oscillation, thereby creating specific vibratory frequencies of energy emission.

Quartz crystals can be used in many different ways to process various types of energy. These functions are numerous and include reception, reflection, refraction, magnification, transduction, amplification, focusing, transmutation, transference, transformation, storage, capacitance, stabilization, modulation, balancing, and transmittance.[8]

Of particular interest to our discussion is the application of these functions of quartz crystals toward subtle energertic healing of human illness. According to crystal researcher Marcel Vogel, a senior scientist with IBM for 27 years:

> The crystal is a neutral object whose inner structure exhibits a state of perfection and balance. When it's cut to the proper form and when the human mind enters into relationship with its structural perfection, the crystal emits a vibration which extends and amplifies the powers of the user's mind. Like a laser, it radiates energy in a coherent, highly concentrated form, and this energy may be transmitted into objects or people at will.

Although the crystal may be used for "mind to mind" communication, its higher purpose. . . is in the service of humanity for the removal of pain and suffering. With proper training, a healer can release negative thoughtforms which have taken shape as disease patterns in a patient's physical body.

As psychics have often pointed out, when a person becomes emotionally distressed, a weakness forms in his subtle energy body and disease may soon follow. With a properly cut crystal, however, a healer can, like a surgeon cutting away a tumor, release negative patterns in the energy body, allowing the physical body to return to a state of wholeness.[9]

The key concept which Dr. Vogel has presented is that the quartz crystal is capable of amplifying and directing the natural energies of the healer. The subtle energies of the healer's field become focused and coherent in a manner similar to a laser. Ordinarily, light is incoherent, with rays of energy moving randomly in many directions at once. In the ruby laser, the crystal creates an amplification effect by organizing rays of light into a coherent, orderly beam that has a tremendously powerful energetic effect. The quartz crystal works similarly with the subtle energies of the healer. To quote Dr. Vogel:

The psychic healer has to deal with the emanations of his hand or of his bioenergy field, which do not have the same levels of coherence one can obtain by using a crystal. The crystal works much the same way that a laser does: it takes scattered rays of energy and makes the energy field so coherent and unidirectional that a tremendous force is generated—one that is much stronger than if the energies were allowed to be emitted without having come into coherence.

The crystal, then, when used with love, makes the energies of mind coherent. It brings these energies into a pattern exactly fitting the life energies of the person seeking to be healed, and then amplifies them for the healing.[10]

A number of healers have adapted the use of the quartz crystal to amplify their natural healing abilities. Dr. Dolores Krieger, the creator of Therapeutic Touch, has also worked with augmenting healing energies by utilizing quartz crystals. She was shown this technique by Oh Shinnah, who is a trained psychologist, a crystal healer, and a Native American Indian. It is interesting to note that many Native American healers, especially the tribal shamans of cultures throughout the world, have quartz crystals among their collections of power objects. In such widely separated peoples as the Jivaro in South America and the tribes of Australia, the quartz crystal is considered the strongest power object of all.[11]

The quartz crystal can have other energetic abilities besides merely focusing the subtle energies of the healer. When healing energy is focused through the quartz crystal, it is sent into the body of the patient and distributed to the areas most in need of an energy balancing. There is an almost innate intelligence to this focused energy as it is always directed to the body regions where it is needed. The quartz crystal may be held in the hand while touching the patient, and the healing energies sent through the palm chakra. As the energies pass through the crystal, they are both amplified and directed to the part of the subtle anatomy which requires energetic reorganization and healing. Although there is a natural tendency for the crystal to distribute the energies properly, it is still wise to place the crystal over the part of the body which is painful or most affected by illness.

Quartz crystals may be useful for rebalancing and cleansing abnormally functioning or "blocked" chakras. When cleansing a chakra, the crystal is placed over the particular chakra body region and energy is sent through the crystal. The cleansing action may be induced by either the energies of the healer or the individual in need of chakra rebalancing. If the healer is the active energy source, subtle energy is transmitted from the healer's palm chakra, through the crystal, and into the individual's unbalanced chakra, while the healer focuses his/her mind on the task at hand. Conversely, an individual can use the crystal to cleanse his/her own chakras by placing a single terminated crystal over the chakra with the point facing away from the body. In this technique, the individual directs energy from inside the body out through the chakra and the overlying crystal.

A number of visualization techniques can be used in conjunction with this method. With the crystal over the chakra, the individual can imagine breathing in energy of a particular color (although white light is usually the most effective) and then visualize directing this light through the chakra on the exhaling breath. This method can be further augmented with the use of sound and chanting. For instance, while the individual is exhaling energy through the chakra, he or she can chant the "om." The sound energy can be visualized as projected or sung through a window meant to represent the chakra, in addition to directing light energy through the chakra window.

Another method of chakra rebalancing, used by crystal healer Dael Walker, involves having the patient work with the healer. While the healer sends energy through a crystal placed sequentially over each of the major chakras, the patient is instructed to visualize a simple semicircle-type energy meter representing the energy balance of the particular chakra. The meter consists of a single needle that can point anywhere from 0 to 180 degrees. The patient is told to visualize the needle pointing upward at a 90 degree angle to a position representing perfect balance, alignment, and health of the chakra. Starting with the crown chakra, the healer places the crystal at each of the major chakras and has the patient visualize the meter with the needle pointing upward to the perfect balance point. When the image of the needle stabilizes in the vertical position, the patient signals to the healer, who then moves to the next chakra in sequence until each of the chakras have been balanced in this manner.

As a rule, the healing energies transmitted by crystals seem to work at the level of our subtle energetic bodies. They assist the energies of the healer to correct dysfunction at a very primary level. Illness at the physical level is usually preceded by changes which have already occurred at the level of the etheric body. As we have discussed previously, energies from the astral and mental levels also have input into the etheric body. Therefore, dysfunctional emotional patterns may create changes in the astral form which are gradually transformed into energetic pattern changes at the level of the etheric and finally the physical body.

When correction occurs at the level of the astral and etheric bodies via healing energies transmitted through the crystal, the subtle energetic template is repatterned in such a way that normal tissue growth can occur, pain can be relieved, and coordination between the various energetic levels can take place more easily. One of the problems that can occur when healing with crystals, and with subtle energies in general, relates to the problem of disease recurrence. Many times a particular pain or illness stems from a negative thoughtform carried within the subtle energetic field of the individual. This thoughtform is the energy manifestation of some type of weighty or abnormal thought or emotion which has been held by the individual for a long period of time. Sometimes thoughtforms originate at unconscious levels and may relate to problematic issues that the sick individual has never actively addressed nor tried to resolve. Frequently, thoughtforms are charged with a particular emotion. The stronger the associated emotion that created the thoughtform, the more persistent the thoughtform will be in the auric field of the individual. Although one may use the crystal-amplified healing energies to disintegrate a negative thoughtform in an individual's subtle energetic field, the patient may recreate a thoughtform, and eventually the same or a similar illness, unless a correction in the person's emotional and mental patterning has also occurred. This issue was discussed briefly in Chapter 8 in examining the differences between magnetic and spiritual healing.

The implication of disease recurrence following psychic or crystal healing is that there are deeper issues at work relating to factors in the individual's fields of consciousness and subtle bodies which have not yet been appropriately addressed. Many times the best (and most enduring) form of healing is not achieved with a single modality but with a combination of many approaches. In the future, prototype holistic-healing centers will evolve a multidimensional approach to therapy which will utilize physical treatments, including spinal manipulation and proper nutrition; the use of various subtle energetic therapies; and psychotherapy to help the individual deal with maladaptive strategies that have been inappropriately used for coping with stress.

Another interesting application of quartz crystals in healing is the ability of crystals to be programmed with a healing thoughtform. That is, a healer may hold a quartz crystal in his/her hand and imagine sending energy to an absent patient that is in need of healing. The healer may visualize particular types of energy that he or she is sending to a particular organ by visualizing a color or flow of energy going into that area of the body. The healer may also focus on improving the general vitality of the patient by visualizing him/her as healthy, whole, and well. The distant patient may then receive healing energy through two different mechanisms. *Because quartz crystals are thought-energy amplifiers and operate at the level of magnetoelectric energies, the thought-directed energy frequencies of the healer may be intensified and simultaneously broadcast at a distance to the patient.* Alternatively, the quartz crystal seems to be able to act as a kind of thoughtform capacitor in that it is able to absorb a charge of healing energy of very specific frequency characteristics. The healer charges the crystal with the pattern of energy he or she wishes to project into the patient and then gives the crystal to the patient to hold. In the hands of the patient, the crystal is able to discharge its stored energy even in the absence of the healer. In this way, minutes or hours spent in charging a particular crystal can be transformed into a single moment of healing energy release. When the crystal is used in this fashion, it emulates an electrical capacitor which is able to store up weak energetic charges over a period of time and then discharge its contents in a single powerful burst.

In their ability to accept and hold a healing thoughtform, crystals are similar to magnetic recording media like the floppy disk in a computer disk drive. The crystal is programmed with specialized information utilizing the higher dimensional energies of consciousness. The clearer the thought or image can be held in the mind of the healer, the more accurate the energy informational image stored within the crystal will be. Crystals should only be programmed to accomplish one specific energy function at a time. (Large amounts of energy data can be stored in a single crystal, as in a library crystal, but all the data is related to a similar informational function.)

The energy memory of the crystal, like a magnetic recording disk, can only accept one grouping of data at a time. In order to charge a crystal with a new energetic thoughtform or function, it should be cleared first, just as a magnetic disk is erased of old contents before replacing them with new information. In general, when one selects a crystal for personal use or for healing, the crystal should initially be cleansed of old vibrational energies so it will carry out its functions without errors due to old programming. The process of clearing or cleansing a crystal of old energy programming can be accomplished in a variety of ways.

Old methods of cleansing a crystal include placing the crystal in direct sunlight for several days, or packing it in sea salt for one to two days, or burying it underground for two to seven days, or placing it in salt water, or running streams of water over it for one to seven days. One of the fastest methods of cleansing a crystal is accomplished by placing it in a bowl of distilled water or spring water that contains several drops of Pennyroyal flower essence. This procedure takes only a few minutes, compared to hours and days spent in the other procedures. By clearing the crystal of old static energies, one is essentially demagnetizing the crystal so that it may accept new energy functions according to the desire and consciousness of its owner. Most crystals should be cleansed occasionally, as this process assists them in remaining potent in their subtle energetic transformational properties.

The quartz crystals themselves have special energy properties which have healing effects even in the absence of healers. It is believed that crystals are natural purifiers of subtle energies because they absorb negative energies and transmit only those frequencies of a positive, beneficial nature.

The crystals that are used for healing have their own power and energy, and do their work by just being in the proximity of the one in need of healing. When held in the hands, they can be programmed to specific ills. They will magnify the intentions of the healer, and through their purity, combine the forces of nature and spirit to channel healing energies. Yet, the crystals will remove pain, elevate one's vibration, promote clarity, help one to be less emotionally reactive, refract disharmonious energies, release negative ions, collect positive ions, and work with one's dreams, without any help from [people].[12]

Some of the effects quartz crystals are able to have upon humans relate to a particular resonance effect that occurs with our own crystalline structures. As mentioned earlier in this chapter, science has recently begun to recognize a new class of crystals known as liquid crystals. They have a structure which is partially crystalline and partially fluid. Biology is beginning to understand that many substances and membranes within the human body appear to function as liquid crystals. From a subtle-energy perspective, a number of solid and liquid crystalline structures at the physical level are involved in the attunement of subtle energies within the nervous system and the flow of the life-force through the body. To requote from Ryerson's channeled material:

> Midway between the the circulatory and nervous systems, an electromagnetic current is created by the polarity of these two systems. Indeed there is an intimate connection between these two systems in relation to the life-force and consciousness that modern science does not yet understand. *The life-force works more through the blood, and consciousness works more through the brain and nervous system. These two systems contain quartz-like properties and an electromagnetic current.* The blood cells, especially the red and white blood cells, contain more quartz-like properties, and the nervous system contains more an electromagnetic current. The life-force and consciousness use these properties to enter and stimulate the physical body.
>
> There are various quartz-like structures in the physical and subtle bodies that augment the impact of vibrational remedies. In the physical body, these areas include: cells salts, fatty tissue, lymphs, red and white cells, and the pineal gland. These crystalline structures are a complete system in the body but not yet properly isolated and understood by modern medicine.
>
> Crystalline structures work on sympathetic resonancy. There is an attunement between crystalline properties in the physical and subtle bodies, the ethers, and many vibrational remedies, notably flower essences and gems. These properties in the body magnify the life-force of vibrational remedies to a recognizable level to be assimilated. Indeed, these crystalline properties are relay points for most ethereal energies to penetrate the physical body. This allows for a

balanced distribution of various energies in correct frequencies, which stimulates the discharge of toxicity to create health. In a similar fashion, vibrations of radio-wave frequencies strike a crystal in a radio. The crystal resonates with the high frequency in such a way as to absorb it, passing along the audio frequencies which are perceivable by the body.[13] *(italics added)*

An interesting revelation which can be made on the basis of this material is the fact that human beings are, to some extent, living crystals. Certain aspects of the human energy system have the same transformational properties as natural quartz crystals. *When one uses natural quartz crystals to heal the body, energy transference occurs partly because of a resonance effect between the quartz crystal and those cellular crystal systems with quartz-like properties.* These same biocrystalline elements amplify certain aspects of the life-force in special energy circuits that run throughout the body. Biocrystalline systems are intimately involved with mediating the input of higher vibrational energies into the body.

Another method of interacting with the crystalline structures of the body is through the application of gem elixirs. By ingesting a gem elixir, the energy imprint of a particular crystal, in this case quartz, contained within water which has been charged with the crystal in direct sunlight, is transferred directly to the individual's subtle-energy system. The quartz gem elixir, because of its resonant effect on the crystalline structures of the pineal gland and spinal cord which are intimately involved in the kundalini process, seems able to enhance the practice of meditation and to assist the individual in achieving greater spiritual illumination.

In the realm of personal healing, the quartz crystal is an excellent tool to assist the aspirant in meditation. When a crystal is used for gaining spiritual enlightenment through meditative practices, it should be selected for this purpose alone. In other words, the crystal should be used strictly for meditation and not for healing. If healing with crystals is desired, a second crystal should be chosen specifically for this purpose. In general, the individual should not share his/her meditation crystal with anyone else, as the crystal becomes programmed with the specific energetic frequencies of its owner. Allowing others to hold and use one's meditation crystal can cause it to become imprinted or contaminated with undesirable discordant thoughts and energies.

When utilizing a single quartz crystal in meditation, it should be held in the left hand. The reason behind this practice is that the left hand is neurologically connected to the right cerebral hemisphere. The right hemisphere, in turn, seems to be attuned to the higher dimensional fields of consciousness of the Higher Self because the right brain has unique crystalline connections to the pineal gland (see Chapter 7). By holding the crystal in the left hand, incoming crystalline energies have direct input into the subtle-energy circuitry linked with the right brain, which is more closely in tune with the Higher Self. Meditative techniques which employ the use of visualization allow one to utilize natural right-hemispheric abilities to link more directly with the quartz crystal.

Instead of holding a single crystal in the left hand, two quartz crystals may also be utilized, with one held in each hand during the meditative process. When using two single-terminated stones (those ending in one faceted point), the stone in the right hand should point away from the body while the crystal in the left hand should point toward the body. There are natural energy circuits involving the hands which take energy in through the left palm chakra and send energy out through the right.

Double-terminated crystals—those with a natural point at either end —are especially useful for meditative purposes. Double-terminated stones are not only more powerful, but they are better at linking crystals together in subtle energy circuits. Various geometric arrangements utilizing multiple crystals may be explored. Each arrangement can have a particular value and application. For instance, a third, smaller crystal may be taped over the brow chakra region to complete a triangular circuit with the two stones in either hand. Another particularly powerful amplification effect can be created by sitting in a special geometric crystal meditational space. By aligning six crystals in a six-pointed Star of David, composed of two interpenetrating triangles, the meditative aspirant seated in the center is able to draw on invisible energy-grid patterns in the planetary environment as well as on the special subtle fields generated by such crystalline arrangements. These invisible grid patterns represent potentially utilizable energy lines which may be tapped for applications in consciousness, healing, and even industry. The grid pattern may be activated by taking a single crystal in the right hand, termination directed away from the body, and pointing at the crystals in a connect-the-dots type fashion. This process may be augmented if the individual visualizes taking in energy (such as white light) through his/her crown chakra while breathing in. The energy is then directed down through the heart center and out through the right-hand crystal during the outward breath. During this process, the crystals of the grid are connected by the intention and thought energies of the individual. The individual visualizes creating lines of energy or light that connect the crystals until they form the desired geometric pattern. This process is especially augmented if the geometric pattern has a central crystal to anchor and amplify the energy pattern.

Multiple crystals placed in specific geometric patterns produce unified energy fields known as "gridwork systems."[14] These systems blend the energies of multiple crystals together to manifest a powerful synergistic effect. The use of such arrangements of crystals is based upon principles of sacred geometry in conjunction with crystal and human energy dynamics. The basic principle in creating gridwork systems is to place programmed crystals in harmonic patterns, in which each crystal resonates strongly with every other. The frequencies interact with each other like the multiple circular waves that emanate from several pebbles dropped simultaneously into a pond. The intersections of these waves produces a dynamic energy mandala. When utilizing such arrangements of crystals, it is best that the individual in the center hold a "focal crystal" which assists in unifying, focusing, and directing the subtle energies appropriately.

There are numerous variations on the use of these crystal geometric coordination complexes, which also have applications for healing specific illnesses. When attempting to heal via the use of crystalline geometric patterns, clusters of quartz crystals, as opposed to single crystals, may be needed for creating the points along the geometric form. Depending upon the type and severity of the disease one is attempting to heal, clusters of quartz crystals can create an energy grid with a much larger field-strength in order to produce more noticeable therapeutic effects.[15]

Energy grids of different shapes can be created with varying effects upon the consciousness of the individual. Grids can be circular mandalas or even rectangular forms. A simple grid pattern may be achieved by placing crystals in each of the four corners of a meditation room and either setting a fifth crystal on the center of the floor or suspending it from the ceiling. Again, the grids are activated by the individual via the power of active visualization and intention, utilizing an additional crystal. Amplification of meditation's effectiveness is possible by creating unique crystalline geometric grid forms which have specific effects upon the consciousness of the meditator. By sitting in the center of the grid, holding a focal crystal, the individual actually becomes a part of the grid's energy network. In addition to sitting within crystalline grid patterns, there are additional methods, including visualization, which can amplify the effect of the crystal upon the meditative experience.

As mentioned previously, visualization techniques used when meditating with crystals appear to give positive results because of the right hemispheric link with the higher self. There are a number of meditative imagery techniques which are based upon the use of powerful esoteric and archetypal symbols. The inner-directed use of these symbols and images allows the individual aspirant to creatively explore the energies of the meditation crystal. Before attempting any crystal meditative technique or other process of attunement, it is necessary to visualize surrounding oneself within a sphere of protective white light. This helps to seal one's energy field from disturbing outside influences.

One technique which may be effective in exploring the energies of the crystal is to visualize oneself shrinking and entering a door in one of the facets of the crystal. When mentally inside the crystal, various imagery exercises may be utilized. One may explore the natural landscape of the crystalline interior while trying to feel the energies which flow through the crystal. Another interesting variation is to imagine that one sees a number of labelled doors within a crystalline corridor inside the crystal. For example, while in the corridor, imagine yourself standing in front of a door which is labelled Library Room. See yourself entering through this door. When in the room, you see many shelves lining the walls, each shelf containing rows of crystals instead of rows of books. Imagine thinking about a particular subject you wish to know about. As you think about your subject of inquiry, also think about which crystal in the library room will give you further information on this subject. As you look against the walls, a particular crystal will begin to glow. Imagine walking over to this crystal, picking it up, and mentally asking for more information about the subject. The library crystal may supply information about the desired subject matter through feelings, pictures, and even spoken messages mentally transmitted to the inquiring mind.

Although this technique primarily involves the internal manipulation of symbols, much information of value can be obtained about aspects of the personality and the higher dimensional self. The symbolism of visual images, like those utilized in the crystal meditation exercise, unlocks the hidden potential of the right hemisphere, which processes information of a symbolic/metaphoric nature as opposed to the linear/verbal mode of the left hemisphere. The fact that symbols hold great hidden meaning and power explains why dream interpretation holds one of the access keys to our inner psychic potential. Because it activates the right-hemispheric connection to the Higher Self, symbolic imagery used during crystal meditation exercises may allow an individual to gain greater access to the information banks of the soul.

New Perspectives on the Mineral Kingdom: The Energies of Nature & the Seven Crystal Systems

The quartz crystal is but one of many stones and gems that can be used for the purposes of healing, energizing, and gaining access to higher dimensions of consciousness. The quartz we have been discussing up until now is the rock crystal of the quartz family. All crystals in the quartz family are composed of silicon dioxide. There are many different colors and variations of quartz, because within the mixture of silicon dioxide there are also traces of other elements. For instance, amethyst, which is a violet type of quartz, is so colored because there are trace amounts of manganese in its crystalline structure. In addition to amethyst quartz, there is also smoky quartz, citrine or golden quartz, rose quartz, green quartz, blue quartz, and quartz with inclusions, such as rutilated quartz and tourmalinated quartz. Each variety of quartz has its own special subtle energy and healing properties. Quartz is but one type of crystalline form which contributes to the mineral kingdom of the earth.

The mineral kingdom is one of many domains in nature which have both an exoteric or physical side, and an esoteric or spiritual aspect. All kingdoms in nature have their own unique expressions of the divine energies of the Creator's consciousness. In the plant kingdom, the exoteric side can be seen in the numerous multicolored and visually unique flowers that populate the earth. Conversely, through the flowers' subtle energies and the abilities of their essences to transmute and transform human consciousness, we see more of the plant kingdom's esoteric or spiritual side. In the mineral kingdom, this exoteric aspect may be seen in the myriad varieties and colors of crystals and gem stones which can be found throughout the earth. The physical or material aspect of the mineral kingdom is expressed through the many varieties, sizes, and shapes in which crystalline growth may occur in nature. The spiritual aspect is expressed through the inner geometric construction that makes up the crystalline forms. The study of these inner forms—the divine symmetries of atomic structure within crystals—is known as the science of crystallography.

Crystal, gems, and stones have been classified by those studying crystallography into specialized systems of order derived from the unique symmetries of their molecular arrangements. There are seven divisions of order which make up the classification of crystal systems. These seven systems are based upon key differences in the geometries of the crystalline lattice structures. These systems are the triclinic, monoclinic, orthorhombic, tetragonal, hexagonal, cubic, and trigonal systems of crystalline structure. The trigonal classification is frequently considered a part of the hexagonal system by mineralogists. It is listed here as a separate system because the hexagonal and trigonal systems possess uniquely different affinities with levels of higher dimensional energies and matter, much like that demonstrated by the seven major chakras in the etheric body.

Each of the crystalline systems has an affinity or subtle-energy resonance with a particular subplane of energy in the mineral kingdom. It might be said that each mineral subplane represents a type of divine thoughtform or energy pattern within nature that assists in the organization of crystalline form. The physical atomic pattern of the crystal is pre-organized at a subtle level by energies originating at the etheric (and higher) planes. *This coordinating process in crystals is similar to the patterning in the human etheric body which precedes the manifestation of cellular activity and organization in the physical body.* Indeed, crystals demonstrate properties of growth and expansion much like those of living organisms. As the crystal grows, its atoms migrate into appropriate molecular positions as guided by the etheric energies associated with the crystalline kingdom. The concept of an etheric body surrounding and interpenetrating the physical is as true for the mineral kingdom as it is for the human kingdom. Therefore, there is great power within the potential resonance between crystalline and cellular etheric bodies. It is through the etheric structure of the crystal that energy radiates from or is absorbed into the stone. For instance, in uranium ore we have a demonstration of the natural expression of the radiating principle, while in lead we see the ability to absorb.

As discussed briefly at the end of Chapter 4, there is consciousness in all aspects of matter, from the human level on down to the atomic level. The quality and quantity of consciousness differs at each level of existence and manifestation. All matter is an expression of the crystallized light and energy of the Creator, which is itself pure consciousness. Whether or not one accepts a creationist or evolutionist concept is irrelevant to this point. It is merely being suggested that the cosmic energy from which all matter is formed, whether originating from a big bang or from one great divine thought, is the energy of pure consciousness, which is God.

Some esoteric texts refer to the energy of God as *all there is*, for the divine body is the very loom and yarn from which the universal mural is woven. All matter, even at the subatomic level, is formed of tiny drops of frozen light—a kind of focused mini-energy field. There is consciousness in this basic energy unit. It is the prime ingredient forming the basic building blocks of the universe. Its basic energetic properties may be seen reflected in all aspects of creation. All particularizations of this energy, such as atoms or even electrons, have some rudimentary form of consciousness, albeit highly different from what one considers as human consciousness.

If one can accept the premise that every atom possesses a form of consciousness, it may be easier to recognize that when atoms of like consciousness come together and coalesce, as in the form of a crystal, there is created a body of energy which expresses a definite vibrational pattern. In nature this is known as the Law of Attraction, where atoms of similar structure or vibration are gathered together to vibrate in unison, thus producing a physical form, or aggregation of atoms. *Each crystalline vibrational pattern has an energy relationship or correspondence to particular subplanes in other kingdoms of nature.* As will soon be demonstrated, *each of the seven subplanes of the mineral kingdom has an energetic correspondence to the seven major chakras of the human subtle anatomy.*

> Have you ever wondered why there is such a diversity of gems and minerals upon this planet? Could it be there is an endless process of form-building that goes on (as in all kingdoms of nature), whose basic purpose is the development of quality and the expansion of the consciousness? In considering these atoms of mineral substance, can there be an expression of "consciousness" within their corresponding kingdoms in nature? And if so, can we begin to faintly perceive the concept that our solar system is but the aggregate of ALL forms, and the body of a Being who is expressing Himself through it, utilizing it in order to work out a definite purpose and central idea?

> If you will recall the esoteric truism that "we are but the microcosm of a greater macrocosm," (as above, so below) and recognize that the tiny atom is within itself a solar system of expression, differing from other atoms according to the number and arrangement of the electrons around the central charge, you can perceive that this theme is being repeated over and over again in countless forms and expressions, and recognize that we are ALL a part of the ONE

WHOLE.[16]

In a way, this describes not only the basic premise that consciousness evolves through various forms of physical matter and expression, but it is also a rewording of what the Atlanteans referred to as the Law of One. Because we are all composed of the same conscious energy as everything else in creation, we are all expressions of an unseen unifying principle. This concept tells us that we are all different manifestations of a unique, underlying, divine consciousness, and that this consciousness is expressed through special geometric forms and arrangements that are repeated at both the microcosmic and macrocosmic levels. *The levels of order in the construction of all life and matter are governed by unseen laws of form. The subtle energies that determine form exist as repeating geometric patterns and shapes that influence the expression of systems ranging from the tiniest atom to the greatest galaxy.*

The atoms of the mineral kingdom are directed by specialized thought-forms or subtle energetic patterns in nature that exist at particular subplanes of matter. These subplanes are paralleled by the energy levels of the seven major chakras in the human being. Each major chakra is associated with a different frequency and quality of energy. Each chakra also possesses different subtle characteristics and properties of form-building as they relate to the expression of the human vehicle at the physical level. Each of the seven subplanes of the mineral kingdom has a correspondence to the energies of the seven chakras.

The thoughtform of each mineral subplane gives direction and form to the balanced geometric organization of atoms of a similar vibrational nature. As such, all crystals formed by patterns existing at any one subplane will exhibit certain common vibrational and subtle-energy properties. There are, however, slight geometric variations which create subtle differences in the energy qualities of gems of the same crystal subsystem.

In a very general way, minerals belonging to each of the seven crystal systems have special subtle-energy properties associated with particular higher dimensional energies (or rays) and with specific chakras of the subtle bodies. The color rays associated with each crystal system are higher octaves of colors which exist in the visible spectrum, and can only be seen by clairvoyant vision.

In general, stones belonging to a particular system share the qualities listed in Diagram 28. Although different crystals may belong to the same

Diagram 28.
SUBTLE ENERGIES OF
THE SEVEN CRYSTAL SYSTEMS

CRYSTAL SYSTEM	RAY	ENERGETIC NATURE	CHAKRA AFFECTED
TRICLINIC	Yellow	Completion	Crown
MONOCLINIC	Blue Violet	Pulsation Movement	Third Eye
ORTHORHOMBIC	Orange	Protection Encompassing	Throat
TETRAGONAL	Pink	Balancing	Heart
HEXAGONAL	Green	Growth Vitality	Solar Plexus
CUBIC	Cobalt Blue	Fundamental Earth-Nature	Sacral
TRIGONAL	Red	Energizing	Coccygeal

crystalline classification scheme, each crystal will be slightly different than its family members. In addition to its shared properties with stones of the same class (i.e. tetragonal vs. hexagonal), each gemstone possesses unique energy characteristics of its own. The crystal systems in Diagram 28 have been listed in order of their relationship to the seven major chakras of the body.[17] In addition to the resonance of a gemstone with a particular chakra, crystals belonging to each system will usually tend to have energetic effects upon other chakras as well.

The energy qualities of each crystalline system are quite interesting. For instance, crystals of the cubic system (diamonds, garnets, and fluorites) possess qualities of a very fundamental or basic nature. These crystals may be used in meditation or other states of consciousness to deal with bulky problems and things that tend to be more mundane or of an earth-plane nature. These crystals possess a quality that radiates a basic building-block type of energy patterning. Crystals of the cubic system have an energy pattern that can assist in the repair of damaged cellular structures, from the molecular level of DNA on up to the bones of the skeletal system. The cubic system also tends to resonate most with the sacral chakra in the human subtle energetic anatomy. Although diamond, garnet, and fluorite may demonstrate properties of the cubic system of crystals, each also possesses specific subtle energetic qualities which transcend this very basic classification.

Crystals of the hexagonal classification (emeralds and other members of the beryl family of stones, aquamarines, and apatites) are of a more complex nature than those with cubic lattice arrangements. They tend to give off energies, and to encourage processes of growth and vitality. Actually, quartz is considered both hexagonal as well as trigonal, and it demonstrates properties belonging to this crystal class. Crystals of the hexagonal classification can also be used for healing, energy balancing, communicating, and storing information. These crystals have an energy that tends to be associated with service. The applications of the crystals in this area are considerable. They can be helpful in focusing healing energy into the organs and endocrine glands, and also into the acupoints and meridians. They can assist in rebalancing the energies of all the chakras and subtle bodies. Additionally, crystals of this class can have beneficial effects upon consciousness in assisting the development of creativity and intuition, enhancing psychic abilities, deepening meditation, and increasing attunement with the Higher Self. Although crystals of the hexagonal system can influence all of the chakras, they tend to resonate most strongly with the solar-plexus chakra.

Stones such as zircon, wulfenite, and chalcopyrite belong to the tetragonal system, and are "half-giving" and "half-receiving" crystals that are of a balancing nature. Crystals of this class have qualities which allow them to absorb many of the negative qualities of the Earth, yet they are also able to give forth positive vibrations. Following the absorption of negative energies, these stones act to transmute the negativity. As such, they might be referred to as transmuting stones. The tetragonal system also corresponds to the heart chakra in the human. Through the lessons of the heart—both of a positive nurturant aspect as well as of a harsh, negative character— there is a balancing of the soul's nature. Crystals of the tetragonal system channel vibrations into the Earth and create connections between basic structures and higher dimensions. The tetragonal shape forms the basic three-sided pyramid. This basic pyramidal structure and its attunement to sacred geometric forms is one of the reasons that crystals of the tetragonal class can be useful for attunement to higher dimensions.

Stones belonging to the orthorhombic system, including peridot, topaz, and alexandrite, have a unique aspect of encircling and encompassing energy patterns, problems, and thoughtforms. They can bring far things closer, or project near things further away. In other words, they can assist in bringing greater perspective to issues that may seem out of focus. Such crystals help to magnify and clear away that which is irrelevant. They magnify consciousness in a way that allows one to switch from the perspective of the microcosm to the macrocosm and vice-versa. Crystals of the orthorhombic class help an individual isolate problems and contain them until they can be worked out at various levels of experience. Although not well understood, this is a necessary aspect of dealing with problems. Bypassing obstacles does not usually help the student become stronger in problem-solving. Our problems cannot be dissolved, released, or transmuted until their inner meaning has been thoroughly grasped. All problems contain potential lessons for soul growth and are often external reflections of our inner struggles. In addition to qualities of encircling and encompassing, stones of the orthorhombic class can also serve to confer an element of protection. This crystalline system relates best to the throat chakra or center of will in the human, which carries the ability to accept or reject problems.

Azurite, jade, malachite, and moonstone are crystals of the monoclinic system and have a unique, constant pulsating action. Their nature is that of continual expansion and contraction. They possess a system of crystalline growth whereby the crystal expands, then reaches a point where it breaks off, and then expands again. This aspect of pulsation is important to all life. It helps to serve as an impetus to action and growth as well as to the expansion and contraction of consciousness. Because of its continued growth and stepwise expansion, crystals of the monoclinic class also have a directional aspect. They can point the way to go by helping clear away obstructions to our inner vision. These stones can help clear our paths by dissolving trivial problems via their influence at higher energy levels. The monoclinic system corresponds to the third-eye center in the human chakra network. By holding such crystals up to the third-eye chakra, one can be assisted in perceiving self and others on a multidimensional level of spirit.

Crystals of the triclinic system, such as turquoise and rhodonite, possess aspects of completion within their makeup, in that they form a triad. The triad is a repeating form within nature and in the hierarchical structure of the universe. Triclinic crystals have an aspect of totality or completeness. They also help to balance the yin and yang energy within an individual. They assist in merging and harmonizing polarities of any type of energy which is unbalanced. Because of this quality, gemstones of the triclinic classfication can help to balance personalities and attitudes that are too polarized or unbalanced. They allow individuals to attune to higher spiritual dimensions of order. The triclinic system of crystals corresponds to the crown chakra—the highest energetic level in human beings. Through the energies of this system and the crown chakra, there comes the highest form of understanding, of giving and receiving, and of all things that can be accomplished.

Lastly, there is the trigonal system, which is represented by bloodstones, carnelians, agates, and amethysts. The trigonal system contains crystals that continually give off energy. They are always (at a subtle energetic level) in a spinning motion which is of neither a positive nor a negative nature. They give off energy of a balanced nature. As such, crystals belonging to the trigonal class may be useful in balancing the subtle energies of the human body, especially when there is a particular lack of energy in one of the component systems such as the meridians. They can help balance energies of the brain as well as the subtle bodies. Although they are similar to crystals of the hexagonal system and possess certain common energetic qualities, trigonal crystals tend to be more varied in their uses. They are more purposeful in their energetic nature, and they assist in achieving sharper clarity than stones of the hexagonal class, which are both giving and receiving in their qualities. They help to prepare the multilevel energy systems of the body for spiritual work. The trigonal system corresponds to the base or coccygeal chakra, which relates to the kundalini energies. As we will soon see, these qualities belonging to the trigonal system make bloodstone an important crystal in working with the chakras and the kundalini energies.

The seven classes of crystals provide a framework for understanding some of the common subtle energetic properties of gems and stones. However, each gem within the same system has unique yet slight variations on the mathematical symmetry of its class, which give it subtle differences in energetic properties and qualities. The seven crystalline classes are important to understand because they represent a repeating pattern of symmetry and organization that can be found throughout the many kingdoms of nature, including the human kingdom. It is important to recognize that this structure and organization, as well as the subtle energetic properties of crystals, originates at the etheric level of their crystalline forms.

There are subtle correspondences between the levels of energy in the chakras and the levels of substance which help to form the etheric structure of the mineral kingdom. More will be said on the specific energies of the chakra system in the next chapter. Each class of crystal structure assists in transforming the energies of human consciousness in very special and unique ways. More important than the class, however, is the particular crystal or stone itself. Each gem possesses unique spiritual, energetic, and healing properties which may assist us in our search for balance and wholeness.

Hidden Gifts from within the Earth:
The Spiritual & Healing Qualities of Gems & Stones

In order to understand how various gems and stones can be useful in subtle-energy healing, it would be best to examine the properties of individual gems. Although every stone and gem has particular energy qualities, we will examine those which have greatest relevance to the context of this book, such as those which assist in the development of higher consciousness and the balancing of the physical body through the manipulation of human subtle-energy anatomy.

One stone which is of unique importance, and which relates well to our previous discussion of the properties of quartz crystals, is the amethyst. The amethyst is a form of quartz having a wide variety of violet hues owing to traces of manganese and other elements within its structure. It is a stone which has been prized by royalty down through the ages, and many consider it to be a regal stone. Esoteric sources consider amethyst to belong to the divine order of the Violet Flame of Transmutation, because it is a gem which represents the process of alchemy, whether of a physical, emotional, or spiritual nature.

Alchemy has been viewed historically as humanity's search for a process that would transmute base metals into those of a more precious nature. At the physical level, this has been symbolized by the transformation of lead into gold. On a spiritual level, this process represents the transformation of the physical personality into an expression of the Higher Self. Amethyst is powerful in its energizing and transmutational powers because it works at the triune levels of the physical, emotional, and spiritual planes. It can assist in the transformation of habits, speech, thought processes, and emotional feelings, from expressions of the lower personality into manifestations of our inner divine nature.

As a healing stone, the amethyst is quite effective, but like other quartz crystals, it needs the energies of the healer to be directed through the stone. By wearing the amethyst on one's body, an individual can absorb forces that are of both a physical nature and a higher energetic or mental nature. The amethyst can transmute and purify energy from a lower to a higher spiritual level. It repels those energies which would be considered of a negative nature. The quality of the amethyst is to purify and amplify all healing rays of subtle energy If it is worn by an individual who is to be a receiver of healing energy, it can be a focal point for energy reception. If it is worn by the healer, the mental energies of the healer can be directed and focused through the gem to the individual in need of healing. It would be of value for both the sender and receiver to wear an amethyst when healing over great distances.

Because of its higher vibratory rate, the amethyst is more directly connected to the life-force of all things. Because of its violet hue, it is also associated with energies of the ultraviolet spectrum. Researchers have only recently discovered that ultraviolet light has an intimate connection to the process of cellular replication. The spectrum of UV light utilized by life processes at the cellular level is sometimes referred to as mitogenetic radiation. The violet color itself is one of purification, through which many impurities may be filtered out.

Because the amethyst is associated with the flow of the life-force, it is able to affect the blood vessels and arteries which carry this energy through the medium of the bloodstream. It is able to act as a subtle-energy filter for the forces of the bloodstream, especially when placed over a blood vessel such as an artery. In working with the blood, the amethyst works through the etheric body as opposed to a particular chakra. It is often best to place the stone over a particular problem area, but especially near the heart where the blood flows in to become re-energized. The amethyst can be helpful in treating cases of venous thrombosis or thrombophlebitis where it is necessary for the blood clot to be dissolved. If held over the clot, it may assist in the process of dissolution and dispersal in a way that does not create further hazard, as in the case of pulmonary embolism where the clot goes to the lungs. When utilized in this manner, the amethyst should be used over the affected blood vessel and held for a period of about ten minutes, then gently moved towards the heart.

The amethyst is also useful in recharging the energies of the etheric body. This property is of special value to healers, especially those who can work with patients at great distances through the use of the mind. When used to recharge the etheric body, the stone should be held over the top of the head in bright sunlight, allowing the energies of the sun to be focused through the amethyst into the crown chakra. After re-energizing, the healer may then focus this same energy through an amethyst placed over the

third-eye chakra while attempting to send healing energy to a distant patient. This particular technique tends to be of value only to healers, in that
the stone has the ability to allow the healing energies to penetrate and seek
within the body of the patient being worked with. This technique may be
especially helpful for healers working with patients who are trying to mend
fractures and broken bones.

The health, healing and well-being of the total planet are within
the capabilities of this stone of great nobility. Encapsulated within the
core of the amethyst is the vibration of love; it is that which blends
all areas of the body and the being together. It has the ability to transmute pain into pleasure, and break into harmony. It has the ability
to change the molecular structure of things. Light of the sun focused
through the amethyst is also very benefical, as it then enhances the
rays of energies that come from outside the planet. It can also be directed towards the moon and used in a like manner, however it should
be pointed out that light rays reflected from the moon affect the emotional and spiritual bodies, while the sun's rays affect the physical body.

Although the amethyst can be of great benefit to a body, both in
the physical and spiritual sense, it is also important that the purpose
be of a high repute, and that the one who is working with this particular stone should also be above reproach, for stones in themselves,
though not dead, are only as a sending and receiving station, and it
is necessary that the energy be of a vital source.[18]

Another gem which is useful in affecting blood vessels and the flow of
life-force through the bloodstream is the ruby. The ruby is helpful in assisting the flow of blood, not as a purifier, but as an aid to increasing the circulation of blood to different parts of the body. The ruby can also be useful
in working with blood clots, as can the amethyst, but in a different manner.
Whereas the healer would project his/her own energy through the amethyst to dissolve a blood clot, the ruby is best used for this purpose in conjunction with a prism.

The prism is placed on a table near the patient so that incandescent
light or natural sunlight may be refracted through it. From the prism comes
a spectrum of natural rainbow colors which may be allowed to play upon
the walls of the room; the colors need not fall upon the body of the patient.
The ruby is able to pick up the subtle overtones and higher harmonics of
the colors, which are magnified to dissolve clots or cholesterol placques
adherent to blood vessel walls. The ruby which is best used for this type of
work is one which has been faceted similarly to a brilliant-cut diamond.
The point of the stone is used by the healer to go over different main arter-

ies or blood vessels which have blockages. When dealing with blood clots, the ruby is lightly but purposefully stroked over the vein containing the clot in the direction of the heart (similar to the manner in which the amethyst is employed.)

Another interesting application of the ruby is to maintain the stability of failing vision. Although the energies of the ruby will not restore impaired sight, they can be helpful in maintaining the level of function that is already present. The ruby energies are able to have this effect because they sometimes increase local blood flow and microcirculation within and around the eye. The blood vessels are strengthened by stabilizing the cells of the vessel itself. This assists the maintenance of blood flow to the eye at whatever stage of impairment the ruby is used. (The energies of the ruby might be especially helpful for diabetics, who may undergo rapid microvascular deterioration of the retina in the later years of their disease, leading to progressive loss of vision and possible blindness.)

In its effects upon the chakras, the ruby has a cleansing effect upon those centers which are of greatest importance to the flow of blood throughout the body. The centers most affected are the heart chakra, the solar-plexus chakra, and the lower chakras of the body. The ruby may have a very disquieting effect upon the solar-plexus chakra, because it tends to stir up energies of the emotional body (or astral body) which are intimately linked to this center.

From a spiritual perspective, the effect of the ruby upon the heart center is also linked to the inner quality most reflected by this stone: the quality of love. There are particular characteristics of the energy of this gemstone which assist an individual in focusing on issues of love for self and others, as well as in believing in one's own inner potential.

> Love is the quality that is reflected by the ruby; love is the need that can be filled by this particular stone. Those who lack in self-love would do well to meditate on a stone of this color, of this quality. By so doing, they can release within themselves the energy that is necessary to overcome much of the trauma engendered by their lack of self-love.
>
> This stone also encompasses the quality of courage; not the courage of "going into battle," but the courage to be able to seek the truth at all times; courage to be able to stand up for that which is right; courage to be the true part of one's own highest potential. Courage is a very commendable trait with this stone. It also could be termed valor.[19]

Another stone which is able to affect the heart center is the emerald. Whenever the heart has been affected by disease, whether it be at the spiritual, mental, or physical level, the emerald can be effective in strengthening and unifying the energies of the heart center. It has the capacity to unify all the higher energy components associated with this center into a sense of oneness. This is partly because the energies of the emerald have a vibration of love. On the higher planes, love is not only an emotion but also an energy with a certain vibratory rate, which can be within the emerald as well as focused through and projected from the stone. The emerald also affects the physical heart center—not so much the blood in the heart as the actual muscle tissue which propels the blood through the body. There is an energy pull between the emerald and the heart similar to the tidal forces that work between the moon and the waters of the earth.

In addition to its influence on the heart center, the emerald is also useful in working with problems stemming from imbalance in the solar-plexus chakra. As the solar-plexus chakra is tied in with the astral/emotional body, many emotional imbalances can result from dysfunction in this particular center. When the energies of the emerald are given as a gem elixir, they can help to ease hidden fears, to balance the emotions, and to stabilize the personality.

A number of illnesses relate to imbalance in the solar-plexus center. One of these is diabetes, as the pancreas is influenced by this chakra. The emerald can be used to help the body fight off the diabetic tendency. When the emerald is used in this way, it increases the vibratory rate of the body to the point that it is able to fight off the disease. The method for using the emerald in healing diabetes is to hold a large emerald between two fingers and to allow bright sunlight to pass through the stone onto the person in need of healing. When utilizing this procedure, the adrenals are stimulated and enhanced in their effectiveness in dealing with stress, as the adrenals also have an energy link with the solar-plexus chakra.

The emerald also has energy qualities that make it useful for dealing with spinal misalignment and back pains. Individuals who have a tendency toward back problems may receive physical strength from the vibrations of the emerald. The emerald will not correct gross abnormalities of vertebral alignment, but it can sometimes strengthen the existing condition, as it works on the energy substance which makes up the bone. It also has a stimulating effect upon the nerves which emanate from the spinal cord, making it of potential benefit for individuals who suffer from sciatica.

A unique stone which is able to influence nearly all of the chakras of the body is the bloodstone. The bloodstone has held a role in mysticism throughout the ages. It is a particularly powerful stone in its ability to affect the base or coccygeal chakra, the seat of the kundalini forces. When used to stimulate the base chakra, it sends out energy patterns that will also stimulate the higher chakras as well. Its nature is such that it causes the kundalini forces to move up the spinal column in exactly the right order when properly applied. Because the forces being worked with are of a potentially dangerous nature (if aroused inappropriately), the stone must be used only by one who has achieved a level of conscious enlightenment. The healer who works with the bloodstone must be guided by an intuitive sense of how and when to use it.

When used by an adept, the bloodstone is unusually effective in aligning all of the chakras of the etheric body and of the higher dimensional bodies as well. (This stone, as with others, would be useless if used by one who lacks the inner knowledge of its application.)

> The energy vibrations [of the bloodstone] are of a very slow rate. The qualities are not of a physical nature, and it would be difficult to relate the energy possibilities here, but they are of a rate which is important for the coming together of the the various bodies of your "high-self." Do not attempt to judge those things which you do not see. This is on a plane which is not visible to the human eye.
>
> The healing qualities of the bloodstone could be defined as the alignment of the centers, alignment of the being, alignment of the several bodies of the person; the spiritual alignment of many areas which is required for the perfect physical healing to be made manifest. It doesn't work on a specific illness, but it brings everything into line. Although the energy patterns would appear to be dispersing that which is given, it is also acting in the manner which causes these patterns to be energized and drawn together much as a magnet would do with iron filings.[20]

When used in healing, the bloodstone is held in the hand with the patient lying on his/her stomach. The stone is moved in a circular motion over each vertebra of the spinal column as it slowly draws the energy up the spine. The bloodstone, as the name implies, is also useful in dealing with disorders of the blood and, specifically, problems associated with internal bleeding and coagulation. The stone is held in the healer's hand over the chakra in the vicinity of the bleeding. In the case of vaginal hemorrhaging, the stone would be placed over the pelvic/sacral chakras, with the patient lying on her back. Similarly, a bleeding ulcer could be controlled by placing the bloodstone over the solar-plexus chakra. Energy is directed from the healer's hand and focused through the bloodstone into the region of the chakra for a period of time intuited by the healer.

One of the keys to working with the bloodstone may come from feedback given by the patient. One technique that may be used is to have the patient report any local sensations in the area of the healer's hand as well as any visual imagery that is experienced. Frequently, patients will report seeing specific colors and shapes that will undergo gradual change as the energy is directed into the area of dysfunction. Initially, patients may see colors of a muddy nature or with dark or jagged forms, depending upon the individual and the nature of the disorder. As the colors go from dark to progressively lighter and higher frequency levels (i.e., from dark red, through green or yellow, to blue and then violet or white), the healer may move his/her hand up to the next highest chakra region and continue the process. In this way, the intuitive sense of the healer is guided by continuous feedback from the patient, frequently with unexpected results and images. Not all patients are able to report visual imagery in this fashion, but when possible, it greatly assists the healer.

By utilizing this technique, and others like it, the healer's natural energies may be amplified and new qualities added to the healing energies. Much experimentation is needed to confirm the applications of these stones and gems. In the future, it will be necessary for groups to work together in exploring the healing uses of many stones, gems, and crystals because, although much has been written about specific uses, not all persons will achieve the same results. It is important to realize that certain healers and individuals will work best with particular stones and not others. Additionally, it is a key concept to remember that the healing qualities of the stones and gems are often due to a blending of the energies of the particular healer with the subtle energy qualities of the stone.

As with the quartz crystals, different gems may be used in groups of stones to form coordination complexes that have particular resonant features. Special energy gridwork patterns may thus be created that have different qualities for healing as well as meditation. Also, stones and gems may be used in combination. Crystals such as diamonds are natural energy amplifiers that will boost the natural subtle powers of other gems when used with them. Another factor that will affect the energy qualities of a particular stone is its shape. Certain gems may be more effective in healing when they are faceted in a particular fashion or shaped in a special form. Also, slight variations in the color of a particular mineral will bring out special energy qualities and uses. For instance, amethysts can be found in shades ranging from a deep violet to an almost clear purple hue. The energy properties of such different colors of amethyst will be slightly different.

Additional applications of gems and crystals may be obtained by making gem elixirs from the stones. In this way, water is imprinted with particular energy and healing qualities of the crystalline structures. This technique may also be more economical when dealing with semiprecious and precious stones that tend to be quite expensive. Another innovative use of crystalline energies comes from their combination with radionic systems. Specific frequencies of energy which may be needed by the patient for a particular disorder can be determined by the radionic device, and then the appropriate crystal selected and its energies transmitted via radionic therapy. The energies of the crystals may be broadcast to the patient using a witness waveguide[21] without the patient ever having to come in direct contact with the gems.

Crystals hold the key to unlocking a vast new technology based upon the manipulation of etheric energies for healing as well as other applications. Because of their special geometric patterning, crystals are able to tap into universal energy patterns and frequencies that science is only beginning to discover. What scientists have not yet realized is that the ordered patterns of crystals, and their relationship to etheric fields, is similar to the ordered molecular structure of permanent magnets and their associated magnetic fields. Crystals, because of their inherent etheric fields, are a source of what Dr. Tiller would refer to as magnetoelectricity (ME).

> We live in an ocean of frequencies as a fish lives in the water. The fish is unaware of the many possibilities of the medium in which he moves. So Man has been totally unaware of the possibilities of the vast ocean of frequencies in which he lives. The many energy frequencies move in geometrical patterns. When the geometrical patterns are altered, their manifestation is altered. *Crystals are those substances which alter the geometrical pattern of frequencies.* We must realize that these frequency patterns are more or less stable, but that crystals because of their strength of geometrical pattern can modify and reform the frequency pattern. In doing so, energy can be released and directed to Man's purposes.
>
> Crystals are orderly arranged molecularly and magnets have an orderly arrangement of molecules also which makes possible the magnetic lines of force. *The magnet represents the most orderly focus*

*of what we may call the Matter polarity. The crystal represents the
most orderly focus of what we may call the Spirit polarity. The orderly
arrangement of molecules in crystals produces an etheric field. The
etheric field is similar to the magnetic field of force. Just as the magnetic field is a key to electricity, so the etheric field of crystals is the key
to di-electric (ME) energy.*

Magnetism on the physical plane is an equal amount of positive
and negative electricity held in a pattern either permanently or temporarily. A magnet can be separated into its component parts of positive and negative electricity by passing a conductor through the
magnetic field at right angles to the field. A permanent magnet is a
magnetic vortex where positive and negative electricity continue to
mix in equal amounts in an eternal pattern. Crystal is a magnet of di-
electric polarities having equal amounts of positive and negative
energy, which is equal and opposite to electric energy in this relationship. Di-electric energy is Spirit and electrical energy is the Matter
polarity. *Just as metals are keys to electricity, so crystals are keys to
this new development of the use of energy by man.*

The crystalline forms are the key patterns for the way the energies
are built in the universe; and the key to unlocking energy in a construc-
tive way. *The atomic bomb is a destructive way to unlocking energy.*
It may be called the *left-hand-path method. Knowledge of the crystalline forms may be considered the right-hand-path method for unlocking energy by the use of crystalline forms and sound,* in the audible, supersonic and infra-sonic, to manipulate and direct forces. We
have already discovered in the cutting of crystals how to get certain
sound effects at different frequencies. This would also give us different frequencies of energies for use. Man has not yet become basically
creative. His movement into creative fields is close at hand. He will
discover how to use crystalline forms to unlock, direct, and control
energy and to modify and mold substance. Remember the universe
was created by sound. Very shortly the scientists will be saying this.

The magnet is the Matter polarity and crystals are the Spirit
polarity. Creativity takes place always between two polarities. Therefore, the right combination of magnets and crystals will produce the
creative effect of energy. Light on the crystal and magnet, that is, lines
of force from the magnet, are the components of a new energy system. Future lighting will be glowing crystals. Energy systems could
be constructed through the use of crystalline forms, and how much
energy and the kind of energy could be regulated by the kind of crystals. This would not involve the use of wires as in our present methods.
Light produced by such method of energy will be more soft and beautiful to the physical and etheric body of mankind. The basic first product of (ME) energy from an energy unit made of crystals will be light
and this light could be transformed into heat and mechanical mo-

tion. *The discovery of the laser effect is just the beginning of a series of discoveries.*[22] *(italics added)*

We have seen how crystals may be combined with sound in the form of sonopuncture to produce healing effects. The use of various frequencies of sound with crystals for healing is just the beginning of an entirely new approach to healing. The vibrational patterns of sound hold the key to understanding the patterns of manifestation and organization of matter in the physical universe. It has been said, "In the beginning there was the word." A word is an utterance, a sonic vibrational pattern. As scientists begin to understand the relationship between the vibrational patterns of sound and the structure of matter, they will tap into a whole new universe of ideas and applications of energy for healing and technology.

Another important realization is that matter and spirit are fundamental polarities of energy expression. These two manifestations are complementary yet opposite. The matter polarity involves electromagnetic energy, the energy of the physical body. The spirit polarity reflects magnetoelectric energy, the energy of the etheric body. By utilizing crystals, which are a source of magnetoelectric energy as well as a tool for repatterning frequencies of this energy, we will discover new ways to manipulate the energies of spirit in the multidimensional human framework in order to effect healing changes.

There are many variations in the uses of gems and crystals for healing and working with the subtle energies of consciousness. Humankind seems to be undergoing a rebirth in both the interest and application of crystals to manipulate electronic and subtle energies. Could this be due to a cyclic rebirth of the Atlanteans who first brought about the development of sophisticated crystalline technologies? The application of crystalline systems for healing and industry carries tremendous potential benefits as well as inherent dangers.

The legend of Atlantis serves as a reminder that we must maintain a balance of power between ourselves and the natural energies of the planet, as well as a balance between the energies of our lower and higher selves. If we forget our inner connection to the divine energies that work for our potential benefit through the gifts of nature, the natural balance will be shifted in a direction such that our present-day culture will no longer dominate the planet on which we live.

The gifts of the mineral kingdom from within the Earth hold undreamt-of benefits for healing and uplifting the consciousness of humankind, if only these gifts can be used correctly. It will be the challenge of spiritually-oriented scientists and the healer/physicians of the future to conduct research on the use of crystalline energies in an intuitive and responsible manner to develop these potentials. If we can only learn to tap into the wisdom of the Higher Self inherent in all people, we will move toward that new position of peaceful coexistence and spiritual light which the Atlanteans hoped might again grace the face of their planet.

Key Points to Remember

1. The exploration and development of crystalline technologies in electronics, laser development, and information storage has been of critical importance to the scientific revolution of the latter part of the twentieth century.

2. There are legends of an ancient civilization, Atlantis, which developed crystalline technologies to a high degree, but utilized a different aspect of crystal properties than is focused on by modern science. It is said that the Atlanteans used crystalline systems to manipulate subtle energies and the life-force, and were successful in applying these discoveries to both healing and technologic developments.

3. The Atlanteans are said to have developed healing systems based on the use of crystals, flower essences, and homeopathics. They focused on the subtle energetic aspects of disease causation and sought to direct vibrational therapies to correct these imbalances. Those who used allopathic approaches were considered a radical minority.

4. Quartz crystals have unique properties which allow them to transmit, transmute, and store energies of both an electronic and subtle energetic nature. Healers can use crystals to amplify their own healing fields and direct them into the body in a more coherent and organized fashion.

5. Healing energies are affected and directed by the thoughts of the healer. As such, various visualization techniques can be used to direct the crystal-amplified healing energies into specific areas of the body in order to rebalance the different subtle and physiological systems.

6. Quartz crystals amplify, and may be programmed with, subtle energies which operate in the negative space-time frame, i.e. magnetoelectrical energy.

7. Subtle energies transmitted into the body by quartz crystals (and other vibrational healing modalities) are resonantly absorbed and assimilated by the body's own biocrystalline system, a unique network of cellular elements with quartz-like properties.

8. Multiple crystals placed into geometric forms and activated by "directed intention" of thought energies are called "gridwork systems." These crystal grid arrays have unique properties which amplify the energetic potential of the single crystals into more potent healing and meditative tools.

9. The various crystals and minerals of Earth have common geometric symmetries which have been categorized according to the seven crystal systems. Each of the seven systems has energetic characteristics and geometries which resonate with a particular subplane of form-building at the etheric level. Each of the seven crystal systems also has an energy relationship to the seven major chakras.

10. Crystals belonging to a particular system will have subtle energetic properties common to that geometric class, but will also display unique energetic and healing characteristics as well.

11. Because of their effects upon the chakras, as well as other subtle and physiological systems, the different crystals may be capable of bringing about an energetic repatterning at the etheric and higher levels of form in order to assist the healing process.

12. Various crystals may be used directly upon the body or prepared via the sun method as a gem elixir and ingested by the patient.

13. Like the quartz crystals, other gems have their own unique healing properties, but they also can act as transducers and amplifiers of the healer's own energy fields.

14. Magnets have an orderly molecular arrangement which makes possible their generated magnetic fields. Conversely, crystals have a similar orderly geometric arrangement of atoms, but they generate etheric fields. Magnets represent an orderly focus of the matter polarity and are the key to electricity. Crystals represent the most orderly focus of the spirit polarity and are the key to magnetoelectricity.

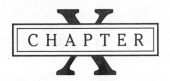

CHAPTER X

The Interconnecting Web of Life:
OUR RELATIONSHIP WITH THE CHAKRAS

In previous chapters we have discussed our true nature as multidimensional beings. The physical body is the densest component of many interactive energy fields. Each of these fields, or higher dimensional light bodies, is connected to the physical cellular structure through a complex network of energy threads. This integral web of life energies allows the higher vibrational forces to manifest in the physical body through their guiding effects upon the patterns of cellular growth and upon the unfolding of human consciousness.

This multidimensional network allows energy of varying vibrational characteristics to flow into the body and influence behavior at both the cellular and organismic level. In order that incoming subtle energies are properly integrated into the cellular matrix, they must first pass through specialized step-down transformers. These unique centers, known as the chakras, process vibrational energy of specific frequencies. The chakras translate the effects of etheric, astral, and higher vibrational inputs into biological manifestations via our unique endocrine system.

The endocrine glands are part of a powerful master control system that affects the physiology of the body from the level of cellular gene activation on up to the functioning of the central nervous system. The chakras are thus able to affect our moods and behavior through hormonal influences on brain activity. Recent scientific research in the field of psychoneuroimmunology has begun to hint at deeper connections between the brain, endocrine, and immune systems than had been previously recognized. The relationships between stress, depression, and immune suppression are only now finding increased recognition.[1] The chakras play a vital role in the regulation of various states of consciousness, especially in regard to people's emotional nature. Because inner emotional balance is partly a function of properly working chakras and integrated subtle bodies, a greater understanding of the chakras will eventually provide explanations as to how different emotional states can create either illness or wellness.

A New Model of Illness & Wellness:
Disease as a Manifestation of Chakra Dysfunction

The chakras are specialized energy centers which connect us to the multidimensional universe. They can be understood at a variety of levels. The chakras are dimensional portals within the subtle bodies which take in and process energy of a higher vibrational nature so that it may be properly assimilated and used to transform the physical body. Although there are many minor chakras throughout the body, we shall only be concerned with the function of the seven major chakras. Each of these major chakras is connected to a major nerve plexus and glandular center within the endocrine system of the body.

Diagram 11.
NEUROPHYSIOLOGICAL & ENDOCRINE ASSOCIATIONS
OF THE CHAKRAS

CHAKRA	NERVE PLEXUS	PHYSIOLOGICAL SYSTEM	ENDOCRINE SYSTEM
COCCYGEAL	Sacral-Coccygeal	Reproductive	Gonads
SACRAL	Sacral	Genitourinary	Leydig
SOLAR PLEXUS	Solar	Digestive	Adrenals
HEART	Heart Plexus	Circulatory	Thymus
THROAT	Cervical Ganglia Medulla	Respiratory	Thyroid
THIRD EYE	Hypothalamus Pituitary	Autonomic Nervous System	Pituitary
HEAD	Cerebral Cortex Pineal	CNS Central Control	Pineal

As can be seen in Diagram 11, each major chakra is also associated with a particular physiologic system. For instance, the heart chakra is associated with the physical heart and circulatory system. The throat chakra is associated with the trachea and thyroid gland, and so on. Proper functioning of each of the major chakras is critical to the balance and cellular health of each organ system. This is not to imply that abnormalities within the chakra system are the only cause of illness. There are also toxic environmental, chemical, bacterial, viral, and other influences which can create disease in the physical body. The chakras help to regulate the flow of vital energy into different organs of the body. With proper functioning, they help to establish strength and balance in a particular physiologic system. Conversely, abnormal chakra function can create weakness in an area of the body. There are many interlocking homeostatic systems within the physical and subtle bodies which cooperate in maintaining the health of the individual. Each system works in harmony with the others along a hierarchical axis of energy flow. Changes in the physical body are merely the observable end result of physiologic events occurring simultaneously on a variety of energy levels. The purpose of this chapter is to focus attention on how imbalances at the level of the chakras can contribute to the manifestation of either health or illness in the physical body.

A key point to understand is that the chakras contribute a type of subtle nutritive energy to specific parts of the physical body. This cosmic energy, sometimes referred to as prana, is a manifestation of the life-force itself. The uninhibited flow of prana through our energy channels and cellular/molecular systems helps to maintain the vitality of the physical body. Although the digestive system takes in biochemical energy and molecular building blocks in the form of physical nutrients, the chakras, in conjunction with the acupuncture meridian system, take in higher vibrational energies that are just as integral to the proper growth and maintenance of physical life. Whereas the physical nutrients are used to promote cellular growth and homeostasis at the molecular level, the subtle-energy currents conveyed by the chakras and meridians assist in promoting stability and organization within the etheric body. The etheric body is the energy growth template for the physical. Energetic changes occur at the etheric level before becoming manifest as physical cellular events. Thus, one can see the importance of maintaining proper organization and health of the etheric body.

Currents of energy are taken into the body through a stream entering the crown chakra on top of the head. Since the chakras are closely linked to the spinal cord and nerve ganglia along the body's central axis, energy flows downward from the crown chakra to the lower chakras, which distribute the subtle currents to the appropriate organs and body parts. Each chakra is associated with a different vibrational frequency. One might envision white light entering a prism and then being split into the seven colors of the rainbow. Inherent within the white light are all seven colors. In a similar fashion, cosmic energies enter the crown chakra, and the seven vibrational currents are then refracted from the single higher stream containing all the colors. Each vibrational "color" is thereby distributed to the appropriate chakra attuned to that specific "color" frequency.

Subtle energies taken in by the chakras are converted to endocrine signals in a manner akin to a step-down transformer. As energy of a higher vibrational or subtle nature enters the chakras, it is stepped down and transmitted as information of a more physiologic nature. Subtle energy is converted into hormonal signals from each of the major endocrine glands that are linked with the chakras. Through the release of small amounts of powerful hormones into the bloodstream, the entire physical body is affected. In addition, each chakra distributes vital energy to a number of different organs that are in the same body location and that tend to resonate at a similar frequency.

Each organ within the body has an energy frequency of its own. Organs of similar frequency tend to be clustered together in the same body region or to be linked together in a special physiologic relationship. For instance, the solar-plexus chakra is intimately connected to organs that lie in the general vicinity of the solar-plexus. These include the stomach, pancreas, gall bladder, and liver. Each organ is involved in the initial process of digestion. Subtle energies distributed to these organs by the solar-plexus chakra help to maintain the health and function of this aspect of digestion. Abnormalities of vital energy flow affecting the solar-plexus chakra will thus manifest as difficulties in the digestive system such as peptic ulcer disease, gallstones, pancreatitis, etc. The reasons for an abnormal chakra function are even more important because they involve emotional, mental, and spiritual issues as well as behavioral patterns linked to the function of the solar-plexus chakra.

As has been mentioned in previous chapters, the chakras are more than passive transducers of subtle energy. They are actually organs of psychic perception in our subtle bodies. Each chakra is associated with a different type of psychic function. For instance, the third-eye or brow chakra is associated with intuitive insight and clairvoyance. The throat chakra functions during the use of clairaudient skills. The heart chakra has an association with clairsentience and so forth. The reason that the chakras are involved with higher perception is that they are points of energy influx from the etheric, astral, mental, and higher spiritual levels. Each chakra is actually a multiplexing of several overlapping energy centers in the subtle bodies. There is a mental, an astral, and an etheric chakra occupying the same area. Subtle energies originating at the mental and higher spiritual / vibrational levels are processed through the mental chakra and stepped down to the astral level. This process is repeated as the stepped-down mental energy and direct astral imputs are processed through the astral chakra. From there the energy is sent through the etheric chakra and then stepped down further until it can be distributed, via the nadis, to special nervous and glandular centers throughout the physical body.

Seventh Chakra

In addition to assisting psychic perception, each chakra is associated with a different emotional and spiritual issue in the development of human consciousness. For instance *the crown or seventh chakra, which is considered one of the highest vibrational centers in the subtle body, is associated with deep inner searching: the so-called spiritual quest.* This chakra is most active when individuals are involved in religious and spiritual quests for the meaning of life and in the inner search for their origins as conscious evolving beings. The opening of the crown chakra allows one to enter into the highest states of consciousness. The conscious activation of this center represents the beginning stage of ascension into a state of spiritual perfection.

On the physical level this chakra is tied to the activity of the cerebral cortex and general nervous system functioning. In addition, the proper activation of the crown chakra influences the synchonization between the left and right hemispheres of the brain. The crown chakra is also closely linked with the pineal gland. For the crown chakra to be fully awakened there must first occur a balancing of body, mind, and spirit. In the individual who has an opened crown chakra, the seventh center is represented by an energy polarity between the pineal gland and the right and left cerebral hemispheres. Abnormalities in energy flow at the level of the crown chakra may manifest as various types of cerebral dysfunction, including psychosis.

Sixth Chakra

The sixth chakra is the brow chakra, sometimes referred to as the "third eye." The past mystical associations of this center with the pineal gland are well known. From an evolutionary standpoint, it is interesting to note that in lower animals such as reptiles the pineal gland is still associated with a rudimentary third eye, complete with lens and retina-like photo-receptor. When the seventh chakra is activated, the sixth or brow chakra is represented by an energy polarity between the pituitary and pineal glands. When the seventh center remains unopened, the brow chakra is represented by the pituitary and the medulla oblongata (part of the brainstem).[2]

The third-eye chakra is the seat of intuition and the subtle organ involved in clairvoyance. The degree of activity of the brow chakra is an indication of an individual's intuitive prowess as well as their conscious level of awareness. The brow chakra is one of the psychic centers that is gradually developed by various types of meditative practices. An individual who has a highly developed third-eye chakra has the ability to "see within," an aspect of consciousness also related to introspection. This type of third-eye vision is an inward focusing of awareness which results in clearer insights and new perspectives on the higher causes of both outer and inner world events. The translation of the term clairvoyance is literally "clear vision." Physically, the brow chakra is associated with the pineal gland, the pituitary gland, and the spinal cord, as well as the eyes, ears, nose, and sinuses. *Diseases caused by dysfunction of the brow chakra may be caused by an individual's not wanting to see something which is important to their soul growth.* Difficulties associated with energy blockages at the level of the third-eye chakra can physically manifest in the form of illnesses as divergent as sinus problems, cataracts, and major endocrine imbalances (because of this center's association with the pituitary gland).

Fifth Chakra

The fifth chakra, or throat center, has influence over the major glands and structures in the neck region. These include the thyroid and parathyroid glands, the mouth, vocal cords, and trachea, as well as the cervical vertebrae. There is also an association between the throat chakra and the parasympathetic nervous system. The greater part of the parasympathetic division of the autonomic nervous system originates in the tenth cranial nerve, also known as the vagus nerve, which leaves the brainstem and travels down the neck to innervate the heart, lungs, and abdominal organs. The parathyroid gland (which is energized by this center) regulates the calcium metabolism in bone cells via the secretion of PTH (parathyroid hormone).

In addition to production of thyroid hormone, which regulates the general metabolic activity of the cells of the body, the thyroid gland also produces thyrocalcitonin, a hormone which affects calcium and bone metabolism in a manner opposite to that of parathyroid hormone. Because the throat chakra energizes both the thyroid and parathyroid glands, each of which differentially regulates calcium metabolism in bone cells, the throat chakra affects general skeletal activity. Symbolic of its position in the vicinity of the mouth and vocal cords, the throat chakra is important in communication. On a psychic level, the throat chakra functions during clairaudience, or hearing at an astral level.

At the physical/emotional level, dysfunction in the throat chakra may reflect difficulties in communication. This is especially evident in individuals who have difficulty in expressing themselves in front of others. Such inability to express oneself may stem from a wide variety of emotional causes. The throat chakra is also a center of higher creativity such as the creation of word and song. Speech and sound are means by which we can vibrationally communicate with one another and verbally express new ideas. *Blockages in the throat chakra may occur in people who do not express themselves creatively or who may have great difficulty in doing so.*

In addition to communication, the throat chakra is sometimes known as the center of the will. Difficulties in self-expression may be seen here as a problem in exerting the will to communicate one's true inner feelings. The will activity of the throat chakra can also affect an individual's ability to consciously recognize his or her own needs. Abnormalities of chakric energy flow may manifest as diseases which involve dysfunctional cell activity in those structures that are energetically dependent upon the throat center. Examples of diseases involving an imbalanced throat chakra include laryngitis, thyroiditis, parathyroid gland tumors, and cancer of the larynx.

The type of disease that may manifest in the physical structures adjacent to the throat center is dependent upon a number of different factors. Although blockage of energy flow through a particular chakra is commonly recognized, the opposite condition can just as easily create imbalance. That is, an excess of energy flow through a particular chakra can also produce illness. Whereas inadequate energy flow due to a chakra blockage might result in a degenerative disease or a problem related to atrophy of function (ex. hypothyroidism), overabundant energy flow can cause inflammation (thyroiditis associated with hyperthyroidism) and cancerous growth (carcinoma of the thyroid). More detail will be given on this aspect of chakra dysfunction later in the chapter.

Fourth Chakra

The fourth chakra is known as the heart center. It is perhaps one of the most important centers in our subtle energy bodies. *The reason that the heart center is so significant is that an open heart chakra is integral to an individual's ability to express love. This includes both self-love as well as the expression of love toward others.* Love may manifest as brotherly love toward friends and neighbors, as emotional love in a love relationship between lovers, and also as spiritual love. The highest form of spiritual love, of course, is unconditional love toward others. *The lessons of love are among the most critical that we must learn during our allotted time upon the physical plane. Difficulties in learning these lessons can manifest as abnormalities in the function of the heart chakra which, in turn, affects the physical heart.*

Because many people experience difficulties in developing the inner potential of the heart chakra, the so-called "inner heart" center, it is not surprising that there is a tremendous mortality due to heart disease in the world today. Although smoking and high cholesterol levels are certainly a contributing factor to the high incidence of heart disease, it is ironic that most doctors and patients fail to recognize the significance of the energetic link between heart disease, the heart chakra, and one's ability to express love. Patients' awareness of this important psychoenergetic relationship could assist physicians in healing the attitudes and consciousness that helped to create the energy imbalances which predisposed them towards heart disease in the first place.

Along with its link to the physical heart, the heart chakra provides nutritive subtle energy to the bronchial tubes, lungs, and breasts, and also affects the function of the entire circulatory system. In addition to contributing toward coronary artery disease and heart attacks, imbalances in the heart chakra can lead to such other circulatory diseases as strokes—an illness which affects thousands of people each year. Reduction of energy coming into the heart chakra can manifest as stagnation of blood flow through a diseased physical heart. Stasis of flow through the chambers of the heart may result in the formation of blood clots. These clots are then propelled through the circulation where they lodge in small cerebral arteries and block the flow of lifegiving oxygen (and prana) to brain tissue, thus causing a stroke. (This is only one example of how energetic dysfunction at the level of the heart center can manifest as a stroke.) The amount of subtle energy flow through the heart chakra is a reflection of the importance of love in an individual's life and the degree to which that individual is meeting his or her needs in this regard.

Given this information, one can look at childhood diseases such as asthma with a new understanding. Children with asthma often come from families where the mother (or father) is overprotective. At both a symbolic and a literal level, the child is smothering from an unbalanced expression of parental love, affecting the heart center. As the heart chakra influences the bronchial tubes, the unbalanced energy creates a tendency toward spasm in the airways and breathing difficulties, especially during periods of inner emotional conflict.

The energies of the lower four chakras are symbolic of the ancient four elements of our planet: earth, water, fire, and air. Because of its association with the heart and lungs, which take in and circulate oxygen throughout the body, the heart chakra is symbolically representative of the element of air. The solar-plexus is linked with the element of fire, the navel chakra represents water, and the root chakra symbolizes the element of earth. Whereas the lower four centers represent the physical plane, the three higher chakras are symbolically linked with the etheric and higher spiritual elements of creation. The heart center is considered a transitional chakra, mediating between the lower earthly energies and the higher spiritual energies. As air, the heart center symbolically occupies a position between heaven and earth.

Since the heart chakra is closely tied to the expression of love and compassion, it is also naturally considered to be an important center of nurturance. Most of the organs associated with the heart chakra help to nurture and promote life and vitality throughout the rest of the body. The lungs take in oxygen and prana from the atmosphere. The heart pumps the blood to the lungs, where oxygen and prana are taken in and distributed to the rest of the body's organs. In the digestive system, more nutrients are added to the bloodstream, where the circulation can distribute them to the rest of the physical body. The breasts are also located at the level of the heart chakra. They are perhaps the only organs in the body which are totally dedicated to the nurturance of another being.

The ability to nurture oneself, as well as other people, is linked to the development of the love nature of the heart center. *As the one becomes*

*more able to unconditionally love oneself and others, the heart chakra
begins to become more open as it increases its nurturing energy flow to the
organs it supplies.* Asthma is a disease related to heart center dysfunction
which can actually be the result of overnurturing by another. If a child is
given too much loving attention, to the point of stifling its ability to become
independent, the lack of balance in the heart center results in abnormal
stimulation of the bronchial tree, cutting off the inflow of life-sustaining
oxygen. Just as inadequate nurturing can have negative effects, too much
of a good thing can also be bad. When a child is overwhelmed by too much
nurturing, however well meaning, the result can be a physical sensation
of smothering through the energetic mechanisms just discussed.

At a psychological level, the heart chakra deals with the emotions that
bind individuals in various loving relationships. People often experience
strong positive feelings toward others as a welling up of energy in the chest
area. When activated by feelings of love, especially romantic love, this sensation is caused by an awareness of energy flow through the heart chakra.
The act of nurturing is fed by the different emotional feelings of love, compassion, and empathy. The ability to nurture another person is a reflection
of love and empathy for others and the recognition of their inherent needs
for physical and spiritual growth. *The development of compassion and em-
pathic feelings for others is one of the first steps on the path toward opening the heart chakra and developing higher consciousness.* When these
elements are lacking in the personality, one can be sure that some blockage
in the heart chakra exists.

*One of the most important links between the heart chakra and a phy-
sical organ is seen in the association of the heart chakra with the thymus
gland.* For years doctors thought that it was normal for the thymus gland
to atrophy in size and function as an individual grew older. As physicians
begin to understand the energy relationship between the heart chakra and
thymus gland, it is likely that this view will undergo considerable revision.
It is possible that the age-related involution of the thymus gland is not a
universal phenomenon. In those who do have thymic atrophy in later years,
there may be a relationship between loneliness, depression, blockage of
the heart chakra, and loss of glandular function. Researchers in the developing
field of psychoneuroimmunology have yet to examine the subtle energetic
links between emotion and immunologic function. They have begun to examine the physiologic links between human emotions and illness, but
there is a deeper esoteric aspect of immunology that has yet to be fully

grasped.

Medical science now acknowledges that the thymus gland plays an important role in the regulation of the immune response. Previously, it was felt that the thymus was primarily functional during childhood, when so-called T-lymphocytes become preprogrammed for special immunologic capabilities. This special activation of lymphocytes takes place during a critical developmental period while they are residing in the young thymus gland. Researchers are now beginning to discover powerful regulatory hormones which are produced by this gland. These thymic hormones, known as thymosins, influence an individual's ability to fight off disease throughout their entire life by enhancing the activity of different types of T-lymphocytes.

Regulation of the thymus gland's hormonal activity can also influence diseases that have an immunologic basis. For instance, rheumatoid arthritis, an autoimmune disease in which the body literally attacks itself, is being experimentally treated by irradiating the thymus gland in order to curb its activity. Although there are many illnesses which are primarily disorders of immune function, doctors are beginning to find evidence of immunologic components to many other diseases not thought to be related to this aspect of bodily function. For instance, scientists have recently discovered evidence of an immunologic contribution to coronary artery disease, a problem thought to be related primarily to cholesterol, diet, hypertension, and smoking. Many diseases of organ hypofunctioning, such as primary ovarian failure, adrenal atrophy, and certain types of childhood diabetes, are now being linked to autoimmune mechanisms of glandular destruction. The important point is that many diverse diseases may be indirectly affected by the immune regulation of the thymus gland, which, in turn, is influenced by the activity of the heart chakra.

Various researchers who have examined the link between emotions and illness have found a strong association between depression, grief, and suppression of immune functioning. A number of psychologists who have studied the life histories of cancer patients have noted interesting similarities. Many patients were found to have experienced depression prior to the development of their malignancies. In studies by LeShan[3], many cancer patients were diagnosed with their illnesses approximately twelve to eighteen months following the death of their spouses. In these patients, it is likely that prolonged grief and depression caused suppression of their normal immunosurveillance activity, which screens and destroys single cancer cells. Thus, the impaired immunity of the grieving patients would have allowed the formation of larger and less immunologically vulnerable masses of tumor cells. Patients with immunosuppression from any cause are known to be at greater risk for developing malignancy. Some cancer researchers have noted that parents who undergo grief reactions following their children's diagnosis of leukemia also manifest indications of immunosuppression in laboratory blood tests. These examples illustrate the powerful negative effects that grief, stress, and depression can produce within the body's immunologic defense systems.

Medical researchers do not yet understand that the subtle energy flow of prana through the heart chakra is an integral factor in the proper functioning of the thymus gland and, thus, the body's immune competence. The thymus gland produces hormonal factors, such as thymopoetin and other thymosins, which regulate the activity of lymphocytes throughout the body. It is primarily a subset of these blood cells, known as T-lymphocytes or T-cells, which are affected by the thymus. T-cells are so named because they acquire their specialized abilities during residence within the thymus gland at an early stage of cellular programming.

Recent scientific advances in immunology have discovered that there are subcategories of T-lymphocytes known as T-helper and T-suppressor cells. T-helper cells assist antibody-producing and other types of defender cells in removing foreign or "non-self" proteins and invaders from the body. There are also other special lymphocytes called killer T-cells which are known to destroy cancer cells. These cells participate in the so-called immunosurveillance function of the immune system, which screens, not only for foreign invaders such as bacteria and viruses, but also for cancer cells. Perhaps the most important of these T-cells are the so-called T- suppressor cells. These cells regulate the intensity of the immune response and keep the other watchdog lymphocytes in check so that only the non-self proteins are attacked. When this self-regulatory function is lost because of decreases in the number and activity of T-suppressor cells, the body actually begins to attack itself. Medicine has begun to recognize an increasing number of these so-called "autoimmune" diseases.

There are a wide variety of diseases which have an autoimmune mechanism as their common link. In these illnesses, the lymphocytes produce antibodies against cellular proteins from various organs, as well as against DNA, causing the body to immunologically attack itself. One of the most common autoimmune diseases is rheumatoid arthritis. Other examples of diseases with autoimmune components are lupus, mysasthenia gravis, multiple sclerosis, Hashimoto's thyroiditis, adrenal failure, primary ovarian failure, and possibly certain types of childhood diabetes.

In some of these diseases there is evidence to suggest a possible viral contributing factor. Some researchers have suggested that particular viruses may alter certain proteins, making them look foreign to the eyes of the immune system. These foreign-appearing proteins may initiate a general immunologic attack against both virally-altered and normal proteins within the body. There is additional evidence pointing toward a predisposition to these viral infections, or at least the autoimmune reactions they initiate. For example, certain individuals with juvenile diabetes were discovered to have evidence of both viral invasion of pancreatic tissue and also autoantibodies against pancreatic tissue. These same diabetic patients were found to have a common genetic background as defined by HLA typing, a measure of immunologic similarity between individuals. Circulating antibodies directed against the insulin-producing cells of the pancreas could be found in these diabetic children.

Other viruses may even take up residence in and destroy the cells of the immune system, impairing the body's ability to defend itself from other invaders. AIDS (Acquired Immune Deficiency Syndrome), one of the most controversial diseases of our time, is associated with immunosuppression, loss of T-lymphocytes, and viral infection. AIDS is a disease which demonstrates convincing evidence of a virus with a predilection for T-lymphocytes. There is now additional information to suggest that there may also be herpes-related viruses with a predilection for the antibody-producing B-lymphocytes.

Regardless of the fact that viruses may physically initiate the disease process, there are various subtle-energy factors which may predispose certain individuals to acquiring an immunologic illness when confronted with such pathogens. Not every person who is exposed to the virus comes down with a severe illness. Individuals with strong immunologic defenses may be able to remove the virus from their system or limit its effects to minimal flu-like symptoms.

A significant energy factor contributing to a strong immune response is a healthy flow of subtle energy through the heart chakra to support the thymus gland. When there is a blockage of pranic flow through the heart chakra because of problems in manifesting love towards self or others, there is a diminution of vital energy flow to the thymus gland. Sometimes this can manifest as a disease in the thymus gland itself. For instance in myasthenia gravis, an autoimmune disease caused by antibodies produced against the neuromuscular junction (thus causing generalized muscular weakness), there is an increased incidence of thymoma, a type of malignant tumor of the thymus gland.

Impaired function of the thymus gland (because of heart chakra blockages) can also result in a higher susceptibility to severe viral infections of any type. Certain types of T-lymphocytes specifically work at removing viruses from the body. It is likely that these cells are distantly influenced by circulating hormonal factors produced not only by lymphocytes (so-called lymphokines), but also by immune regulatory hormones (such as thymosins) which are secreted by the thymus gland. In individuals with immunologically linked illnesses that may be related to a particular virus, blockage in the heart chakra can create a subtle energetic predisposition toward developing such diseases. The viral infections may only play a secondary, albeit important, role in the development of these autoimmune and other immunologically related diseases.

The predisposition toward illness appears to relate to certain emotional imbalances concerning the love nature and the heart chakra. *Blockages in the heart chakra may arise from an inability to express love; but even more importantly, dysfunction frequently arises from a lack of self-love.* The ability to love oneself is far more important than many psychologists realize. Persistant negative self-images and loss of self-worth do more physiologic damage than currently recognized because of the resulting abnormalities which occur along the heart chakra/thymus axis.

In many cases, the sick individual will have multiple chakras which are functioning abnormally. For instance, blockage of energy flow through one chakra may result in too much energy flow to the chakra below. A blockage at the level of the heart chakra might result in too much energy pouring through the solar-plexus center below. Blockage of energy flow can be imagined as a log jam in a river that causes flooding in regions leading into the area of interference. Kundalini energies generated in the root chakra tend to rise up the spine to the crown center and feed energy to chakras in ascending order along the way. Blockage of higher centers can thus result in congestion and overflow of energy in the lower chakras as a means of venting the excess flow. Frequently, illness may be associated with abnormal function in more than one chakra because an individual may have multiple emotional blockages. Each chakra blockage is associated with a particular emotional issue that is not being adequately addressed by the individual. Different emotional and spiritual issues are dealt with at different levels of chakra energy modulation.

Many of the emotional and spiritual issues which are inadequately addressed by individuals with dysfunction at the level of the heart chakra revolve around the opposing emotions of grief and joy. When one's life is filled with grieving, sadness, loneliness, depression, and an inability to express love to those around oneself, imbalances occur within the heart chakra. This is especially true among siblings or spouses facing separation and loss of a family member due to terminal illness. Depression following the death of a loved one may be related to feelings of guilt at not having acted properly or in time to prevent such tragedy. The individual may blame him/herself inappropriately. This is often reflected by an inability to experience joy in one's life. Such emotional and spiritual imbalances result in blockages to energy flow through the heart chakra which can later become manifest as cellular dysfunction at the level of the thymus gland.

Because the thymus can affect many types of disease-fighting cells throughout the body, abnormal thymic function can create a general depression in immune defenses and thus promote susceptibility to a variety of bacterial and viral infections. Because of the effects of the thymus gland on particular types of lymphocytes, especially T-helper and T-suppressor cells, more specific kinds of damage can occur to particular organs of the body. The T-suppressor cells have undergone increasing scrutiny by doctors in attempts to understand their involvement in autoimmune diseases. If the T-suppressor cells fail to keep the body from attacking itself, the immune system can go on a rampage against particular parts of the body that have been deregulated from immune control.

Selective immunosuppression of T-suppressor cell function, caused by various types of heart chakra-thymus gland dysfunction, can affect other endocrine centers throughout the body. Demonstrations of distant autoimmune effects on glandular centers can be seen in such diseases as autoimmune thryroiditis, adrenal failure, and primary ovarian failure. In illnesses where a particular endocrine center is affected by autoimmune destruction, it is likely that the sick individual has subtle-energy imbalances within both the heart chakra and the glandular center that has immunologically impaired hormonal functions. For instance, autoimmune adrenal failure might be associated with chakra dysfunction in the solar-plexus chakra as well as the heart chakra. Primary ovarian failure would likewise tend to be associated with subtle-energy blockage in the heart chakra and also the sacral or gonadal chakra.

Another immune disease which is likely to be associated with blockage of the gonadal chakra is AIDS. One of the early correlations found between AIDS and homosexuals was the great frequency of sexual contacts in those afflicted with the disease, especially among gay men. Going from one sexual one-night-stand to another without feelings of true love would tend to focus too much energy on the gonadal center. This in itself, of course, does not cause AIDS. Frequent sexual contacts do promote greater exposure to the AIDS virus, however. Also, the negative cultural views associated with homosexuality promote a poor self-image in the unconscious mind and a lack of self-love among gays. Over time, this could easily cause an imbalance in the heart chakra. Negative energy changes in the heart chakra lead to decreased thymic function and thus to a greater susceptibility to the AIDS virus.

The way that the AIDS virus contributes to recurrent illness is a function of its effect upon lymphocyte function. Specifically, the virus influences certain types of T-lymphocytes, especially the T-helper cells. One of the criteria for diagnosing AIDS in laboratory tests is the examination of the T-helper to T-suppressor cell ratio. In AIDS there is a reversal in the normal ratio of helper to suppressor cells. With fewer T-helper cells and also diminished numbers of killer T-cells, the body becomes more susceptible to viral and bacterial infections as well as to malignant tumors such as Kaposi's sarcoma. From an esoteric standpoint, the reduction in lymphocyte number is caused not only by the HIV (Human Immunodeficiency Virus or AIDS virus) infection but also by the dysfunction in the heart chakra/thymus gland axis which may have predisposed the individual to the severe infection in the first place. In addition to their association with the HIV infection, it is likely that AIDS victims will eventually be shown to have energy blockages in the heart chakra, the gonadal chakra, and other chakras within the subtle body. Needless to say, subtle energy dysfunction within the heart chakra, and the associated illnesses which reflect imbalances in the expression of love, will be viewed with increasing importance by future healer/physicians.

Third Chakra

The third chakra is the solar-plexus chakra. Imbalances in this center will also generate increasing interest, as it is a common site of energy-blockages. As mentioned previously, the solar-plexus chakra supplies nutritive subtle energy to most of the major organs of digestion and puri- fication. These include the stomach, pancreas, liver, gall bladder, spleen, adrenal glands, lumbar vertebrae, and the general digestive system. (The small intestine and colon are tied to the second chakra.)

From an emotional and spiritual standpoint, the solar-plexus chakra is linked to the issue of personal power. Personal power might be inter- preted as a feeling of control over one's life. Personal power also relates to how people view themselves in relation to others in their lives. Do they see themselves in control of their lives and comfortable with their relation- ships, or are they subject to the whims of others? Individuals with a so- called "victim consciousness," who have no sense of control over their lives and who feel it is inevitable that they will be taken advantage of in the future, will often manifest an imbalance in the solar-plexus chakra. One's sense of comfort with the universe as a nurturing place, as opposed to a feeling that the world is a stage for uneasiness and bad things waiting to happen, directly affects the subtle-energy flow through the solar-plexus chakra.

In a rapidly changing world filled with increasing demands on one's mind, body and spirit, it is easy to see how stress can manifest as illness caused by energy blockage in the solar-plexus center. *Domination, anger, and abuse of others can also be associated with abnormal function of the solar-plexus center.* Oftentimes this anger is an expression of an inner feel- ing of powerlessness that may be discharged towards innocent bystanders, coworkers, or even the children of individuals who have too much unvented energy in the solar-plexus or "adrenal" center. This could be considered a misuse of the solar-plexus energies.

On a symbolic level, the solar-plexus chakra represents the element of fire. Indeed, the solar-plexus region is like a miniature sun, burning energies of chemical oxidation through the digestion of food—a type of inner fire. If the inner flame is improperly regulated, it can actually burn a hole in the wall of the chakra-associated organs, as in the case of duodenal ulcers. The solar-plexus center is also a seat of anger, aggression, and other emotions. These emotions are often connected to an individual's sense of personal power and also to feelings about how much control they seem to have over their lives. If the issues relating to this chakra are not consciously resolved, the individual may be left with an internal conflict, causing a preoccupation with dominance and control over other people. The issue then becomes a conflict between dominance and submission. *Thus, persons who become preoccupied or "stuck" in the lessons of the solar-plexus center may either be tyrannical in their outward aggressiveness and assertiveness, or just the opposite—they may be cowardly, meek and submissive.* Many times, individuals with solar-plexus blockages may alternate between these two modes, depending upon the situation. Interestingly, some psychological studies of ulcer patients reveal that they are often people who force themselves to take on responsibilities of a dominant, controlling position; yet underneath they are often passive, dependent, and submissive.

Imbalances in the solar-plexus chakra can affect any one of the digestive organs of the body which receive energy from this center. Thus, growing stresses in the workplace caused by increasing employer demands, coupled with an inner sense of powerlessness to change one's life, can easily manifest as an ulcer in the lining of the stomach or duodenum. The adrenal glands are also linked to the solar-plexus chakra. (Some esoteric sources view the adrenal glands as having an energy link to the root chakra as well.) The adrenal glands play an important role in hormonal activation of the body systems during times of stress. When there is blockage in the solar-plexus center, diseases may occur which can cause degeneration of the adrenal gland and lead to fatigue and weakness. As such, the solar-plexus chakra is an important energy center of the body which contributes to the outward vitality of the personality.

Another widespread disease that is associated with imbalance in the solar-plexus chakra is diabetes. Although this subtle-energy aspect of diabetes has never been addressed by conventional medical practitioners, it is nonetheless of importance to the pathophysiology of the disease process. It might be said of diabetics that there is a sense of loss of personal power accompanying the disease, linked to a feeling that might be metaphorically expressed as the sweetness having gone out of life. Other reflections of solar-plexus chakra imbalance might be related to a longing for the past or for that which might have been. Sometimes the imbalance may stem from a deep inner need to control. This is not to say that all diabetics are sad and powerless individuals dwelling on the past. Most of the inner emotional conflicts that affect the functioning of the chakras are deep unconscious feelings that usually are not consciously recognized nor verbally expressed to those around them.

Many illnesses which are manifestations of chakra imbalances are the results of faulty data on old memory tapes which have been recorded and programmed into the unconscious mind during early portions of the individual's life. These tapes have been unconsciously playing back messages told to them by others or falsely thought by themselves, which are no longer appropriate to present-day circumstances. Regardless of their inappropriate content, these inner tapes are used as reference material by the unconscious mind to formulate each person's physical self-image and sense of self-worth. In order to change the blockages and imbalances in the chakras, it is necessary to recognize the bad messages we may be sending ourselves and to change the inner programming. One of the most powerful yet simple methods by which this can be accomplished is through the use of conscious verbal affirmations. By repeating the affirmations of positivity over and over, the destructive inner tapes which contain messages of inadequacy, fear and guilt are erased and reprogrammed with new messages of security, self-assuredness, and self-worth.

Second Chakra

The second chakra has been variably referred to as the navel chakra, gonadal chakra, splenic chakra, or sacral chakra. *The sacral or gonadal chakra is the subtle-energy seat of sexuality.* There appears to be some variation in different esoteric sources as to the association of the spleen with the second chakra (as opposed to the third or solar-plexus chakra). Some clairvoyants like Charles Leadbeater have described the second chakra as overlying the splenic region. In reality, there are probably two different major chakras that lie between the solar-plexus and root chakras. The splenic chakra is associated with the physical spleen and is recognized in esoteric literature as a portal through which prana and vital energy are taken into and distributed throughout the subtle body. There is also evidence to suggest that there may be two chakra systems with different organ assocations for those born in the East and the West. When the two chakra systems merge, a new chakra system is created. For the purposes of our discussion, however, we will simply refer to the second center as the sacral chakra.

The sacral chakra is associated with the gonads and reproductive organs, in addition to the urinary bladder, large and small intestines, the appendix, and the lumbar vertebrae. From a psychoenergetic standpoint, the sacral chakra is associated with the expression of sensual emotion and sexuality. The type and adequacy of energy flow through this center is reflective of the degree of involvement with emotional and sexual energy in an individual's life. The nature of one's focus on sensual expression and sexuality can have both positive and negative effects. There are certain schools of Eastern meditative thought (tantric yoga) which look toward the channeling of sexual energies as a source of mystical experience. Conversely, an overfocusing on sexuality to the exclusion of higher spiritual pursuits and other types of creativity can have negative energetic and physiologic effects. Individuals whose energies are centered primarily in this chakra will tend to view relationships for their sexual and sensual aspects and to view people as sexual objects.

The gonadal energies associated with the sacral chakra relate to the hormonal function of the leydig cells within the testes and ovaries. These leydig cells produce testosterone, which is associated with libido and sexual drive in both males and females. At a symbolic level, the navel center is linked with the element of water. The metaphoric symbolism of water in relation to the gonads and genitourinary tract is obvious. During a sexual climax, there is the release of bodily fluids. In addition, the sacral chakra is associated with the genitourinary tract (which excretes urine) and the colon (which is an important site of water absorption).

It is quite probable that women suffering from cervical and uterine cancer may have blockages or other types of imbalances within the gonadal or sacral center, (in addition to other chakras). Other illnesses resulting from dysfunction of the sacral chakra include colitis, irritable bowel syndromes, bladder tumors, malabsorption diseases of the small intestine, various types of sexual dysfunction, prostatitis, and low back pains. Many of these diseases have been found to be associated with various physical factors which contribute to the final pattern of cellular dysfunction. Cigarette smoking, for example, is linked with bladder cancer. However, the abnormal functioning of the sacral chakra creates a subtle-energy predisposition toward manifesting these diseases, especially when combined with constant exposure to known irritants and carcinogens. *When viral and chemical environmental stressors are introduced into the human biological system, the place where they will cause the most damage will be partially determined by the weakest link in the physiologic/subtle energy chain. The most unbalanced major chakra will influence which body site represents the weakest energy link in the chain.*

First Chakra

The first chakra is known as the coccygeal, base, or root chakra. As the name implies, *the root center reflects the degree to which we feel connected to the Earth or are grounded in our activities.* The amount of energy flow through the root chakra is a reflection of one's ability to link with the Earth and to function effectively upon the Earth plane from day to day. On a practical level this refers to the ability to keep one's feet firmly upon the ground. Such rooting or groundedness also relates to how well someone is able to make day-to-day decisions based on their acute needs. At the symbolic level, the root chakra represents the earth element, and is reflected in the denser or lower vibrational aspects of being.

Psychologically speaking, the root chakra is linked to the basic survival instincts. It is connected with primal feelings of fear from physical injury and is the prime mover behind the so-called fight-or-flight response. This connection with survival and fight-or-flight is why some esoteric sources associate the root chakra with the adrenal glands, the body's major source of adrenaline in times of stress. It is possible that the solar-plexus chakra is associated with the adrenal gland's outer cortex, which produces corticosteroids, while the root chakra may be linked with the inner adrenal medullary production of adrenaline and related compounds.

Individuals with too much energy focused in the root chakra may manifest paranoia of the world and a tendency to react defensively to most situations. This type of over-focus upon the root center causes the afflicted individual to operate in a type of jungle mentality. Conversely, underactivity of the root chakra can also be detrimental, as this center is partly responsible for that which has been called "the will to live."

The root chakra is also regarded as the seat of kundalini. The kundalini is symbolized as a coiled serpent within the sacral/coccygeal region. The coiled serpent represents a powerful subtle energy that is poised and waiting to spring into action. Only when the proper meditative and attitudinal changes have occurred does this force become directed upwards through the appropriate spinal pathway and activate each of the major chakras during its ascent to the crown. The kundalini is the creative force of manifestation which assists in the alignment of the chakras, the release of stored stress from the bodily centers, and the lifting of consciousness into higher spiritual levels.

From a physical level, the root chakra is associated with the sacrum, the spine in general, and the external orifices of excretion such as the rectum, the anus, and the urethra. Disorders which affect the anus (hemorrhoids and rectal fissures) and also urethral strictures may be associated with energy dysfunction of the root chakra. The physical structures associated with this center are symbolic of the process of release. As the sacral chakra is associated with the small intestine and colon, there is a close relationship between the first and second chakras. Certain physiologic functions of sacral chakra organs represent the process of absorption, assimilation, and retention. The root-chakra associated organs represent release of previously digested materials. These two functions, assimilation and excretion, must work in harmony for the body to maintain a state of equilibrium. There must be both absorption of needed elements, then a release of unnecessary waste. If waste is not appropriately released, there can be a buildup of toxicity within the system. *At an esoteric level, dysfunction in the lower two chakras may be symbolic of holding onto old outdated thoughts and program tapes—a so-called inability to release the past.* Diseases affecting the colon, rectum, and anal sphincter may be manifestations of dysfunction in the lower two chakras which are symbolized by problems relating to the release of old "garbage." Whereas constipation would represent a disorder in which release of old issues is difficult, diarrhea-associated disorders might be more reflective of "dumping" and rejection without assimilation (usually due to fear).

Some esoteric sources link the root chakra with both the gonads and the cells of leydig. The cells of leydig produce estrogen and testosterone and are found in the male testes and female ovaries as well as in the adrenal cortex. The gonads may be linked to both the first and second chakras, depending upon whether the individual was born in the East or the West. This makes sense because of the dual functions of the gonads. At the root chakra level, the reproductive function of the gonads is seen in sperm and ovum production, the ingredients that unite to form new life. At the sacral chakra level, the hormonal function of the cells of leydig within the gonads can be seen in the way testosterone production affects libido and sexuality.

From an esoteric perspective, the cosmic creative energies which emanate from the root chakra can be funneled either into procreation (the birthing of new life) or artistic creativity via the generation of new thoughts, ideas, and inventions. Creative expression can manifest through writing, painting, sculpture, and the translation of new ideas into physical reality. Thus, the powerful energies of the root chakra can be used to create babies or to write poetry and music. Either expression is a reflection of creativity of one sort or another. The creative kundalini energies which emanate from the root chakra are actually more like the fuel for the furnace. These energies must be channeled upward into higher centers, like the throat chakra, for the refined expression of art and creativity to occur. When released in a controlled fashion, the energies of the kundalini can attune and align the higher chakras so that higher creative expression as well as higher consciousness is possible.

Chakra Dynamics & the
Spiritual Lessons of Personal Evolution

Each of the seven major chakras has its particular emotional and spiritual lesson to be learned. The chakras connect the organs, glands, and nervous centers of the body with the vital forces which animate the physical body. The degree to which an individual is successful in dealing with the particular lessons inherent in each chakra will determine the amount of subtle-energy flow which can move into the body to maintain proper health. When a chakra is functioning abnormally because of improper attitudes, old self-deprecating message tapes, fears, and guilt, the organs which receive vital flow from that chakra become affected. Total avoidance of a particular lesson can result in blockage of the chakra and inadequate vital flow to the associated organs.

The lack of subtle-energy flow due to chakra underactivity may manifest as a degenerative, destructive, or cancerous lesion in the deprived chakra-associated organs. Conversely, overexaggeration and overfocusing on a particular emotional issue to an extreme degree can result in too much energy flow through a chakra. Chakra overactivity can result in overstimulation of the associated glands, overproduction of cells in the form of tumor growth, and inflammation. The lessons of the chakras and their associated energetic function is summarized in Diagram 29.

As can be seen in Diagram 29, *the lower two chakras (root and sacral) are classified as physiologic in nature.* They are related to the basic processes of absorption, assimilation, excretion, and reproduction. The primal issues dealt with at this level are groundedness, connection to the Earth, sexuality, and survival instincts. These might be considered "earthier" issues of spiritual development, which must be adequately addressed and mastered in order for consciousness to rise to higher levels of focus. The subtle-energy forces which are processed through these two centers are the kundalini and general pranic flow. Although prana flows throughout the entire body, the second or splenic chakra is considered to be the central distributor of pranic intake. The kundalini energies are, of course, the

Diagram 29.
ENERGETIC DYNAMICS OF THE CHAKRAS

	CHAKRA	POSITION	INNER ASPECTS	FORCES	NATURE
I	ROOT	Base of Spine	Grounding	Kundalini	PHYSIOLOGIC
II	SACRAL	Below Umbilicus	Emotion Sexuality	Prana	
III	SOLAR PLEXUS	Upper Abdomen	Personal Power	Lower Astral	PERSONAL
IV	HEART	Mid Chest	Love	Higher Astral	
V	THROAT	Neck	Communication Will	Lower Mental	
VI	BROW	Forehead	Intuition Inner Vision	Higher Spiritual Forces	SPIRITUAL
VII	CROWN	Top of Head	Spiritual Seeking		

primal energies of creation, manifestation, and the building of higher consciousness. Kundalini energy and prana are forces which are more closely linked with the physical-etheric interface and the etheric energies in general.

The third, fourth, and fifth chakras (solar-plexus, heart, and throat) are considered to be related more to issues of personal development and individuation. These issues include establishment of a sense of personal power in relation to self and one's external relationships, development of the higher love nature (in expressing love toward self and others), and communication and mastery of the will (discipline). From lowest to highest, these three chakras process energies originating at the lower astral, higher astral, and lower mental levels of vibration, respectively. On a physiologic level, these centers control the processes of digestion and purification, circulation, respiration, immune defenses, and the preservation of the integrity of the self.

The higher major chakras—the brow and crown centers—are primarily spiritual in nature. The brow center helps to direct the higher spiritual forces (from the higher mental, to the causal, and higher vibrational levels) into the third eye. The process of subtle-energy assimilation through the brow chakra assists the individual in intuitive decision-making and in seeing beyond the physical level (clairvoyance). As the name implies, the crown chakra is the highest center. The seventh chakra is especially activated when the individual is attuned toward inner searching for the meaning of life, during the practice of meditation, and through the process of active spiritual seeking.

In reality, the first three centers *(root, sacral, and solar-plexus chakras) form a lower triad of physiologic and grounding functions.* The uppermost three centers *(throat, brow, and crown chakras) form the higher spiritual triad.* (The throat center is also involved in receptivity to higher vibrational influences via the mechanism of clairaudience.) *The heart chakra is the bridge between the lower and the higher triads. It is only through the manifesting of one's higher love nature that one can unite the higher and lower energies. The ultimate expression and the unfoldment of the heart chakra is unconditional love and the active demonstration of the Christ consciousness.* When one learns to develop and manifest the higher spiritual aspects of the heart chakra, one comes closer to eliminating physical disease not only from the heart and associated organs but also from the entire physical body.

The Energies of Kundalini & the Search for Enlightenment: How the Chakras Function in the Development of Higher Consciousness

Up to this point we have examined the subtle-energy pathways which link the major chakras to the normal functioning of the human body. Each main chakra provides nutritive energy for the health and homeostatic maintance of the body's integrated physiologic systems. An individual's level of emotional growth and spiritual development is directly related to the functioning and openness of each major chakra. The amount of chakric energy flow, in turn, affects the physiology of the physical organs of the body. If a chakra is blocked, then there will be an associated difficulty in the organ (or organs) which receive energy from that center. There is a key symbolism behind the location of illness in the body and the emotional blockage that is occuring within the personality. An understanding of how emotional and spiritual difficulties can create disease in the body is based on a broad working knowledge of how the chakras affect physical and mental illness (as discussed in the previous section).

If physicians understood that emotional and spiritual blockages were indirectly responsible for organ dysfunction in the body, there would be more attention directed to dealing with a patient's psychotherapeutic needs and not just with the pharmaceutical and surgical aspects of a patient's care. Conventional medical treatments are necessary at this time to deal with the disease processes that manifest, but vibrational therapies can often augment their effectiveness. The various subtle-energy treatments—flower essences, gem elixirs, crystal and color therapies—work at the level of the chakras and subtle bodies to assist in energy rebalancing. It is physicians' lack of knowledge of the chakras and subtle bodies and their relationship to illness that keeps many practitioners from understanding the great potential of the vibrational remedies that have been discussed throughout this book.

Perhaps one of the simplest but most powerful methods of opening, activating, and cleansing blockages in the chakras is through the techniques of meditation. Although meditation is sought by many as a source of relaxation, it is much more than that. In addition to providing relaxation to the body, meditation opens the mind to the energies of the Higher Self. It helps to clear the mind of day-to-day concerns of the earthly personality, and allows higher information to be processed through the individual's consciousness. Most forms of meditation do this to some degree or another. However, certain meditative techniques are more powerful than others in accelerating this process of inner communication.

One of the input channels for higher information is through the right cerebral hemisphere. Ordinarily, human beings tend to be fairly left-brain dominant throughout their waking life. That is, they tend to be logical, analytical, and verbal. The public school system emphasizes left-brain skills in their curriculums of reading, writing, and arithmetic. When we view reality through left-brain consciousness, objects in the real world are seen in terms of their literal meanings. When we sleep, we usually function in right-brain mode and work at a more symbolic level of meaning. During right-hemispheric processing, objects are taken less at a literal level and seen more for their symbolic significance.

During sleep, when the conscious mind is turned off, the right brain predominates. Dreams are largely symbolic in nature and can be best interpreted from their multiple levels of meaning. During the sleep state, the Higher Self tries to communicate with the physical personality in order to relay helpful information about emotional and spiritual difficulties that are manifesting at the conscious level. When communication from the Higher Self is unsuccessful in reaching the personality directly, information is encoded in the symbolic language of dreams. If people attempt to decipher the symbolic meaning of their dreams, they will discover important messages to themselves that describe their true thoughts and feelings about work, relationships, and in general, life on the physical plane. If people can realize the meaning in their dreams, they may be able to understand how they are functioning at an subconscious level. They can try to change the programming of negative message tapes that may have been running through their cognitive computer for many years.

The problem with such subconscious tapes is that they are unconscious—below the level of waking consciousness—and normally inaccessible to the conscious mind. The subconscious mind operates at a level below the conscious mind. The subconscious is primitive in nature and has the logical thinking of, at most, a six-year-old child. The subconscious mind stores all of our waking experiences and selectively emphasizes certain messages about our personal appearance and our feelings of value and self-worth. Conversely, the Higher Self or superconscious mind operates at a level above the conscious mind. It understands the predicaments of our life even when, consciously, we do not. The Higher Self holds the solutions to many of our problems because it is able to see from a perspective that goes beyond the mundane day-to-day obstacles that we encounter. The Higher Self is also aware when we are holding ourselves back from our true potentials by replaying negative self-image tapes at the level of the subconscious mind. Dreams are one form of symbolic communication through which the Higher Self attempts (often unsuccessfully) to contact the conscious personality. Through the right-brain metaphorical language of the dream state, the superconscious tries to reveal how faulty programming and emotional blockages may be the real causes of our day-to-day problems and illnesses.

Another more powerful form of inner communication with the Higher Self is meditation. Meditation clears the mind of conscious thought programs to allow higher vibrational sources of information to enter into the biocomputer for processing and analysis. In addition to allowing access to the Higher Self, the process of meditation causes gradual changes in the subtle-energy anatomy of the human being over a long period of time. Specifically, the chakras are slowly activated and cleared, and the kundalini energies within the root chakra eventually make their climb up the subtle pathways within the spinal cord to reach the crown chakra.

During the natural course of human development, an individual will gradually open up most of the chakras within the body. The degree to which the chakras are opened will depend on the extent to which each person develops his or her abilities to communicate with others, to express ideas creatively and artistically, to love both self and others, and to strive toward the higher meanings of life. When traumatic emotional events oc-cur which hold back one's growth in a particular needed direction, there is an associated blockage acquired in one of the chakras of the body. This blockage is an impediment to the natural flow of the creative kundalini energies up the spinal cord to higher chakras. To varying degrees, certain stresses which are acquired through the course of one's life become locked into an area of the subtle body and its associated area in the physical mus-culoskeletal system.

The daily practice of meditation, done over a period of many years, results in the gradual upliftment of the kundalini energies, which in turn opens each of the chakras from the root center on up to the crown chakra. As the chakras are opened, subtle stresses that have been incurred throughout the individual's life are slowly dissipated. Releasing of the blockage to energy flow through a chakra is partly due to the cleansing and opening effect of the kundalini forces, but is also related to the gradual realization of the emotional and spiritual lessons necessary to the proper functioning of that chakra. The meditational process assists in the learning of such im-portant life lessons over time as the conscious personality begins to under-stand the reasons for existing blockages. This information comes slowly to the individual through meditation as he or she learns to listen to the inner wisdom of their own Higher Self.

Meditation helps to build subtle energy bridges of learning and com-munication which connect the physical personality to knowledge contained within their own higher vibrational structures of consciousness. Different types of meditation do this to greater or lesser degrees, with resulting variable rates of consciousness development. For instance, the repetition of various sounds and mantras can have powerful effects if done consistently over time. At a simplistic level, mantra repetition helps to clear the mind of conscious thoughts. It causes the left brain to step aside, so to speak, and the mind to be stilled temporarily. On a subtle-energy level, particular man-tras are actually special higher vibrational sonic energy signals which have unique effects in lifting consciousness to higher spiritual levels of being. Certain mantras, when repeated over time, may cause subtle changes within the nervous system. These meditation-associated changes in the brain can result in the evolution of the structures of consciousness to pro-cess higher levels of vibrational input. Repetition of mantras, as in the prac-tice of Transcendental Meditation, might be considered a form of passive meditation.

On the other side are systems and techniques which might be more appropriately referred to as active meditation.[4,5] This system of meditation involves the use of particular types of creative imagery and visualization, including imaging oneself going to a school of higher learning. Oftentimes the advanced meditator, when visualizing him or herself attending classes in a school of higher learning, may actually be working with inner teachers and learning on an astral level. Another type of active meditation involves the individual stilling the mind and body through various relaxation techniques and then addressing their consciousness directly to their Higher Self. One may ask questions of one's Higher Self about particular aspects of one's life (past, present, or future) and listen and observe for meaningful information which may come in the form of words, images, or feelings. Another type of active meditation would be a type of inner dialogue with the Higher Self, dedicating oneself to the pursuit of higher learning. This can be combined with particular types of visual imagery exercises which involve actively cleansing the auric field[6] and the chakras[7] as well as creating a greater alignment between the physical and subtle bodies.

There are other forms of active meditation which combine the art of visualization with quartz crystals. Quartz crystals are amplifiers of the energies of consciousness. The crystals may be held in each hand or over the third-eye center during the meditational process. One may then actively visualize subtle energies in the form of color rays or white light entering into the body through the crystals. The energy thus taken in causes a raising of the vibrational rate of the body and an upliftment of consciousness to higher frequency levels. Visualization exercises (such as those mentioned in the chapter on crystals) can be used in conjunction with meditation, the individual seeing him or herself shrinking and actually entering into the crystal. Depending upon the choice of visual metaphors, one may decide to visualize entering a hall of knowledge within the inner structure of the crystal.[8] This hall of knowledge can be set up like a library. Only this unique library allows one access to information about oneself in present and past lives, as well as allowing one to obtain general information about any number of historical subjects. The visual metaphor of the library allows one to use imagination to tap into higher levels of cognitive processing. The technique of visualization itself, when used in conjunction with the meditational process, allows human beings to not only reprogram their own biocomputers (as in biofeedback and autonomic control) but also to access levels of inner potential not ordinarily available to waking consciousness.

Visualization and imagery holds the key to unlocking the hidden reserves of human thoughtpower.

Visual images like the crystal library scenario are powerful tools that may be used to unlock the hidden potentials and resources available to higher levels of consciousness. Imagination is far more important to people than most psychotherapists and educators even dream. Behind imagination lie the doors to higher levels of reality. The ability to use symbolic imagery also holds the key to tapping into vast inner sources of creativity and insight. Meditation offers us a way to access our own Higher Selves and higher levels of knowledge. By consistently turning within through the meditational process, we can begin to know ourselves and our relationships to others in a clearer light.

Learning about the obstacles we have chosen to overcome and the necessary activation energy needed to achieve these goals can make life on the physical plane much easier for us. Humans need only learn that they already possess the required equipment and energy to realize these goals. It has often been said that it is unfortunate that human beings do not come with an "Owner's Maintenance Manual." In a sense, meditation allows one to enter into states of consciousness that allow access to information equivalent to an "Owner's Consciousness Maintenance Manual."

This information is already stored in our higher memory banks, but it is locked up and inaccessible to the waking personality unless special codes are entered through the biocomputer of the human mind. By entering these special codes into the mechanism of consciousness, meditation allows one to access both subconscious and superconscious memory banks to gain a greater understanding of the hidden aspects of oneself. The use of symbolic imagery in meditation allows one to utilize the gateway of the right cerebral hemisphere to tap into higher levels of human awareness. These methods can be used to acquire a greater understanding of the reasons behind various obstacles or stresses that may be occuring at a particular period in the lifepath.

As the obstacles of life are overcome, especially those blockages that we ourselves have created, the impediments to inner creative energy flow are dissolved and the kundalini's path of ascension is made easier to climb. Most of the time the obstacles that have been created are not in the external world, but exist only within the faulty perception of the self. Removing the blocks to the perception of truth brings human beings closer to the realization that they are manifestations of light, love, and the energies of the

Creator. Meditation is one of those powerful tools that can bring each individual, in time, to a realization of these higher truths and a better understanding of the seeming life struggle that is being played out upon the physical plane.

Meditation, Reincarnation, & Human Illness: The Chakras as Repositories of Karmic Energy

During the reincarnational cycle, we human beings incarnate into the so-called "Earth School" to learn special lessons about the higher qualities of life and to act in service to help our fellow humans. Along the way we encounter obstacles in our path which are, quite frequently, the products of our own ways of thinking. We create obstacles and stumbling blocks along our lifepaths which reflect our faulty perception of reality. The errors in our perception which keep us from existing harmoniously with our fellow beings often manifest as illnesses within the physical body.

Depending upon the specific impediment to perception, disease will manifest in the organ system that most closely resonates with the chakra ruling the particular difficult lesson. The expression and acceptance of love is perhaps one of the most difficult lessons to learn. Often the problem is an error in perception which blocks an individual's awareness of the existence of love's presence in the world. That is, an individual may be surrounded by those who love him or her, but their inner fears of the world projected outward onto others may make the world seem threatening, thus blocking the perception of the presence of love. When the difficult lesson being learned by the personality involves being able to love others and feel love for oneself, blockages of energy flow through the heart chakra can manifest as physical afflictions of the heart, thymus gland, bronchial tubes and lungs.

Interestingly, the unlearned lesson may not originate within the present lifetime. Diseases may also be related to past-life carryovers. These include both physical and mental disorders. Hypnotic past-life regression of individuals with unusual phobias have helped them unlock the real traumatizing emotional events which caused the phobias. When the individual remembers the traumatizing incident from the past life, the phobia usually disappears. In the case of physical illnesses relating to past-life difficulties, there are different energetic pathways involved. The chakras are also an important mechanism behind the karmic expression of illness. For instance, an individual who has not yet learned the important life lessons of the heart chakra in one lifetime will carry over these unbalanced energies into future lives.

During embryogenesis, the subtle-energy bodies, including the etheric and astral templates, are formed before the physical body develops. The chakras that develop in the fetus's etheric and astral form are affected by the energies carried over from the previous lives of the incarnating soul. If the chakras in the fetal body do not provide the necessary sustaining energies to the developing organs, there can be underdevelopment of particular cellular structures at the physical level. Thus, a severe blockage in the heart center relating to either an inability to express love or to too much negativity (i.e., "hard heartedness") in a past life may manifest as a congenital heart defect in the newborn.[9] Karmic illnesses may appear as developmental abnormalities in the infant or they may occur later in the life of the individual. The chakras are the energy repositories of karma. One might say that the chakras are like batteries which store "karmic energy charges." Chakras absorb the subtle energies which relate to the development of the soul in previous lives, and assist in the transformation of the physical body to express unlearned spiritual lessons in the form of physical illnesses. These diseases pose problems and obstacles for the personality to overcome during the present lifetime. Such obstacles can serve as either stumbling blocks or points of personal and spiritual transformation, depending upon whether the individual can discover the esoteric meaning behind his or her "dis-ease."[10]

Although illnesses relating to experiences in a past life are hard to understand, it is only through a true comprehension of human subtle-energy anatomy and the reality of reincarnation that the meaning of disease may be entirely understood and remedied. Meditation is a powerful tool by which individuals may come to understand the meaning behind their illnesses and the lessons which must be learned before they can truly be well. Meditation holds the key to understanding the interlocking nature of the physical, astral, mental, and higher spiritual selves. Each integral energetic element works to assist the soul in developing its many facets and to understand its own true higher nature.

In its earthly sojourns and experiences, the soul comes to comprehend its own higher spiritual qualities through selfless acts of love, service, and caring. When the physical personality has difficulty in expressing these most basic lessons of soul development, physical diseases may be acquired as learning experiences. Depending upon the blockage of expression within the personality, dysfunctions will appear in various chakras. The abnormal flow of subtle energies through the chakras is then translated into physical illness in a particular organ. Through meditation, the personality may come to discover the true meaning behind the physical illness with which it is afflicted. If the person can then correct that problematic emotional and spiritual dysfunction, the disease will often improve or completely abate. Of course, there are additional karmic factors which enter into the equation which make the issue somewhat more complex. But the basic idea still applies.

The real reason to meditate is to achieve enlightenment. Enlightenment might be defined here as a more cosmic or energetic perspective of the structures of consciousness, a feeling of unity with all lifeforms, and an understanding of the spiritual workings behind physical reality. This higher level of perception will ultimately allow the individual to comprehend the meaning of his or her life in relationship to others and to the universe in general. This is what is referred to as a more cosmic perspective. Meditation may ultimately allow humans to come into closer relationship and greater comprehension of God the Creator.

In human beings the process of enlightenment is intimately tied to the proper alignment and normal functioning of the major chakras of the body. When all of the major chakras are open and active and when there is adequate etheric vitality in the body, the human being begins to function at optimal levels of health and higher consciousness. Attunement of the personality toward seeking higher spiritual meanings in life, whether it is through Christianity, Judaism, Hinduism, Buddhism, or any other world religion, ultimately results in an awakening of the seven major chakras. Meditation merely amplifies this gradual process of awakening. It accelerates the opening of the chakras and their alignment with the physical and subtle bodies in special ways that devotion and prayer alone do not achieve as quickly and directly.

Physiologic Concepts of Meditation & Enlightenment: Bentov's Model of Heart-Brain Resonance & the Physio-Kundalini Syndrome

In addition to the subtle-energy activation of the various chakras, meditation causes physiologic effects in the body that have been documented by researchers in various centers. Scientists at the Maharishi European Research University have shown that long-term meditators demonstrate greater coherence of brain wave activity between the left and right cerebral hemispheres while practicing the TM meditative technique.[11] Electrical wave activities generated by the two hemispheres of such meditators are more in step, and function with greater coordination, than in non-meditators.

In an indirect way, brain waves reflect ongoing cerebral activity. Greater coherence of brain wave activity may be understood by examining the difference between the coherent light of lasers and the incoherent light of a candle. When light waves are induced to move in step, as in a laser beam, the amplification of energy is tremendous. Increased coherence of brain wave activity may reflect similar changes in the more coherent and directed application of mind energy. Greater interplay and coordination between left and right hemispheres, as seen in long-term meditators, has also been associated with greater creativity and flexibility of thought.

Long-term practice of yogic types of meditation has been correlated with greater control of the autonomic nervous system. Yogis such as Swami Rama and others have demonstrated to Western scientists their ability to selectively regulate heart activity, skin temperature, and blood flow. More recent studies have shown that particular yogic meditative practices have positive therapeutic benefits to individuals with various illnesses such as asthma. Asthmatic patients practicing pranayama (a special breathing technique) and other yogic meditative techniques have demonstrated fewer asthma attacks, less shortness of breath, and greater control over their breathing.

Meditation in general causes unique changes in the body both acutely and over time that have been confirmed by various scientists. One particular researcher who has brought about new levels of insight into the physiology of meditation is Itzhak Bentov. As a long-term transcendental meditator himself, Bentov sought to understand how the body changes during the practice of meditation. Utilizing a special electrical measuring device known as a ballistocardiograph, Bentov found that there were unique changes that occurred in heart and brain activity during deep states of meditation.[12] From his research findings, he began to piece together a model of how meditation, through a specialized link between the heart and brain, could eventually cause lasting changes in brain and bodily functioning. Bentov referred to this as the "physio-kundalini" model.

Bentov discovered a special system of tuned rhythmic oscillators in the mechanism of the physical body which, in meditation, were driven by circulatory pulses coming from the heart. When the body entered a state of deep meditation, Bentov noted that there was a rhythmic, up and down pulsation of the body as measured on the ballistocardiograph. During meditation, the slow, rhythmic micro-oscillation of the entire body up and down becomes regular and pronounced. As the cycle of breathing changes during meditation, so does the rhythm of heart activity.

It is known that when the heart contracts, it sends out a pressure wave of blood through the aorta (the largest artery in the body, which carries blood away from the heart). When the pressure wave front hits the aortic bifurcation (the place where the great artery splits into two smaller arteries going into the legs), there is a reflected wave that travels back up the aorta in the reverse direction. Bentov discovered an unusual internal feedback loop between the aortic bifurcation and the heart which, during deep meditation, regulated the cycles of pumping activity as well as the rhythmic activity of breathing. When the pressure wave coming from the heart reached the aortic bifurcation, a signal was sent to the heart to initiate its next beat at the precise moment that the reflected wave front reached the aortic valve. This meant that there would be a wave front simultaneously coming and going at the same point. When the timing of the pressure pulses travelling down the aorta coincides or is in phase with the reflected pressure pulses, a standing wave is achieved. This wave activity coincides with a frequency of about seven Hertz (cycles per second). This special oscillating system of circulatory waves caused the up and down rhythmic motion that Bentov detected in advanced meditators with his ballistocardiograph arrangement.

This up and down micromotion of the body, caused by standing waves within the heart-aorta oscillator system, is the first in a series of tuned oscillators in the physical body which becomes activated during the process of meditation. The oscillators are set up in series in such a fashion that when the first is activated, the remaining oscillators are resonantly driven as well. The up and down motion of the body causes the cranial vault within the skull to oscillate up and down also. Although the micromovement of the body is quite small (approximately 0.003 to 0.009 mm), the up and down motion is enough to induce measureable changes in the nervous system. Movement of the head up and down creates a small impact of the brain against the cranial vault in both directions. This motion creates acoustical (and possibly electrical) plane waves reverberating within the closed space of the brain's skull cavity.

The acoustical plane waves set up within the cranial vault become focused upon the hollow, fluid-filled ventricular cavities inside the brain. Within the lateral and third ventricles, acoustical standing waves are created by the reflected motion of the plane waves. The fundamental frequencies of these standing waves are a function of the shape and length of the ventricles in the brain. Interestingly, the resulting vibrations transmitted to the surrounding brain tissue are conducted to the nerves of the middle ear and result in the "inner sounds" frequently heard by meditators. Identification of the frequencies of inner sounds heard during meditation by a large group of meditators showed striking similarities to Bentov's frequency predictions (based on his oscillator model).

Most important in this series of oscillator loops is the last in the sequence. The final reverberating loop in Bentov's model is in the brain tissue of the cerebral cortex. The acoustical standing waves created within the hollow ventricular system of the brain create an up and down motion on the large nerve bundle connecting the right and left cerebral hemispheres (the corpus callosum). Acoustical energy from the ventricles is translated into electrical activity within brain tissue. From the corpus callosum, the nerve activity follows a circular loop along the sensory cortex.

In the brain the sensory cortex is mapped out such that areas of brain tissue correspond to various parts of the body. The body parts are arranged in sequence so that the area of gray matter processing sensation from the feet is adjacent to the area corresponding to the legs and so on up through the entire body. Areas of the body which are involved with intricate types of sensory processing of tactile stimuli, such as the hands and fingers, face and tongue, are associated with correspondingly larger areas of gray matter along this strip of tissue in the cerebral cortex. There is a strip of sensory cortex in each hemisphere which processes sensation from the opposite side of the body. The right hemisphere processes sensory input from the left side of the body and vice versa. Direct stimulation of cortical tissue in the sensory cortex (as was originally used to map brain function by neuro-researchers) creates the sensation that the corresponding part of the body has been touched.

In Bentov's model, sonic vibrations which are created within the deep, hollow, fluid-filled ventricles of the brain by pulsations transmitted from the heart, cause a mechanical and electrical stimulation of the overlying nervous tissue. Directly above the third and lateral ventricles lies the corpus callosum (the nerve bundle bridge between the two cerebral hemispheres), as well as the lower portion of the sensory cortex. Just above the corpus callosum is the part of the sensory strip of cortex corresponding to the toes. Mechanical stimulation of brain tissue by sonic vibrations creates electrical depolarization (nerve firing) within the sensory cortex. The wave of electrical firing moves up through the sensory cortex from the toes to the ankle, knee, hip, trunk, on up to the head, eventually returning in cyclical fashion to its point of origin over the corpus callosum.

Bentov postulates that in advanced meditators, meditation produces a cyclic stimulus loop of electrical activity which reverberates in a circular path through the sensory cortex. As the electrical wave moves through the gray matter, Bentov suggests that the gray matter becomes polarized in the direction of stimulus flow. The polarization of brain tissue causes various sensations to occur in sequence throughout the body, starting with the toes and working up toward the head. Because the meditational process appears to affect the right hemisphere more than the left, these sensations often begin in the left side of the body.

Diagram 30.
NEUROSENSORY BASIS FOR
THE PHYSIO-KUNDALINI SYNDROME

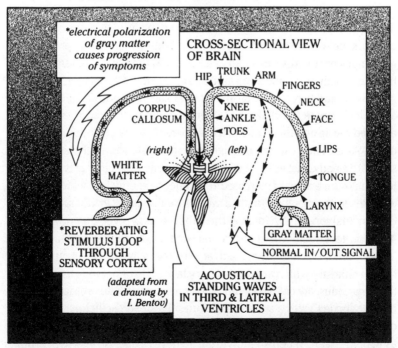

Actually, Bentov's model was formed to help explain progressive left-sided bodily symptoms that were occuring in various meditators. Lee Sanella, M.D., studied numerous individuals, mostly long-term meditators, who complained of pains that would often begin in their left foot and travel up their body as time went by. In many, strange sensations and sharp pains would run from the feet, up the legs, and over the back to the neck. A number of individuals described roaring sounds and high pitched whistles in the head, followed by a brilliant sensation of light flooding their entire being and then a feeling of total bliss. Dr. Sanella refers to this progression of symptoms as the physio-kundalini syndrome or complex. In some instances, individuals who were not necessarily long-term meditators, but who were having powerful psychic experiences as a result of "spontaneous" kundalini awakening, also experienced these same left-sided pains and abnormal sensations. Sanella felt that the adverse symptoms, experienced by meditators and others with this syndrome, were somehow related to the activation of their kundalini energies. Bentov was able to piece together the reasons for this unusual symptom complex by studying the way the brain was affected during the meditational process.

Bentov's model of heart-brain resonance during meditation and its effect upon the sensory cortex was used to explain how pains in the feet could actually be a by-product of the kundalini energies. The progression of symptoms is partly due to an awakening of the kundalini forces in the root chakra. In reality, the kundalini energy ascends the inner paths through the spinal cord to reach the crown chakra. During this process, impurities and blockages in the chakras are released and burned away. Some have likened the kundalini to an electrical current passing through a thin filament. As the energy moves through areas of resistance, a light and burning heat are created just as in an electric light bulb. Blockages at the levels of the chakras are areas of increased resistance to energy flow which must be cleansed in order for the current to travel the entire circuit to the crown chakra.

In addition to movement at the subtle-energy level, Bentov theorizes that there are additional changes that occur in the central nervous system when the kundalini forces are activated by the daily practice of meditation. These changes, which are related to polarization of nervous tissue in the cerebral cortex, are created by the vibrational waves in the ventricular cavity. Meditation activates a system of resonantly tuned oscillators, which are acoustically powered by vibrational energy derived from the pumping action of the heart. When an individual achieves a deep state of meditation, breathing becomes slow and shallow and heart activity becomes synchronized so as to create a resonant vibrational link between the heart and the brain. The oscillating electrical circuit within the brain becomes established only after grey matter along the sensory cortex has been completely polarized in a circular stimulus loop.

Diagram 31.
CREATION OF THE NEURAL STIMULUS LOOP

MEDITATION ASSOCIATED RESONANCE OF
HEART-AORTA SYSTEM
▼
UP AND DOWN OSCILLATION
OF CRANIAL VAULT
▼
ACOUSTICAL PLANE WAVES
IN BRAIN
▼
STANDING WAVES IN
3RD AND LATERAL VENTRICLES
▼
MECHANOELECTRIC STIMULATION
OF SENSORY CORTEX
▼
REVERBERATING STIMULUS LOOP
▼
REPETITIVE CIRCULAR
NEURAL CURRENTS
▼
POLARIZATION OF CORTICAL TISSUE
IN DIRECTION OF CURRENT
▼
RELEASE OF STORED-UP STRESSES
IN SENSORIMOTOR CORTEX

It is suggested that, in addition to lifelong emotional stresses being locked into various chakras and bodily regions, there is a corresponding energy blockage within the tissue of the brain itself.[13] As the vibrationally induced current moves through the reverberating circuit, gray matter is gradually polarized along the direction of energy flow. As the slow current meets areas of resistance to energy flow within the brain tissue of the sensory cortex, the signal hammers away until it is able to pass through to the next area. This process continues until the circular brain loop has been freed of old stress points and blockages to energy flow. When the slow current meets such an area of stress and blockage, a corresponding sensation of pain is experienced by the individual in the associated area of the body. Although the sensation originates at the level of the sensory cortex, the pain feels like it is coming from the physical body.

Since the first area of cortical tissue encountered by the induced cur rent is associated with the feet and toes, unusual sensations would be experienced in the feet by those meditators with blocks in this area of the brain. Sanella and Bentov have found that a number of meditators with the physio-kundalini syndrome describe pains beginning in their feet, and especially in the left big toe. As the hammering current is able to release the stress from that area of the sensory cortex, higher levels of resistance in the sensory cortex are encountered and released from blockage. This explains why the sensation of pain beginning in the feet or toes would then ascend up the back of the leg, to the spine, and so on.

The motor cortex of the brain, an area which controls voluntary muscle movement in the body, is a strip of cerebral tissue directly adjacent to the sensory cortex. Sometimes these regions of the brain are referred to collectively as the sensorimotor cortex. Quite often, individuals experiencing progressive symptoms of the physio-kundalini syndrome will feel spasms of muscles as well as unconscious muscle movements in the head and body. This may be explained by electrical cross-stimulation of the motor cortex by the hammering away of the current at the adjacent sensory cortex along the reverberating stimulus loop.

As the stored-up stresses within the sensory cortices of the cerebral hemispheres are released, the current is gradually able to complete the entire stimulus loop through the brain. Continued meditation helps to complete this loop over time. Once the loop becomes cyclic and repetitive, the current becomes stronger. Areas of brain tissue just adjacent to the path of current flow lie in the limbic system, which includes areas known to be pleasure centers. These are deep areas of brain tissue which, if artificially stimulated, produce sensations of extreme pleasure. Bentov theorizes that when the current loop through the sensory cortex is completed and all stresses are released from the circuit, energy flow through the circular path stimulates the adjacent pleasure centers. He suggests that this may be the reason for the sensations of pleasure and bliss experienced by long-term meditators following many years of daily meditative effort.

Relevant to our discussion of meditation-induced reverberating circuits in the cerebral cortex and adjacent limbic system is the phenomenon of "kindling". Kindling refers to the effects of repeated low-intensity electrical stimulation of the limbic system, an important center of emotion and spatial memory within the brain. As the name implies, kindling acts like small pieces of wood that help to start a fire. In this case, the fire is the rapid fire of neurons along specialized paths in the limbic brain. Although kindling was originally a laboratory phenomenon which was theorized as a possible model for epilepsy, later biochemical data suggested that this supposition was incorrect. Scientists found that taurine, an amino acid, could suppress epileptic seizure activity, but later discovered that taurine had no effect on neurological phenomena known to be caused by kindling. In spite of being thrown out as a model for epilepsy, some scientists have suggested that kindling may have relevance to the phenomenon of kundalini.[14]

Repetitive stimulation of certain limbic structures eventually causes bursts of electrical activity along special paths within the limbic system. Over the course of time, these bursts of electrical activity "kindle" similar patterns in adjacent brain regions. Also, kindling causes the threshold for nerve cell depolarization (activation) along this path to become progressively lowered, so that a smaller stimulus can cause the "epileptic" discharge. Epilepsy is caused by a small fire or burst of energy from certain electrically unstable nerve cells, which spreads like wildfire to create a diffuse electrical storm of activity. In the case of kundalini, the electrical storm is thought to move strictly along well defined pathways within the limbic brain, after it is activated by specially entrained neurons.

Kindling appears to occur only within structures of the limbic system, and not within the cerebral cortex, thalamus, or brainstem. Some researchers have suggested that resonant stimulation of the limbic brain might be an important phenomenon underlying the effects of kundalini. In reference to Bentov's model of meditative brain stimulation, kindling may come into play after the circular stimulus loop through the sensory cortex has already become established. As the sensory cortical loop becomes a reverberating pattern, it is suggested that the loop becomes larger and generalizes to involve key structures of the limbic system within the temporal lobe of the brain, such as the amygdaloid complex.

Repetitive stimulation of limbic structures such as the amygdala, which is a site of pleasure and emotional control adjacent to the sensory cortex stimulus loop, may trigger discharges along a special path in the limbic system. The repeated stimulation of the amygdala (and other limbic structures) produces a kindling effect which decreases the energy threshold for further activation. Thus, the energy paths through the limbic brain and the pleasure centers become more easily stimulated during later meditative attempts once the loop has been completed through the sensory cortex. In essence, kindling of the limbic brain by meditation (through the effects of heart-brain resonance) may result in the establishment of new circuitry in the hard wiring of the brain.

In addition to stimulating the pleasure centers of the limbic system, kindling also induces discharge patterns which activate both sides of the brain. For instance, stimulation of the amygdala in one hemisphere results in the travelling of afterdischarges to the amygdala on the opposite side of the brain. From there the discharge pattern follows an orderly sequence to the hippocampus (an important limbic structure which is involved with spatial memory), then to the occipital cortex (a site of visual processing), and finally to the frontal cortex (an area involved in decision making and future projection of events). Thus, stimulation of this unique limbic circuit by the initial sensory cortical loop could evoke unusual visual phenomena by activation of the occipital cortex. Meditators who have worked through the physio-kundalini syndrome often describe sensations of brilliant light accompanying the so-called state of bliss.

According to Bentov's model, the energy circuit induced in the sensory cortex is a physiologic means by which meditation and the energies of kundalini can discharge stored-up stresses from the human nervous system. As discussed earlier, meditation appears to involve the intuitive, symbolic right hemisphere more than the analytical, logical left brain. Correspondingly, changes tend to occur in the reverberating loop of the right hemisphere earlier than in the left. This would explain why most meditators with the physio-kundalini syndrome experience left-sided pains and sensations, as the right hemisphere controls the left side of the body. These pains and sensations are not experienced by everyone who meditates— just those individuals who have stored up large amounts of stress in their bodies and nervous systems. Individuals who have accumulated only minor stresses in the brain and body may feel minor abnormal sensations in various parts of their bodies due to physio-kundalini activation, and are less profoundly affected by this meditation-activated sequence of stress-release.

Bentov also suggests that cases of spontaneous activation of the physio-kundalini process may occur, partly because the affected individual is chronically exposed to acoustical, mechanical, or electrical and magnetic field stimulation in the key, brain-stimulating frequencies produced by the natural meditative process (in the range of four to seven cycles per second). Such environmental vibratory energies may be generated by electrical equipment, poorly-tuned car suspensions, or even air conditioning ducts. The cumulative effect of this vibratory stimulation may be to trigger a spontaneous physio-kundalini sequence *in susceptible people who have a particularly sensitive nervous system.* Besides those cases due to stimulation by environmental energies, spontaneous kundalini activation may also occur because of premature opening and activation of the chakras with the ascent of the kundalini energy, before the nervous system has had a chance to integrate the stepped-up energy input as normally occurs during long-term meditation. Bentov feels that individuals with this type of spontaneous kundalini activation, as opposed to meditators, are the ones more likely to experience severe, long-standing symptoms.

Kundalini, as a developmental process of daily meditation, is a natural means by which human beings may release the stresses that have been stored within the physical and subtle bodies over a lifetime, and by which they may open their channels to creative expression and attunement with higher levels of subtle vibrational input. Not only are stresses released, but once the cortical loop has been completed, the brain and body become more efficient at handling stress. Through its transformational effects on the nervous system, kundalini eliminates stresses from the body/mind as rapidly as they occur, thus preventing the accumulation of new stress. As old, accumulated stresses are discharged, new pathways of neural activity are created within the brain. Stated another way, the old brain is reorganized in such a fashion as to create new ways of processing energy and information. New circuitry paths are established in the system which open up new abilities and potentials.

The limbic brain, which is affected by stimulation from the current of the sensory cortical loop, appears to be closely tied to the functioning of the autonomic nervous system. Bentov theorizes that the connections created by meditation and the physio-kundalini process result in a stronger and more conscious linkage between the cerebrospinal and autonomic nervous systems. Unconscious autonomic processes such as breathing, heart activity, etc., are brought under potential control by the cerebral cortex and the conscious thinking mind. This has been demonstrated to scientists in the West by yogis who can control heart activity, blood flow, etc.

In addition to releasing stress from the brain and body, the energies released by the kundalini process move through the body and up the subtle paths within the spinal cord while progressively activating the chakras. Bentov describes a pathway of kundalini energy which starts in the toes, travels up the legs to the spine, moves up the neck and over the face, and continues down the front of the body. As it travels up the spine, the energy stimulates the inner roots of the chakras, which link with nerve plexuses along the spinal cord. As the energy travels over the head and down the front of the chest and abdomen, the frontal parts of the chakras are stimulated. As these frontal chakra regions are stimulated, the individual may report tingling or other sensations in the chakra-associated areas of the body. The path of kundalini energy flow through the body is mirrored by the path of polarizing current moving through the circular loop within the sensorimotor cortex in the brain, as both become activated by the meditative process.

Interestingly, Bentov's description of the flow of energy is different from the classical path of kundalini described in Indian yogic literature. But it is similar to the Microcosmic Orbit, a path of acupuncture-meridian energy flow described in esoteric Taoist yoga texts.[15] In time, as more sophisticated subtle-energy measuring devices are developed and used in conjunction with clairvoyant observation, much more will be understood about the physiological and vibrational changes which are produced by daily meditation and the activation of the kundalini forces. Perhaps future research will substantiate much of Bentov's model as it relates to measurable changes in the human brain.

It is important to realize, however, that meditation causes many changes to occur at both the physical and higher vibrational levels of human multidimensional anatomy. Bentov's model provides a "physical" description of brain function and an understanding of some of the phenomena produced by the natural stress-release mechanisms inherent within the nervous system. His model also gives us an unusual perspective on the unique energy relationship between the physical heart and brain, such as when vibrational resonance occurs during deep meditation.

Aside from its effects in changing brain circuitry, synchronizing heart and lung activity, and activating the chakras, meditation has a much more profound effect on the evolution of human consciousness. Through meditation, many secrets withheld from the conscious mind may be discovered. Among these secrets are the hidden lessons which the individual has chosen to learn during his or her particular lifetime. By revealing these lessons and the blockages to understanding which the physical personality has had to cope with, each individual may come to learn better ways in which to deal with their emotional, mental, and spiritual dimensions of being. When blockages in perception are dissolved and dysfunctional behavior is changed, the illnesses which have been created at higher vibrational levels may be healed or lessened considerably. As humanity begins to pay greater attention to the function of the chakras and their relationship to the development and expression of human consciousness, much will be revealed which will change the way in which human illness is conceptualized and treated by the healer/physicians of the future.

Key Points to Remember

1. The major chakras are specialized energy transformers which take in subtle energy and distribute it to the major glands, nerve centers, and organs of the body.

2. The function of the chakras is related to various aspects of consciousness, especially the emotions, which affect the flow of energy through these centers. When the emotional body of the individual has a field disturbance related to emotional problems, that emotional disturbance becomes translated into an altered flow of subtle energy through a particular chakra.

3. Each of the seven major chakras has a particular emotional and spiritual issue which affects its proper functioning. When an individual has significant unresolved emotional issues in any one of these areas, chakra dysfunction may occur. Such dysfunction leads to deprivation of nutritive subtle-energy flow to the bodily region and associated organs and glands supplied by that impaired chakra. If the chakra blockage is chronic, cellular imbalance and disease may eventually occur.

4. Altered subtle energetic flow through the various chakras is one mechanism by which chronic stress can negatively affect the physical body.

5. Perhaps the most critical chakra imbalance is one that affects the heart chakra, as this is the center involved with the issue of self-love and love toward others. The heart chakra supplies nutritive subtle energy to the physical heart and the general circulation, the lungs, and the thymus gland. Thus, chronic heart-chakra dysfunction can contribute to heart disease, strokes, lung disease, and various types of im-

munological impairment which may open the body up to bacterial, viral, and cancerous invasion.

6. Because the chakras feed energy to the developing organs of the fetus, as well as the adult, past-life carry-overs of severe unresolved emotional blockages can sometimes result in karmically-related congenital illnesses. Such karmic illnesses may occur in childhood or manifest as a delayed effect in later life.

7. Meditation is an important method of opening, activating, and cleansing the chakras of the body, especially when practiced in conjunction with active forms of visualization.

8. The root or base chakra is the storehouse for a natural, yet powerful, energy, called the kundalini. This kundalini energy has the potential to activate and align all of the major chakras with the higher centers, bringing illumination and spiritual enlightenment with the proper sequence of chakra unfoldment. The kundalini energy is naturally released over time as a result of daily meditation.

9. Itzhak Bentov, Dr. Lee Sanella, and others have characterized a series of physical problems which relate to unresolved stresses and their effect upon the natural unfoldment of the kundalini process. They have termed this bodily disturbance the physio-kundalini syndrome. It is most frequently observed in meditators, but can occur spontaneously as well.

10. Bentov discovered a series of serially tuned oscillators within the body which become operational during meditation. Via a unique feedback system between the heart and aorta, micro-oscillations of the body produced during meditation are translated into electro-acoustical stimulation of certain pathways within the brain.

11. According to Bentov's model, with repeated meditative attempts over many years time, a circulating current in the sensorimotor cortex is eventually established which gradually releases old stresses locked into the brain tissue itself. It is likely that the symptoms experienced by meditators with the physio-kundalini syndrome are due to the release of these stored stresses from the brain.

12. Over time and with repeated meditation, new neural pathways are established which prevent the reaccumulation of stress effects and actually promote inner stimulation of pleasure centers within the brain. Thus, the meditative and kundalini process, as envisioned by Bentov, is a natural stress release mechanism.

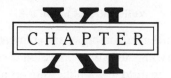

CHAPTER XI

Holistic Healing & Paradigm Shifts:
THE EMERGENCE OF MEDICINE FOR THE NEW AGE

We are poised at a unique point in human history. Humanity is literally at the dawning of a New Age. Within the last 30 to 40 years the acquisition of knowledge and information has accelerated to a tremendous pace, beyond that seen upon this planet in all of recorded human history. Because of new information systems and the widespread availability of books, the accumulated wealth of knowledge that we have amassed through the ages has become more readily available to all people. Science has evolved to the point where computers and similar instrumentation have given us the power to not only store and transmit information to many serious seekers, but also to integrate old data and to reach new levels of comprehension of phenomena which were already known but incompletely understood.

These same computer technologies have also given us the tools to advance into new realms of exploration and to extend our vision into literally unseen realms. Nowhere is this new vision becoming more important than in the understanding of the innermost workings of the human mind and body. Because of new diagnostic imaging systems, such as the electron microscope, the CAT scanner, and the MRI scanner, doctors have new tools with which to probe human anatomy and physiology. Perhaps more importantly, these same imaging systems are beginning to tell us new things about the functioning of the brain, the seat of human consciousness. For the first time in our recorded history, we are on the verge of understanding the inner workings of the human brain, and comprehending how internal neurological structures relate to the expression of consciousness.

Also at this time in history, scientific thinkers of different disciplines have begun to synthesize their findings and uncover new relationships between basic chemistry, physics, and human physiology. Nobel prize winner Ilya Prigogine and other pioneering thinkers have found mathematical relationships that govern the way many systems behave. Applying Prigogine's theory of dissipative structures to various areas of science has demonstrated fascinating similarities between phenomena as simple as the behavior of chemical reactions and as complex as the creation of higher order in the neurological organization of the brain.[1] Other theorists, including neuroscientist Karl Pribram, have also found that discoveries in the fields of laser physics and holography may give us new ways of understanding how the brain may store information.[2] Insights in the areas of high-energy particle physics concerning the energetic substructure of all matter have given scientists a greater understanding of the underlying unity of nature and the physical world. Because human beings function through a physical body, the discovery by particle physicists that matter is a form of frozen energy has significant implications for science's ability to understand the subtle energetic intricacies of human physiology.

As modern thinkers sift through all of this rapidly accumulating scientific data, many scientists have begun to change their views about the underlying meaning of humans as sentient beings and their position in the universe. Many new and radical ideas are evolving which look at human beings quite differently than did the old mechanistic reductionist ideas of Newtonian physics. The quantum physicists and holographic theorists are just the first of a new breed of scientists who have begun to explore some of the complex energy relationships between people and their environment. As many popular books of the last decade have stated, we are in the midst of a massive paradigm shift from the older mechanical worldview of the Newtonian pragmatists to the new perspective of an interconnected holistic universe as envisioned by the Einsteinian thinkers.

As new views evolve about the nature of the world around us, and as we begin to understand human function in terms of complex energetic models, many scientific researchers have stumbled into the realization that there is an underlying unity of structure which connects us to the universe. The more advanced quantum and particle physicists are now coming to the same conclusions about the underlying unity of humanity and nature that ancient Chinese and Indian philosophers described in their writings depicting subtle human relationships with the cosmos.[3] The only difference in approach between the ancient and modern viewpoints is that the old Oriental and Vedic teachers came to their insights through meditation and inner psychic probing of the universe, while modern scientists have arrived at their conclusions through a more mechanistic, electronic, and empirical approach. Whether it is through inner meditative journeys or outer instrumented searching, the ultimate realizations of modern scientist and ancient philosopher have shown striking similarities.

The holographic model of the universe gives a new foundation for comprehending the unseen energy interconnections between all things. This integral relationship between human beings and their environment was always something that was intuitively sensed by the Eastern teachers of ancient times. It is only now that there has evolved a scientific theoretical foundation for this profound inner perception. The Einsteinian viewpoint of matter as particularized energy shows us that we are all constructed from the same subatomic building blocks. At a microcosmic level, we are each complex yet uniquely arranged aggregates of the same particularized universal energy. As scientists and religious scholars start to view the universe from the new perspective of its being an evolving energy in many forms, the two fields may gradually find common ground.[4] In a way, we are seeing the earliest attempt at reintegration of religion and science, as both disciplines again begin to understand the world through a unified vision.

All living and inorganic things are shaped from the same matter that exists throughout the physical universe. Astrophysicists have now surmised that the matter from which the Earth and its inhabitants have evolved was born in the cosmic incubators of second and third generation stars similar to our own nearby sun. The vast array of physical elements on our planet have their origin in the building up of matter from molecular evolution. The solar fusion of hydrogen to form helium, the triple alpha process of helium recombining to form carbon, and so on up the elemental ladder have provided the primal ingredients for planetary evolution and the emergence of life on Earth. We are all made from the same "star stuff," the basic building blocks of the universe. And whether that material comes from aggregates of cosmic dust, reformed primordial hydrogen, or even astral matter, its basic nature is that of particularized, frozen energy. All matter is energy and light in its myriad forms and manifestations.

The last ingredient to understanding these cosmic processes is the realization that consciousness somehow participates in this entire process of evolution on both a planetary and organismic scale. This final piece of the puzzle has been the hardest to swallow for most, but it is a most important motivating force behind the evolutionary process. In fact, *consciousness itself is a form of energy*. It is the highest form of energy and is integrally involved with the life process. If we consider consciousness as a fundamental quality and expression of life energy, we come closer to understanding how spirit interacts with and manifests through the many forms of physical matter. *It is, in fact, the journey of spirit through the worlds of matter that provides the strongest driving force for the evolutionary process.*

As we begin to glimpse this greatest of truths about our hidden spiritual heritage, only then will we truly understand the higher dimensional aspects of the life processes of human beings. Simple chemistry and physics alone do not hold all the answers to piecing together the puzzle of human physiology, as the pragmatic Newtonian scientists would like to believe. It is only when the higher dimensional components of physics and chemistry are added to the equation of life that we can make sense of the open-ended energy system that constitutes the multidimensional human being. The realities of spirit do not negate the laws of science. They only extend existing laws to include the higher frequency dimensions of matter, even as Einsteinian physics incorporated the earlier discoveries of Newtonian mechanics but went far beyond.

As our vision of light has extended to understanding not only inorganic physical matter but also the behavior of organic living matter from a subtle energy perspective, we are creating the foundations for a new medicine and a new psychology of human beings. Society has just begun to witness the earliest glimmerings of understanding of these principles by the medical profession. As yet, only a handful of pioneering physicians have turned to explore the profound importance of the true relationship between energy, matter, and consciousness. The old guard of scientists and doctors have long held onto their mechanistic view of bodily and mental function. They are reluctant to accept new models of understanding without hard scientific facts and experimental evidence. However, the time has finally arrived when New Age technologies are being created which will validate the hypotheses of the evolving new guard of physician/healers.

As more physicians, nurses, and other health care practitioners become interested and involved in the field of "holistic medicine," there will come a greater understanding of what "holistic" really means. The term holistic, in reference to the health and wellness of human beings, implies not only a balance between the aspects of body and mind but also between the multidimensional forces of spirit that until now have been only poorly understood by the vast majority. *For truly, it is the endowing power of spirit that moves, inspires, and breathes life into that vehicle we perceive as the physical body. A system of medicine which denies or ignores its existence will be incomplete, because it leaves out the most fundamental quality of human existence—the spiritual dimension.* As doctors see themselves more as healers and less as practitioners, spirit will be more appreciated as a motivating factor in health.

Throughout progressive chapters of this book, I have endeavored to construct an image of humans as entities who consist of more than physical nerves, muscles, and bones. We are multidimensional beings of energy and light, whose physical body is but a single component of a larger dynamic system. Put another way, humans are mind/body/spirit complexes which exist in continuous dynamic equilibrium with higher energy dimensions of reality. The tissues which compose our physical form are fed not only by oxygen, glucose, and chemical nutrients, but also by higher vibrational energies which endow the physical frame with the properties of life and creative expression.

These subtle energies are hierarchical in nature, and work from higher levels downward until they become manifest at the level of the physical body. The higher vibrational energies represent the organizing structures of consciousness which utilize the physical body as a vehicle of expression within our physical space/time universe. Each physical body and personality is an extension of a higher spiritual consciousness which seeks to evolve through learning experiences encountered in the school of Earth life. The drive of spirit to evolve toward a higher quality of consciousness is the motivating force behind the reincarnational system. This increased quality of consciousness can only be achieved through individual experiences and many lives within the physical body. Thus, spirit uses the physical form as a teaching and learning tool. While the physical body may be transitory, the experience and knowledge gained while in physical form is everlasting.

The integral mechanism which regulates the flow of higher energies into the physical form consists mainly of the chakra-nadi system and the physical-etheric interface. The physical-etheric interface is a unique bridge of subtle energies which includes the acupuncture meridian system. It connects the organic/molecular form with the organizational energies of the etheric body. The etheric body is a holographic energy field or growth template which maintains order and determines structural patterning within the cellular matrix of the physical body. The etheric energies provide a waveguide upon which to organize cellular structure and function. They synergistically coordinate life activities through vibrational, genetic and other subtle molecular mechanisms.

Diagram 32.
THE HUMAN BIOENERGETIC SYSTEM

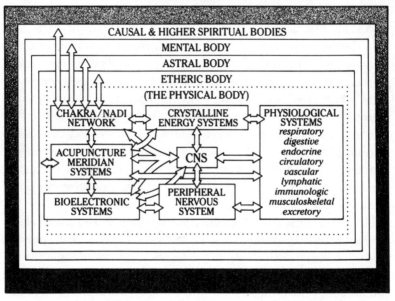

In addition, high-frequency energies entering through the chakras are distributed to the appropriate organs of the body by the fine network of nadis. This higher vibrational input provides a subtle nutritional and organizational influence to the cells of the physical body, helping to maintain balance and order at the molecular level of expression. The total balance and health of the human organism is a product of a balanced and coordinated functioning of both physical and higher dimensional homeostatic regulatory systems. If there is a system failure at any level of the physioenergetic hierarchy, physical breakdown and illness may occur. Health is therefore a function of proper alignment, balance, and coordination of the higher subtle-energy forms and forces with the physical vehicle. When energetic disturbances occur at the etheric and higher frequency levels of structure, pathologic changes eventually manifest at the physical/cellular level.

From a reincarnational perspective, illness or disease can be viewed as an Earth learning experience. The location and nature of many illnesses often contain symbolic information which, if properly decoded, can assist the individual in understanding certain emotional and mental blockages of which he or she may not be aware. These blockages are occasionally karmic, and represent deficiencies in the quality of the incarnating emotional/mental matrix that have been incurred by negative or traumatizing experiences from past lives. Correction of an energy dysfunction occuring at emotional, mental, and spiritual levels of organization will result in a restructuring of the etheric template and improved functioning of the chakras. Thus the physical body will be healed from a more primary level of causation.

The realization by physicists that at a quantum level, all substance is particularized frozen light, gives credence to the concept that matter of different frequencies can coexist in the same space. This is similar to the observation that energy of different frequencies, such as radio and TV waves, can coexist nondestructively within the same space. In the case of human subtle anatomy, the interpenetrating structures of varying frequencies of matter are the physical, etheric, astral, and higher vibrational vehicles. The argument for this idea was discussed in Chapter 1, in which we examined the similarity between holographic images and the structure of the etheric body.

Also inherent within the holographic model is its application for dealing with the universe as one large, dynamically changing energy interference pattern—a gigantic real-time hologram. The holographic model teaches us how vibrational patterns of universal energy can hold unseen levels of structured information that may be tapped, understood, and even manipulated if properly approached. The human body, if considered as such an energy pattern, can be comprehended as a teaching tool which holds within it many lessons about the true nature of self, one's larger reality, and even the structure of the universe.

If humans can be seen from the perspective of their multidimensional anatomy, consisting of higher vibrational bodies, chakras, nadis, and meridians, then much can be comprehended in the evolving field of alternative methods of healing. It is only when this larger picture is fully appreciated that many seemingly "unscientific" methods of treatment will be shown to have viable explanations of efficacy.

The purpose of this book has been to elaborate on many different methods of healing which are, at present, looked upon with great skepticism by the conventional medical community. Many of the explanations given for the various vibrational treatments will likely be viewed with as much skeptical dogmatism and closed-mindedness as has characterized the scientific establishment in times past. It is the hope of the author that this book may be read by enough scientists with an open mind and perhaps a more spiritual orientation, so that a groundwork for extending the present level of medical practice to greater levels of achievement and healing may be provided.

Vibrational Healing & Holistic Medicine: The Gradual Shift from Reductionism to Holism

Vibrational healing methods represent new ways of dealing with illness. Practitioners of subtle-energy medicine attempt to correct dysfunction in the human organism by manipulating invisible yet integral levels of human structure and function. Healing at the level of human subtle-energy anatomy is predicated upon the New Physics understanding that all matter is, in fact, a manifestation of energy. As science and technology evolve to make that which was formerly unseen visible, more scientists and physicians will be forced to change their viewpoint about the extended nature of human beings, just as the development of the microscope forced many a skeptical medical society to follow the admonitions of Lister and other pioneering thinkers who claimed that "invisible germs" were the cause of much illness and suffering.

In the early days of medical science, understanding of human structure and function was quite limited. The human body was understood as an intricate machine of pumps, pistons, gears and pulleys. The only models which existed at that time were mechanistic, and so it was natural that human beings should be compared to what was then state-of-the-art science. Treatment of illness was based on cookbook repetition of previous time-honored methods of drugs, poultices, cathartics, and surgery. Occasionally, pioneering attempts were made at trying new things. Most often, those doctors who tried different or unorthodox treatments were considered quacks and charlatans by their contemporaries. If, however, enough research accumulated to show that their new treatment methods were efficacious, these scientists formerly held to be quacks (Lister, Pasteur, and others) were eventually elevated to the position of "pioneer" and "innovator."

Through the empirical method of trial and error, various treatments were shown to be either effective or dangerous, and were thus either widely adopted or abandoned. Much of medical practice through the years has been based upon what might be known as the scientific medical consensus. Whatever models and philosophy of practice became the accepted body of knowledge of the current medical establishment was taken to be gospel by its practitioners. Various treatments of one kind or another, including bleeding, cathartics, and the even the use of leeches, have had their day.

As scientific thinking has become more sophisticated, new models of function have arisen. Unfortunately, the predominant viewpoint of the human body as an intricate machine has persisted to this day. Only the "gears and pulleys" of the great mechanism have become progressively smaller and smaller. *Even though we have advanced far in scientific understanding, doctors still think of human beings as machines.* For instance, the human heart, the center of our being, is considered to be a tireless pump beating blood throughout the body with unceasing rhythm and regularity. Yet some occult sources consider the heart to be the seat of the soul, the site through which the life-force is anchored in the physical body.[5]

Mechanistically, physicians see the heart as a physical engine of strength and precision. Simplistically, they have tried to duplicate its function through the creation of the artificial heart. Attempts at replacing the human heart with an artificial one have been fraught with problems. The most frequent problem appears to be recurrent strokes and subsequent neurological dysfunction. This complication has occurred with nearly every recipient of the artificial heart, with severity varying among patients. Stroke occurs frequently enough that the FDA is only allowing the use of the artificial heart as a temporary measure prior to human heart transplantation. The mechanistic model would suggest that the reason for this recurrent failure of the artifical heart is due to the formation of blood clots that travel to the brain due to some clot-producing factor in the mechanical pump. In attempts to prevent this complication, cardiac surgeons place their patients on blood-thinning anticoagulants; yet strokes still occur.

An alternative explanation to consider is that the heart chakra, which supplies the physical heart with nutritive etheric energy, may be the higher energetic source of dysfunction that contributed to the degeneration of the heart in the first place. It is interesting to note that dysfunction of the heart chakra, due to emotional blockages in being able to express love to self and others, is associated not only with physical diseases of the heart, including coronary artery disease and various cardiomyopathies, but also with strokes related to stasis of circulation. Perhaps the abnormally functioning heart chakra in mechanical heart transplant recipients is the overriding subtle-energy factor that keeps causing recurrent strokes, and not any physical defect within the device.

This would also suggest that the ability of human heart transplant recipients to accept and live comfortably with their new heart would tend to be assisted by psychoenergetic approaches aimed at correcting dysfunction in the heart chakra. By psychoenergetic, we mean not only the psychological therapies of meditation, imagery, and psychotherapy, but also the subtle-energy therapies of homeopathy, flower essences, gem elixirs, and a variety of other spiritual healing modalities. Interestingly, here is a case where a conventional surgical approach—heart transplantation—might be combined with both allopathic drug therapies (including Cyclosporin—an immunosuppressive drug to prevent rejection) and subtle-energy modalities that deal with a life-threatening illness at a variety of energy levels simultaneously.

Obviously, the mechanistic model can be limiting in being able to provide treatment approaches. When one is faced with a diseased heart, there are only so many physio-mechanical approaches available. Heart disease provides a perfect model of an illness which contrasts the therapeutic methods of orthodox medical practitioners with that of holistic physicians. A conventional doctor, when faced with a patient with serious heart disease, has a number of different diagnostic and therapeutic approaches available in his/her repertoire. These range from the accepted to the more experimental approaches. Noninvasive tests such as thallium blood-flow scans, echocardiograms, and stress tests can be performed. But ultimately the gold standard eventually becomes the cardiac catheterization. Dye injected into the heart through a catheter guided by a fluoroscope gives the ultimate physical visualization of the beating heart, its subtle wall motion, and the patency or narrowing of its nutrient coronary arteries.

If cholesterol blockages are found narrowing the coronary arteries, various medical, mechanical, and surgical methods may be tried to correct the defect. The patient may be placed on drugs that will hopefully dilate the narrowed arteries to their maximum possible diameter in order to reestablish the flow of needed oxygen to the muscular walls of the heart. If drugs are ineffective in relieving the problem of angina pectoris or chest pain, a number of physical methods may be attempted in a hospital setting.

Originally, the next answer for angina after drug therapy was coronary bypass surgery. Now there are newer "physical" treatment methods available. Perhaps the technique which is gaining most in popularity is a system known as balloon angioplasty. In coronary angioplasty, a balloon-tipped catheter is inserted under fluoroscopic observation into the diseased coronary artery, and the balloon is then inflated under pressure. The walls of the thin tubular balloon press back against the cholesterol plaques and widen the opening to allow more blood to pass the blockage. This technique has had various success rates, and complications ranging from chest pain to production of heart attacks that require emergency coronary bypass surgery. Still, this is a less invasive technique than bypass surgery itself.

The other more experimental method of destroying cholesterol plaques in the coronary arteries is through laser angioplasty. The laser beam is transmitted through a thin fiber-optic catheter, called an angioscope, which allows the surgeon to peer into the center of the diseased artery. The laser is used to selectively vaporize cholesterol blockages that occlude portions of the coronary arteries. This technique has had various levels of success, but is a unique approach because it is using pure energy to treat disease. However, the approach is still based upon a mechanistic model of physiology. That is, the laser is being used as a high powered roto-router to remove the offending cholesterol.

Another technique which is considered even more experimental than laser angioplasty is called laser myocardial revascularization (LMR).[6] Tiny holes are blasted in an area of the wall of failing heart muscle while the heart is cooled and held motionless as in typical open-heart/bypass surgery. The prevailing theory is that the externally healed laser holes produce internal sinuses and channels in the myocardium which allow for greater circulation and oxygenation of dysfunctional heart muscle.

LMR and laser angioplasty demonstrate unusual cases where pure energy (laser light) is being used (albeit in a somewhat mechanistic approach) to treat illness. These types of approaches, in which the laser is being used as a surgical instrument, might be considered transitional in the gradual introduction of energy medicine into traditional medicine. The development of laser technologies in healing will continue to evolve in the future, especially in the field of subtle-energy approaches. Notable in this area will be laserpuncture, or the use of low-energy lasers to stimulate acupuncture points for the promotion of healing. These and other advanced vibrational healing techniques will become more widely accepted when orthodox physicians begin to approach human beings not just as closed physiologic boxes but as open energy systems in dynamic equilibrium with a multidimensional electromagnetic environment.

Returning to our conventional physician's approach to heart disease, we have considered drug therapy, angioplasty, and bypass surgery. Laser therapy is still considered highly experimental and is only available in certain unique research centers around the world. If the heart disease results in irreparable damage, as in the case of a massive heart attack caused by coronary thrombosis and occlusion, and if the remaining heart muscle is too weak, then the only alternative is mechanical assistance using either the aortic balloon pump or total heart replacement. As discussed, this includes either temporary artificial heart placement or human heart transplantation after a suitable donor organ has been found.

Up until now this combined medical and surgical armamentarium has defined the state of the art in treating heart disease. In addition to the treatments already mentioned, there are also various drugs which can be given to dilate arteries and increase coronary blood flow. Other drugs can be prescribed which assist in strengthening weakened heart muscle or in preventing chaotic and life-threatening cardiac rhythms. Beyond that, conventional medicine has little left to offer. What can the future bring? It is doubtful that the creation of new heart-strengthening medicines will be the key to treating heart disease. Once the physical heart has degenerated in function beyond a certain point, there is little that can be done to strengthen it. The phrase, "you can't beat a dying horse," has sometimes been used by cardiologists who feel they are beating their heads against the wall trying vainly to improve the function of a hopelessly failing heart. The only other alternative is a heart transplantation, either artificial or from a human donor, neither of which are readily available in all medical centers.

Holistic physicans have found a number of alternatives in treating heart disease. Perhaps the most controversial of these techniques is chelation therapy.[7] Chelation therapy is not quite the chemical roto-router that its opponents claim it to be. This type of therapy consists of giving multiple intravenous infusions of a chemical chelating agent called EDTA over a period of weeks and months. This chemical complexes calcium ions from the circulation and leaches out calcium from the rigid, narrowed walls of arteriosclerotic blood vessels such as diseased coronary arteries.

What most critics fail to understand, however, is that chelation therapy is also a hormonal manipulation. The EDTA infusion seems to cause a secondary release of a calcium-regulating substance called parathyroid hormone, which causes continued opening of arteriosclerotic blood vessels days and weeks after chelation therapy has been completed. For instance, it is well known among chelation therapists that drugs like propranolol, which impair parathyroid hormone response, blunt the therapeutic effectiveness of chelation therapy. Patients are typically weaned off these and similar beta-blocker drugs prior to the initiation of chelation therapy.

There are also oral forms of chelating agents which have been touted as alternatives to intravenous therapy, but most holistic physicians feel that the EDTA therapy is the more potent of the two approaches. Interestingly, some holistic physicians have reported improvements in cardiac function following multiple chelation treatments, as measured by nuclear heart scanning. Unfortunately, studies such as these rarely make it into conventional medical journals and are limited to publication in holistic literature and alternative medical journals.

Chelation therapy is not considered a vibrational therapy but is an innovative chemical or drug therapy. Instead of blasting away cholesterol and calcium deposits with laser beams or pushing them aside with balloon-tipped catheters, chelation chemically and hormonally reverses the hardening of the arteries to improve flow through the coronary arteries. Its effectiveness is limited in many cases to the chronological point at which intervention occurs. The older and longer standing the arterial disease, the less likely any benefit is to occur. To the holistic doctors, chelation is a kind of chemical last resort to dealing with coronary artery disease.

An even more important approach to heart disease that is only now being actively addressed by conventional physicians is diet therapy. It was believed by only a few orthodox doctors that changing diet could reverse atherosclerosis. Yet when diet proponent Nathan Pritikin died, his autopsy substantiated his claims. Pritikin had been diagnosed as having coronary artery disease earlier in his life. Coronary catherization had substantiated the degree of narrowing in his blood vessels. Yet after several decades of stringent dietary modification, his autopsy revealed that Pritikin's coronaries were open and clear of blockages. In addition, his cholesterol level was extremely low for his age. This resulted from his low fat, low cholesterol diet.

In reality, Pritikin advised dietary changes which severely limited the amount of fat intake. He also maintained that exercise was similarly important in improving circulation in the heart. Yet it is often difficult for people to modify their diet and exercise patterns. Often, it takes a first or second heart attack to make an individual adopt better health habits.

Utilizing lifestyle modification to treat and prevent illness is one of the few approaches that has begun to make inroads into conventional medicine. The fact that many physicians are now advising patients to make changes in the area of diet and physical activity demonstrates how traditional medicine is slowly moving into areas formerly held to be the province of the holistic therapist.

However, the future of holistic medicine will depend on the integration of vibrational medical therapies into everyday practice. Holistic physicians accept the concept of wellness in human beings as being a function of properly integrating the physical, emotional, mental, and spiritual elements of life. At present, many practitioners have addressed the emotional and spiritual dimensions largely through psychotherapy and counseling. What needs greater clarification, however, is the true relationship of the spiritual dimension to the balanced flow of the life-force itself. This is an area which has been touched upon but which needs further elaboration, especially as to how holistic physicians of the future will be able to impact upon the energy aspects of these subtle dimensions in order to promote health and healing.

As we mentioned earlier, a vibrational approach to healing heart disease would include applying those subtle-energy modalities that would strengthen the heart chakra. The heart chakra supplies the physical heart with nutritive subtle energies. Therefore, it would be appropriate to work with heart disease by strengthening weaknesses and establishing proper energy flow through the heart center. Energetic influences such as the chakras, nadis, and the acupuncture meridians affect the health of bodily organs at an etheric or "pre-physical" level. Changes occur at these higher vibrational levels much sooner than at the cellular level. This is what is meant by dealing with illness at a more primary level of causation.

The ultimate approach to healing will be to remove the abnormalities at the subtle-energy level which led to the manifestation of illness in the first place. This will be the greatest difference in approach between the traditional medicine of today and the spiritual/holistic medicine of the future. In applying the mechanistic model of illness, most conventional physicians attempt to treat only the aftereffects of illness. They try to modify an already failing heart to provide it with greater function by pharmacological and surgical means. In more recent years, there have been attempts made at creating a better metabolic environment for the heart through dietary changes to promote lower cholesterol and weight loss, cessation of smoking, and exercise rehabilitation programs. In and of themselves, these are healthy steps in the right direction. However, there are additional energy factors which can be modified to stimulate healing of the heart beyond that which conventional methods have achieved.

The vibrational approach seeks to provide the heart with a more stable, less destructive subtle-energy environment which may hopefully assist in the recovery of function through more natural means. There are various vibrational approaches that might be used in the case of heart disease. As we mentioned, the use of flower essences, gem elixirs, or possibly homeopathic remedies might be indicated, depending upon the expertise of the individual practitioner. Energy imbalances in the meridian circuitry of the body might be analyzed using the Voll Machine and other diagnostic equipment. Appropriate vibrational remedies could be matched to the patient's specific frequency needs. The appropriateness of specific gem elixirs, flower essences, or other remedies could also be checked on the Voll Machine to ensure correct vibrational matching between patient and therapy.

On the more esoteric levels of treatment, specific color energies might be directed to the chest area in an attempt to strengthen the heart chakra. Additionally, particular crystals known to be beneficial to the heart center, such as the ruby, might be applied to the heart region for positive energy effects. Psychic or spiritual healing could also be utilized, either alone or in conjunction with specific crystals, to try to modify the subtle-energy qualities of the diseased heart. Heart disease might be associated with energy dysfunction in other centers besides the heart chakra. A clairvoyant could be used in diagnosis to describe the function and energy patterns of the individual chakras.

An examination of negative thoughtforms in the patient's auric field might be sought as contributory data which could provide information as to the psychospiritual origins of the patient's illness. It has been suggested that thought patterns have subtle magnetic properties which allow them to be dealt with using not only psychotherapy but also by applying treatments which work primarily at the subtle-energy level. There are certain experimental systems employing inert gas beams which can actually dissolve negative thoughtforms in a patient's auric field. However, treatment with such systems must often be repeated many times. This is because the same pervasive thought patterns which created the original thought-forms will often recreate that identical energy pattern, even after it has been dissolved, if the consciousness of the individual has not changed. In addition to clairvoyant observation, radionic systems might be used (by an appropriately trained radionic specialist) to diagnose problems at a variety of subtle-energy levels, starting with an evaluation of individual chakras and ascending to an investigation of the quality of underlying etheric structures.

Perhaps the most powerful of all healing modalities is the patient's own mind. Positive, spiritually uplifting verbal affirmations may be used to change negative message tapes that may be playing through the subconscious mind. Transformational healing images are also of benefit, especially when visual imagery is combined with the use of affirmations. As we discussed in the previous chapter, abnormal functioning of the chakras often relates to psychological and spiritual blockages in the thinking patterns of the sick individual. The particular chakra that is affected during illness is often a clue to the type of emotional blockage that is contributing to the manifestation of disease.

Trying to modify the negative or faulty perceptions that are contributing to chakra dysfunction may be one of the most important adjunctive treatments to any vibrational therapy. One must change the predisposing subtle-energy conditions behind illness in order for any treatment to have lasting effectiveness. When the patient's consciousness is engaged to assist with any type of therapy, such as the use of visualization to augment a treatment, positive amplifying effects are bound to occur. This applies to both traditional as well as alternative medical approaches. Patients who use relaxation and visualization techniques in conjunction with drug or surgical therapies have faster healing and more positive treatment outcomes.

Specific programs of active visualization and affirmation may be helpful in rebalancing blocked chakras by changing the patterns of thinking that originally led to psychoenergetic, and thus physical, imbalance. By trying to correct chakra dysfunction, we are attempting to heal illness at a more primary level of causation. This contrasts with the traditional medical approach of treating individual symptoms and trying to modify patterns of disease only at the physical level through pharmacologic and surgical manipulations. By working backward through the etheric, astral, and higher levels of dysfunction, illness may be corrected before it has even manifested at the physical level. Of course, proving that one has cured an illness before it became physical will ultimately depend upon the development of diagnostic imaging equipment that can visualize pathologic changes in the etheric organ structures of the body.

Ultimately, this will be the direction that medicine must take in the future. Health will be maintained by diagnosing energy predispositions to illness long before disease has actually manifested at the physical level. It is only through subtle-energy technologies like the Voll Machine, radionic devices, and other systems, that this level of diagnostic accuracy may be approached. Of course, *the effectiveness of these devices is primarily a function of the psychospiritual development of the health practitioner, for systems such as radionic devices are actually extensions of the consciousness mechanisms of the vibrational diagnostician.*

The keys to treating illness will ultimately be determined by our ability to comprehend how illness occurs in the first place. Conventional physicians are slowly making inroads toward understanding the concept of predisposition toward, and participation in, illness. Illness does not necessarily come from outside ourselves, but may have its origins in our own physical and bioenergetic makeup. Traditional medicine has begun to comprehend that illness may not be strictly a function of coming in contact with a particular noxious agent. In other words, illness may not necessarily come from outside ourselves. Sickness has its roots at the level of our own inner being. Only now are doctors addressing the concept of host resistance and the many factors which contribute to an individual's susceptibility to illness.

For centuries, pathogenesis of illness was poorly understood. Infectious diseases provided the first models of illness which were based upon the harmful effects of "invisible" germs. For many physicians, the idea of unseen malefic influences was hard to grasp. Doctors' inability to believe that germs caused sickness made cleanliness and sterility in the operating room a difficult thing to achieve. Doctors would operate on patients using their bare hands, after having handled cadavers or other ill patients. Strict handwashing procedures were uncommon. Lack of sterilization would often result in mysterious wound infections and other complications. It was only after the new technology of the microscope had revealed the presence of "invisible" bacteria that their existence was confirmed. Following years of laborious experimentation by Pasteur, Lister and other medical pioneers, the participation of microbes in illness was hesitantly acknowledged. This eventually led to the widespread adoption of handwashing and sterilization procedures in medical and surgical practice.

Today, we understand that the total picture of infectious disease is actually a two component equation. An illness may be caused not only by contact with an infectious agent but also by the exposure of that agent to an individual who, at that time, is unable to immunologically defend him or herself from attack. To be considered, of course, is the magnitude of the toxic stimulus with which a person is presented. The larger the external stress, the greater the likelihood of illness. In the case of a toxic chemical, the induction of illness would be determined by the total amount ingested compared to the known safety standards of exposure. It is also possible to induce toxic biological effects through chronic exposure to microdoses of harmful chemicals well within current safety standards; these effects are mediated by the same energy principles that operate in homeopathy. This raises questions about the conventional safety standards that exist for toxic exposure to chemicals. However, we will address that issue later in this chapter. In the case of infectious diseases, the more virulent the organism and the larger the size of the innoculum (number of organisms ingested), the greater the probability of illness.

Conversely, the immune status of the individual contributes to the illness equation even more disproportionately. For example, individuals who are known to have severely suppressed immune function, including patients on high-dose steroids, cancer chemotherapy drugs, and AIDS sufferers, are susceptible to overwhelming infections from microorganisms that are indigenous to the environment and harmless to most individuals. In the immunocompromised host, any infection is a potentially life-threatening one. The degree of host resistance impairment stretches across a wide spectrum, with AIDS and chemotherapy patients existing at the most extreme end of the curve. There are a great many factors, both on the physical and subtle-energy levels, which contribute to the total picture of immune competence.

To truly comprehend the issue of host resistance, one must first have some appreciation for the structural elements that endow us with our immunologic defenses. At the physical level, host resistance is a cellular phenomenon mediated by lymphocytes, lymphatic organs, and the reticuloendothelial network of the body. T- and B-lymphocytes and tissue histiocytes are the body's own marines. In actuality, they are closer to the marine shore patrol. They actively patrol our internal borders to keep dangerous intruders from attacking home shores, but they also police their own troops and try to keep the more aggressive types from wrecking the place and getting too out of control.

The immune system is a cohesive network of tireless workers which modulates the cellular environment of the body. The immune network continually samples the internal environment of the body, sensing foreign proteins and elements that are identified as non-self. These abnormal proteins may be the external coats of viruses, the walls of bacteria, or even the outer membranes of cancer cells. In this fashion, the immune system is constantly screening the cellular boundaries of the self to maintain both an internal quality control operation as well as a strategic defense system.

On a vibrational level, the quality of immune function and the body's ability to defend and maintain self is greatly affected by the degree of subtle-energy flow through the heart chakra/thymus gland axis. The heart chakra, in turn, is affected by the psychoenergetic balance within the consciousness of the individual. The heart chakra is affected by one's ability to feel love towards self as well as towards others in daily relationships. We sometimes refer to individuals who cannot express love to others as having a "hardened heart." On a subtle-energy level, this would also refer to a closed or blocked heart chakra, which might actually contribute to hardening of the arteries within the physical heart.

At a symbolic level, the circulation of blood is metaphysically tied to the circulation of love towards oneself, and between self and others. The heart chakra, and the organs it supplies subtle energy to, are strongly affected by the love nature of the individual. When there are negative self-images and self-messages that are unconsciously being replayed by an individual's biocomputer memory banks, the internal image of self and the balance and openness of the heart chakra are affected. Because the heart chakra has an energy link to the thymus gland, and thus the immune system, the psychospiritual elements of self and self-love are intimately tied into the cellular expression and maintenance of bodily self integrity.

When there are unconscious emotional conflicts that negatively affect the heart chakra, as in states of depression and bereavement, there is an associated immunosuppression which causes a greater susceptibility to disease of any kind. When the immune system is suppressed by emotional stress and the personality is overwhelmed by feelings of helplessness and hopelessness, the body becomes more open to attack from viruses, bacteria, and even cancer cells. Occasionally, stress may knock out selective policing factions of immune defender cells. The immune system may turn against the body by attacking itself in the form of autoimmune diseases.

Physiologic and psychological stresses play an important role in the body's capacity for maximal immunocompetence. Over the last 25 years, traditional physicians have begun to recognize the powerful physiologic effects of chronic stress, thanks to early pioneers such as Hans Selye and others. Stress research has been one of the areas where holistic medicine and conventional medicine have found some convergence in thinking. Both factions have acknowledged that stress has significant negative effects upon the mind and body. It is now known that stress induces temporary suppression of immune functioning. Perhaps the most dramatic illustration of the attention toward stress and the mind/body relationship has been in the recognition of stress-related disorders. Doctors have become increasingly aware that stress-linked illnesses occur frequently among a large part of their patient population.

In spite of the fact that many traditional physicians have acknowledged that stress contributes to asthma, peptic ulcer disease, ulcerative colitis, and other diseases, there have been very few attempts to directly address the psychological factors affecting these illnesses. Even though some physicians might recommend psychotherapy to their patients with stress-related disorders, the physical treatment of the illness by conventional pharmacologic methods has been given the greatest attention. The increasing recognition that stress contributes to disease exacerbation has led to a search by drug companies for better and more potent antianxiety agents, exemplified by Valium and its many new relatives.

Admittedly, these drugs may be useful in short-term treatment of acutely stressful situations, but they may only mask the primary problem while ignoring the reasons for the stress reaction. Better therapeutic methods of dealing with psychological stress include biofeedback, meditative practices, imagery techniques, and progressive relaxation exercises. Alternative approaches commonly employed by holistic doctors give the individual greater control over self and the manifestations of stress in the physical body, as opposed to dependence on drugs for relief of anxiety.

The mechanistic model of traditional medicine can provide new pharmacologic treatments to suppress our feelings of anxiety, dread and panic; but is this really therapeutic from a holistic viewpoint? The aim of the holistic practitioner is to integrate and rebalance the elements of mind and body with the element of spirit. Drugs like Valium may make it easier for time-limited physicians to deal with stressful patients, but such drugs do little to accomplish the higher goals of the holistic model.

Throughout the twentieth century, physicians have looked at the body and mind as separate and distinct components of human beings and, based upon this assumption, have dealt primarily with the body in trying to treat illness. Gradually, evidence has accumulated which has shown that the mind and body are less separate than previously thought. A greater understanding of the negative effects of psychological stress on the mind and body in promoting illness has provided the impetus for this reevaluation in medical thinking. In spite of physicians' changes in thinking about stress and illness, treatment approaches within traditional medicine have tended to remain focused on only the bodily components of illness. Conventional doctors tend to direct therapeutic strategies toward particular organ systems instead of treating the whole person.

There has been a gradual evolution of medical thought, moving physicians' thinking toward an appreciation of human beings as complex systems of physical, mental, emotional, and even spiritual characteristics. The progressive shift toward a more humanistic medicine has been responsible for the holistic movement in health care. The reductionist model of the human machine as the sum of its component parts has not been entirely successful in providing therapeutic insights into treating disease, nor in understanding the greater nature of human health. For in reality, humans are greater than the sum of their physical organs and nervous systems, because the physical body is not a simple closed system.

Humans are beings whose sum total is only partly represented by those integrated physiologic mechanisms known as physical bodies. The physical body interfaces with complex subtle structures and networks that mediate the flow of the energies of consciousness and the life-force into it, thereby nurturing and maintaining its existence upon the physical plane. The multidimensional human is a manifestation of the evolving soul which incarnates through the vehicles of the physical and higher vibrational bodies. This energetic stream of consciousness works through the synergistic mechanisms of the subtle and physical bodies to express itself creatively and to learn more about its true nature through its actions upon the physical plane. In the near future, spiritual physicians will begin to understand human beings from this expanded perspective and to help treat the diseases that humanity has often brought upon itself. To truly help people in distress, doctors must begin to understand that illness is partly due to a blockage within the human energy system, and especially within the individual's structure of emotional expression. This blockage can impede the flow of spirit and of the individual's higher consciousness into the conscious waking life.

In order to comprehend why people become ill and to understand how to treat those illnesses, one must have an intricate knowledge of the complex regulatory systems of the human body as well as a greater awareness of the subtle vehicles of consciousness which interact with the physical form. The holistic approach to health and illness is a great step forward in medical thinking. Holism allows us to integrate our understanding of the effects of emotion into the larger picture of human functioning, and helps us to visualize the subtle unseen connections between stress and disease. By utilizing a systems approach to human physiology that incorporates the interrelationships between the many component structures of mind, body, and spirit, the healing professions will gradually evolve toward the use of various subtle-energy treatment methods that will be successful in healing disease and in promoting health, happiness, and continued spiritual growth.

Stress, Illness & Wellness:
Creating New Definitions of Health & Wholeness

To better understand some of the differences in therapeutic approach between the traditional and holistic practitioner, one must first appreciate that the end points of treatment between these two health-care provider groups differ significantly. The reason for this discrepancy is that there are significant differences in the ways that holistic and traditional physicians define health, dysfunction, and illness.

The typical orthodox physician has a busy practice of patients who come to him or her for various types of medical assistance. Most people who go to the doctor are motivated by the search for relief of a particular symptom or group of symptoms which are causing dysfunction and distress in their normal daily lives. People seek medical attention because of aches and pains, coughs and colds, fatigue, and various other problems that create feelings of dis-ease. Because orthodox medicine has become extremely time-limited, due largely to financially imposed restrictions, the traditional physician seeks to quickly treat particular health problems brought to his or her attention, and to return patients to their previous state of functioning.

In recent years, modern medical education has become focused upon what is referred to as the "problem-oriented management approach." Using this style of health management, physicians address their attention to specific identifiable problems that patients bring to their attention. The endpoint of therapy is thus the resolution of those problems. If something is not discussed with the physician as being problematic, it is not entered in the list of problems to be dealt with; thus many other potentially important aspects of the patient's life are often ignored. Although this particular model of practice has benefits in a time-limited system of health care, it is often less than an ideal system.

In addition to the history, the patient's physical exam may bring the physician to identify problems of which the patient is unaware, such as an elevated blood pressure, an enlarged liver, or possibly signs of anemia. Therefore, the problem-oriented approach is not strictly limited to patient complaints, but also to the physician's assessment of the patient from both the history taken and from his or her physical diagnostic acumen. This system of information gathering is a good starting point from which to approach patient care. But it may ignore other pertinent aspects of the patient's life which are not identified as problematic.

Most traditional physicians seek to assist patients in returning to a state of health where there are no further identifiable problems. This means that when the patient is asked how he or she is feeling, or if he/she has any problems, the person states that "everything is OK." If no physical abnormalities can be defined by examination or blood testing, the patient is pronounced "OK" and told to return for yearly exams. The state of "OK" is, in reality, often a state of neutrality. That is, "OK" is defined as a state of "no symptoms." This is the goal of traditional medicine—to get the patient to a state of no symptoms or to a state of no identifiable problems.

Indeed, *that which is defined as a problem is truly in the "eye of the beholder": the physician assessor. It is only within the consciousness of the physician that things are given weight and labelled as problems.* Thus, it is within the scope of questions asked by the physician during patient histories, and within the attention given to particular areas of the patient's life, that problems are identified and focused upon. Beyond history taking, the identification of other problems is dependent upon the physical examination skills of the physician and the sensitivity of laboratory tests which might be ordered.

In reality, health and illness exist along a spectrum of varying degrees of dysfunction. The midpoint of the spectrum is the "OK" point or the state of neutrality. The neutral state is the endpoint of therapy for most busy traditional physicians. When symptoms arise, a shift in health occurs from the neutral midpoint toward the eventual production of illness. If illness is serious and left to progress untreated, the endpoint of this process can be death. Within traditional medicine, such limited definitions of health and illness seem to have prevailed. Orthodox practitioners see human beings existing between the opposite poles of "life" and "death," with illness and disability occuring somewhere in between. But can life merely be a function of existing without physical symptoms? Surely there must be something beyond living in a state of neutrality. In holistic medicine, the aim of therapy is not the achievement of neutrality but rather the achievement of what has been defined as a state of optimal health or "wellness."

Diagram 33.
THE ILLNESS/WELLNESS CONTINUUM

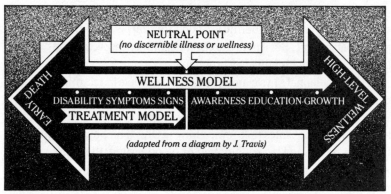

NEUTRAL POINT
(no discernible illness or wellness)

DEATH

EARLY

HIGH-LEVEL

WELLNESS

WELLNESS MODEL

DISABILITY SYMPTOMS SIGNS | AWARENESS EDUCATION GROWTH

TREATMENT MODEL

(adapted from a diagram by J. Travis)

There is a great difference between "OK" and wellness. We would define wellness as a state in which a human being functions at an optimal level of integration between the elements of body, mind and spirit. The well individual is one who is happy, healthy, and whole, and who perceives his or her life as one with meaning and purpose. Implicit within the definition of health and wellness is a shift in consciousness that assists learning of new ideas, aids in finding new meaning in understanding of self, and in general, supports continued psychological and spiritual growth of the individual.

From a treatment perspective, the focus on wellness means that holistic physicians direct attention to health problems that affect both the body and the mind. Included in the issues of mind's effect on the body are emotional reactions to physical illness as well as psychological factors that may be contributing to the expression or exacerbation of disease. The holistic physician is not only a healer and psychotherapist but also a teacher. Patients are instructed in some of the intricacies of the mind/body relationship and taught how seemingly unconnected events, such as emotions and physical symptoms, can be integrally related.

It is well known, even by traditional physicians, that the body and mind greatly influence each other. That which negatively affects the body also produces accompanying emotional distress as well. Thus, physical illness creates emotional stress. Conversely, primary emotional disturbances contribute to bodily symptoms such as in somatization of depression or the expression of stress-related disorders. Holistic physicians tend to be more attentive toward the emotional aspects of somatic dysfunction than are their traditional counterparts. The holistic practitioner questions patients about their emotional health and well-being in relation to various types of stress that may be affecting them at home, at work, or in their relationships. Unfortunately, such important questions are often left unasked by many traditional physicians.

The push toward large, organized networks of salaried health-care workers in clinic-type settings tends to promote time-limited interviews and patient interactions in the face of busy scheduling and financial demands. The brief time spent with patients in these clinics, usually with different doctors each time, focuses attention on specific physical problems only. The proliferation of health maintenance organizations and of similar organizational structures which offer the so-called "benefits" of paying for regular checkups, are actually promoting briefer and more cursory examinations in the name of lower cost. The aim of many of these newer health-care systems is the maintenance of the "no symptom" state of their clinic populations; nothing more, nothing less.

Not to be entirely critical of orthodox medicine, there are many traditional practitioners who do attend to the emotional needs of their patients. With increasing frequency, educational seminars are being conducted for physicians to emphasize the importance of early diagnosis and treatment of depression in their patients. The link between stress and illness is recognized by most traditional physicians. In recent years, medical science has gained a greater awareness of the psychophysiologic pathways by which stress can manifest as illness in the body. Although traditional physicians do recognize the stress-illness link, they tend to approach patients differently than their holistic counterparts. There are significant differences in both the methods of diagnosis as well as the therapeutic modalities employed by each group of health-care providers. Perhaps one of the most important ways that traditional and holistic physicians differ is in their identification of particular stressors that may be contributing to illness and disease.

There are actually many types of stress which can influence human beings. Psychological stress has been given the most press of late and is perhaps the most omnipresent. It is important to understand, however, that to some degree, stress is in the eye of the beholder. That is, the stress reaction is based upon the individual's perception of some type of threat to their personal well-being. The threat may be real or it may be something which is either consciously or unconsciously perceived as threatening.

The degree of stress symptoms that manifests in an individual depends upon the effectiveness of the coping strategies for dealing with stress. Individuals who are good copers have fewer stress-related physical symptoms and have recently been found to have higher levels of immunologic function. The better the immune system is working, the less likelihood of falling ill to coughs, colds, and other types of common infectious diseases.

An important point to be understood is that a certain amount of stress is necessary for growth. For instance, the bones of the body become stressed by supporting the body's weight in Earth's gravitational field. The distribution of this stress along the skeletal structure is necessary for proper bone formation. Microscopic examination of weight-bearing bones shows calcification along lines of force. The cellular crystallization pattern in these bones is due to the piezoelectric translation of gravitational pressure into electrical potentials, which shape the bone into an optimal stress-bearing structure. If gravitational stress is removed, as when astronauts are on prolonged space journeys or when an individual remains in bed for a lengthy period of time, calcium is reabsorbed and the bones become weaker.

So a certain amount of stress is functional to maintaining optimal health. Hans Selye, the pioneering stress researcher, referred to this optimal level of stress as *eustress*. If this level of stress is exceeded, causing dysfunction in the system, the individual experiences *distress*. Therefore, it is not necessary nor desirable to have an environment that is totally without stress. Some level of stress and obstacles provides the impetus for growth and the creation of strategies to deal with new and demanding situations. The formation of successful coping strategies to deal with stress helps to minimize the dysfunctional effects on the system, and allows the individual to function at an optimal level in a variety of demanding environmental situations. The key here is the use of *successful* coping strategies.

Most people acquire defense mechanisms and coping strategies by hit or miss. They tend to repeat old responses to new challenges which have somehow gotten them through situations in the past. Unless they learn new strategies, they will continue to use the old ones, regardless of how beneficial or destructive they might be. For instance, in the face of stress, some people just turn inward, or else they may flee. Schizophrenia and psychosis might be seen as adaptive strategies used by some people to escape from environmental and psychological stresses. Other people lock themselves away and eat to relieve their stresses. Some merely weather the stresses but worry themselves sick with neurotic fantasies that amplify the perceived threats beyond their true weights. Strategies for coping may be a means of adapting, but in many cases, these methods are more maladaptive and destructive than beneficial.

From a therapeutic standpoint, stress reduction techniques offer a method of teaching patients new strategies for dealing with stress. Many people truly do not know how to relax. Everyone has the potential of benefitting from practicing these stress reduction techniques on a daily basis. Individuals with stress-related disorders may tend to benefit the most from using these approaches, but everyone who uses them will find greater emotional health and well-being. Relaxation techniques, especially meditative practices, are perhaps the best educational tools we can offer to people to promote a preventative approach to psychological and physical health.

There are numerous systems of relaxation, from mantra repetition to progressive muscle relaxation and verbally guided imagery techniques. Another less cognitive method of stress reduction is vigorous physical exercise. Exercise is a recognized method of releasing pent-up muscle stress that is left over from the day's thoughts and activities. However, exercise alone does not necessarily prevent further worry and anxiety throughout the rest of the day. Another effective method of releasing muscle tension acquired by stress and worry is massage therapy. Unfortunately, this is not something that can easily be done when one is alone.

One of the better aspects of self-taught relaxation approaches is the establishment of new patterns of neurological response following long periods of technique repetition. Practicing such inner quieting methods in the tranquility of one's home allows the nervous system to become conditioned in such as a way as to turn on the "relaxation response" when there are no distractions. After neural pathways have become well established, such relaxation techniques become effective in helping people at work dissolve muscular tension or abort headaches before the symptoms of stress become full blown.

As discussed in the previous chapter, daily meditation is extremely effective in helping people to become more relaxed and less likely to manifest the severe effects of psychological stress. Activation of the kundalini energies through years of daily meditation becomes the ultimate stress release mechanism available to human beings. After the kundalini has been activated, the circuitry of the brain may become reorganized in a way that will prevent the accumulation of smaller stresses and traumas over a period of time. *Perhaps more individuals would practice meditation if they were aware that the stress release system of the kundalini cycle was built into their inner biocircuitry.* Also, meditation allows us to tap into that vast resource of creativity, knowledge, guidance, and inspiration which we call the Higher Self.

In addition to vigorous physical activity and the various meditative and relaxation techniques, proper nutrition is also important in conditioning the body to respond optimally to stressful situations. Although vitamin supplementation is an area of controversy and disagreement between the holistic and traditional medical communities, this aspect of nutrition can greatly assist the body and mind to better deal with stress. High doses of vitamin C and B-complex, and a balanced multivitamin containing trace elements and minerals, may be of great assistance in strengthening the nervous system to prevent exaggerated stress responses.[8]

Speaking from personal experience, I would probably not have survived my medical residency had it not been for the effectiveness of the vitamins I took in a preventative fashion. In spite of long shifts lasting 36 hours with no sleep, I was awake and fairly alert as long as I kept up with my vitamin regimen. If I forgot to bring along my vitamins for the morning after being on call, I had pronounced feelings of fatigue and exhaustion at the end of the shift. I have been convinced of the efficacy of megadose vitamin therapy for preventing stress reactions by my own personal experience as well as through feedback from the many patients I have placed on similar regimens.

Many vitamins (in appropriately high dosages) not only allow the physical body to function at an optimal level but may also strengthen the etheric body, making the physical and subtle energetic systems more resistant to stress and illness. Orthomolecular proponents have noted significant augmentation of the immune response by vitamin C, especially in treating certain viral illnesses such as infectious mononucleosis and viral pneumonias for which orthodox medicine has little to offer. Vitamins are known to be cofactors in many physiological reactions which involve energy utilization throughout the body. In addition to assisting in chemical enzyme reactions, many vitamins contain metallic ions at their active sites which make them important in electron transfers at the cellular level. Vitamins facilitate proper energy flow through the electron switching mechanisms of the cell. These bioelectronic systems control the basic processes of growth, replication, and repair. There has also been some suggestion that the effect of vitamins on electron flow at the cellular level may help strengthen important interactions between the etheric and physical body. For this reason, vitamin therapy is relevant to the topic of vibrational medicine, because vitamins assist the body in promoting cellular health and wellness at a vibrational or bioenergetic level.

Part of the controversy over vitamins within the medical establishment stems from differing views between holistic and traditional physicians as to their usage. Orthodox medicine has long thought that all the vitamins an individual needs are provided by a balanced diet. Vitamin supplements have been downplayed in most medical education programs around the country until quite recently. Traditional physicians have tended to criticize the overuse of vitamins by holistic practitioners and lay people as contributing to their status as a panacea for many illnesses. The controversy over vitamin efficacy is also a reflection of the differing views between the orthodox medical standard of neutrality, and the therapeutic goal of wellness.

Traditional physicians quote the much touted RDA (Recommended Daily Allowance) as their source of information telling them that a balanced American diet provides all the nutrients necessary for health. Orthodox physicians and hospital nutritionists proclaim that the RDA of vitamins provides all that is needed, and since that amount occurs naturally in a balanced diet, no vitamin supplements are required. The RDA is based upon studies which have determined the minimum amount of each vitamin that will prevent a vitamin deficiency disorder from occurring. If a person takes 50 milligrams of vitamin C a day, then that individual will not get scurvy. A state of "no scurvy," or neutrality, is actually a far cry from a state of optimal health and wellness.

This was an important issue many years ago when first discussed by

Albert Szent-Gyorgi, who was the discoverer of vitamin C and a proponent of bioelectronic mechanisms of cellular replication and repair. Orthodox medical scientists have continued to have great difficulty in understanding that there is more to the use of vitamin C than the treatment of deficiency disorders such as scurvy. Some surgeons do give their post-operative patients vitamin C to promote collagen production, which assists in wound healing, but too few employ this practice on a regular basis.

The reason that conventional physicians do not prescribe vitamins, except in cases of overt vitamin deficiency, is that they are satisfied with keeping patients in a state of neutrality. There are definite benefits to taking higher doses of vitamin C and other vitamins to optimize one's immune response and other physiological functions. When the physical system is nutritionally primed to handle stress, there is less likelihood of immunosuppression, infection, and illness.

Orthomolecular physicians treat particular health disorders with individual nutrients in high doses in a way that demonstrates the difference between using vitamins in a physiologic versus a pharmacologic manner. Conventional doctors only consider the physiologic value of vitamin doses to promote baseline cellular functioning. Alternatively, holistic practitioners prescribe megadoses of individual vitamins to achieve pharmacologic effects. In other words, vitamins given at high doses are like giving conventional drugs to treat illness. If too low a dose of a particular drug is given to a patient, then the therapeutic benefits of that drug will not be achieved. Vitamins are only now being considered for use in the same fashion.

For instance, intravenous magnesium sulfate has long been given to pregnant women with toxemia in order to prevent seizures. Magnesium given in pharmacologic doses has the effect of decreasing neuromuscular excitability. Because it is a nutrient, magnesium is considered safer to give to pregnant women than anticonvulsant medications. Many holistic physicians, and now certain cardiologists, are beginning to catch on to other uses of magnesium. For instance, magnesium has recently been recognized to be of use in preventing abnormal heart rhythms during the acute phase of a heart attack. Some nutritional physicians even use oral magnesium to treat long-term arrhythmias in patients other than those with heart attacks.

More recently, there has been evidence suggesting that giving high doses of folic acid and vitamin B-12 to smokers and women with premalignant cellular pathology reverses the lesions.[9,10] Early reports by Dr. Charles E.

Butterworth, chairman of nutrition sciences at University of Alabama, suggest that abnormal (metaplastic) sputum cytology in smokers, and precancerous pap smears in women, revert to normal if patients are maintained on 10 milligrams of folic acid and 500 micrograms of B-12 daily. These amounts are 25 and 166 times the RDA of folate and B-12, respectively.

Obviously, there are still limits to the maximal amount of a particular vitamin that one should consume, and even the orthomolecular nutritionists have guidelines for megadose usage. Orthodox physicians warn that the ingestion of vitamin C can increase urinary oxalate excretion and may produce oxalate kidney stones if megadoses are used. This manifestation of kidney stones from megadose vitamin C usage has rarely been seen in normal individuals, mainly because most people take vitamin C with vitamin B-complex, which contains high doses of pyridoxine (vitamin B-6). Linus Pauling and others have found that 25 to 50 milligrams of vitamin B-6 taken daily will decrease urinary oxalate excretion, thus negating the potential threat of oxalate stone formation.[11] This also reinforces the point that high doses of single vitamins should not be used alone, but in combination with other vitamins in a balanced proportion. High doses of vitamin C can actually cause decreases in other trace elements such as copper. So the use of a mineral and trace-element-containing multivitamin is important. There are many good sources on vitamin therapy which elaborate further on the specifics of this type of treatment. Vitamin therapy is a simple step that can be taken along with the aforementioned stress reduc-

Diagram 34.

THE VARIETY OF BIOLOGICAL STRESSES

PSYCHOLOGICAL STRESS
NUTRITIONAL DEFICIENCY
ALLERGENIC OVERLOAD
ENVIRONMENTAL POLLUTANTS
PHYSICAL OVEREXHAUSTION
EXTREME TEMPERATURE VARIATION
MICROBIOLOGIC CONTAMINATION
DRUG SIDE EFFECTS
LOW LEVEL RADIATION
ELECTROMAGNETIC POLLUTION
GEOPATHIC STRESS
NEGATIVE THOUGHT ENERGIES

tion techniques to equip the body/mind in better dealing with the stresses of everyday life.

What many do not realize is that there are actually many types of stressors besides emotional stress which can negatively affect the human bioenergetic system by inducing abnormal physiological reactions and eventually illness. Psychological stress is only one of many subtle influences in our modern civilized society which promotes the manifestation of disease states.

Diagram 34 lists a variety of internal and external factors which many would not ordinarily consider as stress. Nonetheless, each of these is a stress which pushes the body/mind from its normal state of physiological functioning and, depending upon its intensity over time, can result in states of illness and disease. Many different types of stress have a common effect in that they decrease the general vitality of the body. In addition, these stresses eventually affect the performance of the immune system and other regulatory mechanisms, making the body more susceptible to attack from a variety of outer and inner threats to well-being. The differing views between traditional and holistic practitioners may be seen in regard to the significance which physicians give to each of the above-mentioned stresses for their potential contribution to everyday illness. Many of the above-listed stressors would not even be considered as such by the orthodox medical establishment. We shall go through each of these, from the more recognized and "physical," to the more subtle and less well-known stress factors, and examine how they might be considered as potential threats to our health and well being.

Psychological Stress

We have already discussed the effects of emotional stress. It is known that emotional depression and other negative cognitive states may be associated with relative immunosuppression which opens up the body to various types of illnesses. Also, specific types of emotional imbalances relate to individual chakras of the body (as discussed in Chapter 10) and may later express themselves as particular types of illnesses relative to the level of energetic blockage being produced.

Stressful Climatic & Working Conditions

Pure physical sources of stress, such as overexhaustion from putting in too many hours at work with too little sleep, are a common source of emotional and physical imbalance, and may place the individual in a state of greater disease susceptibility. Also, constant changing of working schedules from day to night shift and vice-versa places unusual stress on the body's adaptation mechanisms, similarly leading to increased fatigue, decreased vitality, and a greater likelihood of illness. There are many other physical stress factors that are recognized as contributing to the production of illness. Extreme variation in temperature can produce instability in the body which contributes to illness. The ancient Chinese recognized conditions of excessive dampness or coolness as significant disease-associated environmental factors. Asthmatics often experience acute asthmatic attacks when constantly going from hot summer outdoor weather to chilly air-conditioned places.

Drug-Related Stresses

Other sources of physiological stress include side effects from the many drugs we ingest, either through prescriptions or from the many over-the-counter drugs we now have available. In addition, there is now a widespread use of cocaine, heroin, LSD, amphetamines, marijuana, and other illicit recreational drugs which are sources of much distress and illness for chronic users. These drugs also produce long-term effects upon the physical nervous system and subtle bodies which modern medicine has not yet discovered. The emotional and psychiatric disturbances associated with the use of many of these mind-altering chemicals are keys to understanding the potency of their negative effects upon the human subtle-energy system. There are also many potentially disturbing side effects from prescription drugs which can result in the production of silent or overt illness. This area is one that is well recognized by the traditional medical community, but remains a considerable source of unrecognized stress to everyone who relies on medicines in our increasingly drug-oriented society.

Nutritional Stresses Due to Deficiencies & Sensitivities

States of nutritional deficiency are also stressful because they force the body to work without all the necessary ingredients for optimal functioning. Relative nutritional deficiency states exist more and more today in our fast food society. Older individuals who may be ill, or are afflicted with arthritis or neurological impairment from strokes, have less mobility and are often not able to cook for themselves. This makes seniors especially prone to true vitamin-deficiency states. The use of various prescription drugs also results in the depletion of particular vitamins.

As orthodox medicine has increased the sensitivity of specific tests, traditional physicians have slowly begun to acknowledge an even longer list of vitamin-like substances, including trace elements and minerals, that are necessary for the maintenance of health. But there are still many essential elements which need to be added to this list. Through the use of vibrational measuring devices, science will confirm that trace amounts of certain substances, such as gold, are also necessary for optimal health. It is probable that many of the more esoteric trace metals are involved in vibrational and bioelectronic systems throughout the bodily organs and central nervous system. The Edgar Cayce readings often mentioned gold deficiency as an importance etiologic factor in multiple sclerosis. Gold deficiency was linked with a defect in the assimilation or digestive system which led to glandular imbalance and later to dysfunction within the nervous system. Thus, nutritional deficiency states may include deprivation of not only vitamins and minerals, but also of necessary metals and trace elements like gold, silver, silicon, carbon, and others that have not yet been recognized as being important for optimal health.

In addition to vitamins and trace elements that may be missing from our diets, there are also naturally-occurring substances within food that may be considered an additional source of physiological stress. Unrecognized allergies or cerebral sensitivities to phenolic derivatives in common foods can produce a wide variety of dysfunctional symptoms. Such sensitivity reactions may be caused by disturbances of the immune system along less well studied paths of expression. The recognition of these subtle sensitivities to elements in food and our environment has resulted in the newly developing field of clinical ecology. The majority of orthodox medical practitioners do not consider food allergies in many of their patients. The reason for this is that, aside from itching, hives, or asthmatic attacks, most traditional physicians do not believe that food allergies, or cerebral sensitivity to foods, can cause changes in mood, emotional depression, extreme fatigue, muscular aches and pains, and a variety of other symptoms. Most do not even acknowledge a belief that cerebral sensitivity disorders exist, mainly because they do not understand how such reactions could occur outside of conventionally recognized immunologic pathways.

One of the difficulties in diagnosing food allergies is that patients are often unaware of their particular allergies, and conventional skin testing is typically of little use. Also, the symptoms patients may be experiencing are not associated in their mind with the ingestion of particular foods. Because the area of clinical ecology is still largely unrecognized by the traditional medical community, a food allergy diagnosis will not often be considered. Therefore, patients are given standard medical workups for their symptoms. When all testing comes back negative, patients are either sent on a roundabout trial of various medical specialists or are referred to psychiatrists. It is difficult to believe that the food we eat may be producing physiologic stress, but it is an idea whose time has come.

The difficulty in diagnosing environmental sensitivities is that most methods of detection are laboriously slow and painstaking. One system which has been able to provide rapid diagnosis in detecting allergenic materials is the Voll Machine, which employs electroacupuncture methods of measurement (see Chapter 6). This system is more sensitive than conventional blood or skin tests because it interfaces directly with the bioenergetic network of the acupuncture meridian system.

The Voll Machine allows one to test an individual for sensitivities or dysfunctional responses to many different materials. Practitioners who utilize the Voll system of electrodermal diagnosis are able to test patients for a wide variety of allergic sensitivities in a short period of time. More importantly, the Voll Machine is able to determine the exact strength of homeopathic remedy which will neutralize the allergic symptoms.

Because the Voll Machine and other similar electrodermal diagnostic systems interface directly with the acupuncture meridian system, they allow one to tap into the physical-etheric interface. This means that they are able to measure energy dysfunction which may not have yet become manifest in the physical body as chronic or acute illness.

The problems with detecting many of these allergies is that there are few conventional tests available which have the sensitivity of the Voll system in detecting the abnormal reactions. The Voll system primarily determines an abnormal energy response, and not something that would necessarily show up in a blood or skin test. In fact, the sensitivity reactions are to some extent an energetic as well as a physio-chemical annoyance to the body. Much of the problem with the inability of orthodox medicine to recognize many of these stresses is that some of the body/mind disturbances may be extremely hard to detect. The reactions may be too subtle, in fact, to be picked up by the gross tests employed by the medical community at this point in its evolution. Unfortunately, it has been the opinion of many physicians that if a patient complains of a problem that does not bear substantiation by some type of abnormal lab test, x-ray, or scan, then the problem is probably all in the patient's head.

In other words, *problems are defined by their measurement through orthodox medical testing.* When we examine the list of contemporary stresses, most doctors might be afraid to employ more sensitive testing, such as the Voll Machine, for fear of results which would show the widespread influence of modern environmental stress. If the traditional physician has no way to objectively measure any abnormality in the patient's physiology either through physical examination or testing, then in his or her mind the problem does not physically exist. There are obviously serious consequences to this type of fallacious reasoning. We are confronted by a common illustration of this problem when we deal with the stress of environmental pollution.

Environmental Stress, Pollution & Miasmatic Illness

There are an increasing number of substances which have recently been added to the list of potentially harmful environmental pollutants. More often than not, the definition of a harmful substance is based upon giving massive quantities of a particular suspect chemical to rats and then slicing them open at autopsy to look for cancers or other physical abnormalities. The Ames test for detecting potential carcinogens looks at the ability of a chemical to cause genetic mutations in bacteria to determine its carcinogenicity. Even the tobacco companies and their lobbyists still proclaim that there is no definite link between cigarette smoking and such illnesses as heart disease and lung cancer. However, the current medical establishment does acknowledge a strong association of various types of cancer with cigarette smoking. It is only recently that doctors have begun to study the more subtle effects of cigarette smoke on passive smokers, and the potential danger to developing unborn children. Yet, most people in our culture tend to focus only on the more overt, negative side-effects of the chemicals in cigarette smoke, such as the production of cancer.

One of the problems with this limited definition of toxic side effects is that it is extremely hard to determine whether environmental chemicals are causing any adverse effects upon human health. Conventional medicine's ability to measure the effects of various pollutants is limited by the sensitivity of current medical testing. This is the same argument we find ourselves up against when trying to prove the negative effects of various food allergies. Doctors' willingness to recognize a substance as harmful is dependent upon them seeing evidence that the agent produces ill effects. The quality of evidence that scientists use to substantiate the negative effects of a substance is largely a function of the sensitivity of their tools for measuring abnormal physiologic reactions. Conventional laboratory tests are too gross to measure subtle abnormalities like those produced by food allergies and sensitivities to other common environmental agents. This is one of the reasons why the development of vibrational medicine and subtle-energy diagnostic systems is so important. If we are to be able to really assess the health consequences of a whole system of new food additives, new drugs, and new chemicals in the workplace, we must support more sensitive testing.

There are so many unseen negative influences on human health that are missed by conventional medical practitioners that many sources of human suffering remain undetected. It is recognized that sulfur dioxide and carbon monoxide are airborne pollutants which are harmful to human health. These chemicals place abnormal stresses on the body's physiology and lead to the manifestation of illness in certain susceptible individuals. *Disease susceptibility as a consequence of exposure to environmental pollutants is partly a function of the strength of the body's immunologic, physiologic, and energetic defense mechanisms.*

The production of environmental illness is not strictly related to exposure to levels of harmful substances that are higher than FDA safety limits. *Conventional safety limits of exposure do not take into account the subtle vibrational effects of toxic substances.* Because of their inability to comprehend vibrational levels of toxicity, the orthodox scientific community is more lenient in defining safe levels of exposure to many harmful substances. The inadequacy of conventional scientific testing to measure subtle negative disturbances to human physiology also limits the FDA's ability to define exactly which substances are really harmful to human beings, let alone the concentration necessary for toxic effects.

In Chapter 2 we discussed how homeopathic remedies are produced by creating infinitessimally small dilutions of physical substances in order to extract the energy essence of that substance for therapeutic application. By the same token, infinitessimally small amounts of environmental materials can have subtle effects that are not easily measured by gross laboratory tests. An interesting case in point is the metal aluminum, and the potential threat of aluminum toxicity. Because of its easy workability and low cost, aluminum cookware has found its way into many of our homes and kitchens. When these pots are scrubbed and cleaned, or stirred while cooking, infinitessimally small amounts of aluminum metal are liberated, dissolved, and later ingested. Recent evidence suggests that even larger amounts of aluminum are released during cooking and stirring food in aluminum pots if fluoridated water is used.

Some recent research into Alzheimer's disease, an increasing cause of dementia in the population, has shown that a significant number of patients with this disorder have high aluminum levels in brain tissue. Although it may not necessarily be true that aluminum cookware is directly causing Alzheimer's disease, the metal may somehow be participating in the expression of the disease process. The possible linkage of aluminum toxicity with Alzheimer's dementia raises the question of how safe it is to cook with aluminum.

This type of subtle aluminum toxicity may be a function of people's ability to absorb or excrete aluminum taken in through the gastrointestinal tract. For example, researchers studying Parkinson's disease at the Bob Hope Parkinson Research Center utilized Motoyama's AMI electroacupuncture diagnostic system and discovered energetic imbalances in the intestinal meridians of many Parkinsonian patients. It is possible that the common imbalances in the nervous system and digestive system of Parkinson patients are due to an abnormal link between the bowel and brain. The link may be indirect, in that the disease may be dependent upon exposure to a third factor which operates upon the preexisting physiological weaknesses. *Abnormalities in the normal functions of absorption and excretion by the intestines may result in a buildup of certain toxic elements in the nervous system.* Excessive accumulation of toxic agents in the brain could lead to neurological dysfunction in the form of Parkinson's disease. This link between abnormal digestive tract functioning and neurological disease has also been mentioned in many of the Edgar Cayce readings. If this speculation is correct, then some types of aluminum and heavy-metal toxicity may be more pronounced in certain susceptible individuals (i.e., Alzheimer's patients) with intestinal meridian imbalances.

It is likely that conventional medical research techniques are too insensitive to give adequate information to either support or reject this theory. What is needed is more research into various illnesses like Alzheimer's disease, Parkinson's disease, and many others that are poorly understood at this time. Subtle-energy measuring devices, such as the Voll Machine and AMI system, must be utilized to expand on our database of information. With a new pool of information, it is possible that we might also discover viable therapeutic modalities which would make a difference in similar "incurable" illnesses.

There are many substances in our environment including asbestos,

PCB's, dioxin, and formaldehyde, which orthodox scientists have only begun to acknowledge as harmful or stressful to human beings. There are probably many more unknown than known harmful substances in our man-made environment which have yet to be defined as being detrimental to human health. Again, the ability to define chemical stress to our human systems depends upon the sensitivity of one's measuring devices. By utilizing the Voll Machine and other new sensitive measuring systems, scientists will begin to find that many substances formerly thought to be safe at current environmental levels may actually be causing untold silent illness and distress. Aluminum is only one such potential toxin in our everyday environment.

Another potentially harmful metal is mercury, as used in the mercury amalgams of dental fillings. There is a growing body of information to suggest that mercury in dental fillings may be responsible for a signficant amount of undiagnosed chronic illness.[12] Radionic practitioners, who work at a much more subtle level of energy diagnosis, have also found a link between aluminum, mercury, and physical disorders.

> It is also relevant to note that physical and etheric imbalances do not only arise from conventional infections, but can be produced by unsuspected influences from the environment which are inimicable to the human organism. The most important of these is the prevalent use of aluminum utensils both for cooking and in the preparation of processed foods. This has a detrimental influence which does not arise from any chemical reaction within the body, but from the absorption by the food of certain energies in the aluminum which are incompatible with bodily harmony. This form of aluminum poisoning or toxicity is not recognized by the orthodoxy, but its influence is widespread and often found as a major toxin when completing a radionic analysis.
>
> Prolonged absorption of aluminum and other noxious toxins, such as mercury and silver from amalgam fillings in the teeth, have far reaching effects on the physical and etheric form. These many noxious influences in fact are the unsuspecting cause of many ills, some specific in symptoms, others merely resulting in a general lowering of vitality.[13]

In addition to subtle toxic effects of common heavy metals, there are additional harmful environmental influences which have been neglected by orthodox medicine. In Chapter 7 we discussed the importance of certain illness-producing energy states known as miasms. Unlike the conventional physician, homeopathic doctors have long suspected that miasms are caused by subtle-energy disturbances in the human biofield. Kevin Ryerson, the psychic source of technical information in Gurudas' book *Flower Essences and Vibrational Healing,* has suggested that we are beginning to see new types of these illness-producing states. Most significant of these new miasms are the heavy metal, petrochemical, and radiation miasms. Although the medical community expresses some concern for radiation hazards due to diagnostic x-rays, background environmental radiation has largely been downplayed. The subtle effects of radiation, aside from the production of leukemia and certain cancers by very high exposure levels, is not well understood; nor is it considered to be a common source of illness. Similarly, petrochemicals and their many derivatives are an increasing source of undiagnosed toxicities that have been finding their way into our environment.

Miasmatic conditions place the organism in an energy state of potential system breakdown or illness susceptibility. Miasms tend to impede the flow of the life-force into the human bioenergetic system, and also create a greater potential for the manifestation of many different types of illnesses. These miasms can be treated with various vibrational modalities that restore an energy equilibrium with the life-force. Particular flower essences, gem elixirs, and homeopathic remedies are good examples of vibrational rebalancers. However, miasms cannot be treated unless they are recognized as a cause of illness. The traditional medical community has failed to acknowledge either the existence of miasms or their significance as a source of human suffering.

Miasms represent energy patterns which have been incorporated into the human bioenergetic system from the level of the subtle bodies, through the auric field, and down to the molecular and genetic levels. Some miasms are primarily stored in the cellular memory of the physical body. Albeit unknowingly, orthodox medical researchers have started probing the cellular mechanisms of certain miasmatic illnesses through their studies of the phenomena of "slow virus" infections.

Scientists have begun to recognize that it is possible to have an infection with a particular virus, have the symptoms of the illness subside, and yet have a portion of the virus's DNA incorporated into the genetic makeup of the cells of the infected individual. This viral genetic material is incorporated into the existing human chromosomal DNA of the cells. If this viral genome is carried in the reproductive cells of the body, it may even be transmitted to future generations. Some type of unidentified physiologic stress is suggested to cause an activation of the dormant viral DNA.

In examining existing illnesses which might serve as a model for "acquired" miasms (due to an infection acquired earlier in life), it is known that certain childhood viral infections (ex. measles) may become activated decades later, and sometimes result in a rare but devastating neurological disease such as SSPE (subacute sclerosing panencephalitis). Whether it is a form of dormant intact virus or merely a hidden virus DNA that is carried in the host's cells is unclear at this time, but the toxicity of the original viral infection persists at some molecular level to cause a different type of disease at a later time.

Multiple sclerosis may be another illness related to delayed toxic effects from a previous latent viral infection. One model suggests that an earlier viral infection causes some type of alteration in the myelin sheath of nerves, which later leads to a production of antibodies against both the altered and normal myelin surrounding the nerves. The result is a type of autoimmune destruction of myelin throughout the nervous system, which eventually interferes with nerve transmission. Scientists have referred to these types of latent virus-activated illnesses as "slow virus" infections. Most of the recognized slow viral diseases are related to dementia and disorders of the central and peripheral nervous system.

This principle of delayed toxicity from viruses demonstrates one route by which miasms are acquired through exposure to an infectious agent. However, *miasmatic tendencies are caused by bodily changes not only at the cellular level but also at the higher vibrational levels of human structure.* Stresses that release miasmatic potentials into the physical body to create illness may be psychological, environmental, or occasionally karmic. The state of energetic and physiological dysfunction induced by stress allows the molecular and subtle patterns of the miasms to become activated at the genetic and cellular levels. Miasmatic illness then occurs when this subtle-energy time bomb is exploded through the expression of the tainted genetic material. *Miasmatic diseases only become manifest in the physical body when our normal subtle energetic and physiologic watchdog mechanisms fail to suppress their expression.* In the case of slow viruses, some breakdown in the body's immune defenses may trigger the viral DNA's deadly latent potential. These miasmatic traits may lie dormant in the subtle bodies for many years, only to become manifest at a later time when stressful or karmic patterns have created a bioenergetic environment more conducive to their expression at the physical level. As the miasmatic energy tendencies move from the subtle bodies to the level of the physical cell and its nuclear DNA, illness results.

In addition to acquired miasms due to infectious agents, today's homeopaths understand that chronic exposure to environmental pollutants (petroleum derivatives, heavy metals, and radiation) can also result in the production of miasmatic/energetic tendencies toward illness. Of the heavy metals that can result in miasms, aluminum and mercury figure prominently along with lead, arsenic, radium, and fluoride. There is an increasing amount of lead in our environment due to the prevalence of the leaded gasolines which power our cars. Overt mercury poisoning has also become more widespread due to the concentration of mercury in certain types of fishes in our aquatic food chain. This is in addition to the widespread use of mercury amalgams in dental fillings, which may be causing subtle illness. Although minute quantities of many of these minerals existed in our environment for thousands of years, we have been able to build up a tolerance to their presence. It is only within the last century that toxic levels began to build up in the atmosphere and water supply. This has led to the production of acute illnesses from overt poisonings as well as to delayed side effects from the acquired miasms.

The heavy-metal and petrochemical miasms can result in allergies, hair loss, fluid retention, problems with calcium absorption, as well as greater susceptibility to viral infections. Miasmatic tendencies due to radiation contribute to premature aging, endocrine deterioration, weakening of bone structure, anemia, arthritis, lupus, as well as various types of cancer such as leukemia and skin cancer. The problem with the recognition of these miasms is that their effects are subtle, and difficult to measure with conventional laboratory tests. Yet their effects on the production of illness are beginning to be seen in increasing numbers. Miasms contribute to the many subtle causes of illness that go unrecognized by the traditional medical community. Vibrational remedies are one form of therapy which can often be effective in releasing the negative energy patterns of miasms. In view of the increasing pollution in the world today, vibrational medicine and its ability to provide answers to the problems caused by subtle toxicities will be of greater importance in the years to come.

In a way, these diseases may also be considered as spiritual maladies. Miasms and their "dis-ease" producing tendencies may be related to the struggle of the human spirit to recognize its own divinity through the expression of particular illnesses at the physical level. The radiation, petrochemical, and heavy-metal miasms may indicate a spiritual need for ecological evolution. We have said in earlier chapters that diseases often arise when there are chronic emotional and psychospiritual blockages that create difficulties in allowing the Higher Self to manifest through the ego or conscious personality. Miasms tie into this schema of emotional and spiritual blockage in an integral way.

> *The miasms collectively reflect peoples' wish to return to spirit in that diseases arise from blockages in accepting and acknowledging being Divine.* This, of course, may lead to various levels of stress that may activate the miasms and create disease. *Miasms crystallize mankind's struggle toward spiritual evolution.* First there is the need to rise above base sexuality, which includes overcoming syphilis and gonorrhea. Next, there is the use of the breath to draw upward and overcome tuberculosis. Finally, there is the need or attempt to overcome and master the environment. Thus, there is now the radiation, petrochemical, and soon the heavy metal miasms. Miasms reflect blockages in conscious growth that mankind has not yet overcome.[14]
> *(italics added)*

Although it is not always recognized, the divine essence of our Higher Self pushes us onward through the many obstacles and learning experiences that life has to offer. Negative or self-deprecating feelings that inhibit the flow of spiritual energies into physical reality create problems within not only the ego but also the physical body. Dysfunctional patterns of thinking and feeling inhibit energy movement through the chakras and ultimately disturb the physiological balance of the physical body. As we fall victim to our faulty belief systems, we create perceptual blockages that impede the flow of divine higher consciousness into our lives. These faulty perceptions of ourselves and the world around us create disharmony and stress at unconscious levels.

As we become disconnected from our spiritual roots, we fall prey to the untold forms of "dis-ease" that civilization has created. Many of these illnesses are reflections of the struggle taking place within the human race as we seek to rediscover our divine nature. Each disease represents a different hurdle that must be conquered to ascend the ladder of spiritual evolution. Infectious and toxic environmental factors are important negative influences that must be dealt with, but the susceptibility to these agents is often a reflection of an individual's level of conscious evolution and spiritual balance. Our ability to resist subtle and overt attack by microorganisms and noxious substances, and to tolerate living in a potentially threatening environment, is a reflection of how connected we feel to our divine Higher Selves.

It is critical that we begin to understand the importance of our connectivity to our spiritual roots. The spiritual element is an important aspect of health and wellness that is left out of the human equation by most traditional physicians. As the quote above states, there are important symbolic patterns to the kinds of illnesses and miasms to which people have become susceptible. *The miasms represent key issues or learning experiences which impede humanity's progress in its struggle toward spiritual evolution and enlightenment.* We are moving through a period in history when the tendency toward immediate self-gratification and sex without love has begun to have significant emotional and physical impacts upon our culture. From a spiritual perspective, it is interesting to see how sexually-associated diseases such as herpes and AIDS have become more prevalent at a time when human beings needed to take a closer look at relationships of the heart. The widespread concern over sexually-transmitted illnesses has created a new awareness about the over-expression of lower chakra energies. Sexually-related diseases will begin to focus new attention on the emotional and spiritual issues which relate to the energy blockages predisposing people to these illnesses.

Along with these spiritual imbalances, the negative influences of environmentally produced miasms have created difficulties in the immune systems of many people. These miasms have made individuals more susceptible to illnesses from a variety of infectious agents including the AIDS virus. The use of vibrational healing modalities to correct disturbances within the human energy system involves a process of not only rebalancing the physical body, but also of lifting the consciousness of the individual to new levels of spiritual attunement and awareness. This is a fundamental difference between vibrational and traditional medicine. Unlike drugs, which act solely on the physical body, vibrational treatments, especially flower essences and gem elixirs, work through their effects upon higher levels of consciousness, the subtle bodies, the chakras and the meridians, as well as the physical biomolecular form. While the chemical agents of modern medicine may treat the symptoms of disease, vibrational remedies create energy changes at multiple levels in order to produce a more lasting healing. Of course, the permanence of any healing will depend upon changing the subtle inner and outer factors which contributed to the creation of the illness. Vibrational healers attempt to assist patients in correcting their inner dysfunction by introducing lifestyle and mindstyle changes which may help to change negative habits and old perceptual patterns. Additionally, toxic environmental influences must be removed or vibrationally neutralized.

Electromagnetic Pollution

In addition to those already mentioned, there are other subtle forms of stress which can potentially affect the health and well-being of human beings. One of these stresses is electromagnetic radiation itself. As we have seen from our discussion of the unseen subtle toxicities of harmful environmental substances, established safety levels of various chemical and mineral pollutants, background radioactivity, and electromagnetic radiation are based solely on the measurement of gross negative biological effects such as the production of cancer or fetal abnormalities. Subtle biological effects cannot be measured by current detection systems because the systems are too insensitive. Thus, environmental dangers may be wrongly underemphasized. Living in an environment of high-voltage transmission lines, microwave ovens, cathode ray tubes, and other powerful electrical devices probably produces unseen negative biological effects that have yet to be determined. Recent studies have hinted at an increased incidence of childhood cancers in children of families living close to high-voltage transmission lines.[15] Other research indicates that pregnant rats, as well as their fetuses, develop learning deficits when exposed to ELF (extremely low frequency) electromagnetic fields. There has also been some evidence to suggest that constant exposure to microwave radiation from common microwave ovens may slightly increase the risk of developing cataracts. The Soviets, who have done much research into the subtle biological effects of microwave radiation on living organisms, have more stringent criteria for defining safety levels of microwave exposure than do our own American environmental agencies.

Geopathic Stress

In addition to environmental energy hazards from electromagnetic pollution, research suggests that there are additional threats to health from abnormal energy fields generated by the Earth itself. All living systems exist within a planetary energy field. It is likely that there are specialized energy rhythms within all organisms which have been entrained by living within the Earth's own field of natural energetic oscillations. Just as it is known that our biological clocks are affected by cyclic, diurnal rhythms of light, so is it probable that we have a bioenergy field entrainment with other energetic rhythms and energies associated with the planetary field.

The energy characteristics of the Earth's electromagnetic, gravitational, and subtle energetic fields are not homogeneous, but vary with geographical location. For instance, satellite detectors have mapped areas of gravitational fluctuation over certain geographic areas. In addition, the presence of large mineral deposits, such as quartz, and of underground flowing streams, can also affect the electromagnetic fields in the overlying regions. There is evidence to suggest that the Earth has its own meridian system made up of a planetary gridwork of subtle energy channels called ley lines. Just as metals can conduct subtle-energies, as in the Voll testing system, so can man-made metallic building structures conduct these energies, thus changing the pattern of energetic flow.

If, in fact, living organisms are entrained by the planetary field that they live in, there are probably beneficial as well as detrimental effects of particular patterns and types of local energy fields. It is apparent that the ancient Chinese were aware of these patterns of energy flow within the environment. And in the Orient today, as in the ancient past, the selection of favorable energetic sites for the construction of homes and businesses is assisted by the knowledge of these earth energy patterns via a form of geomancy called "feng-shui."[16]

Conversely, one might ask, "What is the effect of living in a field that is radically different from the beneficial field environment?" *Stressful effects upon human health, caused by abnormal fields associated with a particular geographical region, are referred to as "geopathic stress."* Studies in Germany and England have produced evidence which suggests that geopathic stress may not only contribute to the production of illness, but that such stresses may hinder the effective treatment of diseases as well.[17]

Researchers using the Vegatest system, an electroacupuncture diagnostic device similar to the Voll Machine, have discovered that there are subtle energetic patterns associated with blood which are analogous to the phenomenon of optical rotation polarity. It is known that certain molecules exist in both right and left-handed forms, and that each species of molecule, when dissolved in a transparent solution, will rotate the plane of polarized light in either a clockwise (right-handed) or counterclockwise (left-handed) direction. In general, living systems tend to favor the use of one handed form of molecules over another, such as with the amino acids associated with cellular processes. Using the Vegatest device, coupled with a system known as the Rotation Tester, researchers discovered that *the blood of normal individuals had a subtle energetic quality associated with the clockwise rotation or polarity.* It has been found that *individuals living in regions associated with geopathic stress tended to have a counterclockwise rotational polarity in their blood.* When such individuals moved their living quarters away from these abnormal areas, their blood eventually returned to normal clockwise polarity.

There are two interesting discoveries which relate to the presence of this counterclockwise polarity of the blood. Firstly, it has been found that *individuals with this abnormal polarity who are ill are usually resistant to any form of subtle energetic or vibrational medicine intervention.* Thus, geopathic stress may induce an energy state in the individual which opposes therapeutic attempts at vibrational rebalancing. In addition, clinical experience with the Vegatest system has shown that *a majority of patients with cancer possess this counterclockwise blood polarity.*

Such findings raise new questions as to the meaning of epidemiologic studies which link a high incidence of cancer to particular geographical regions and to certain family groupings. It is possible that the common factor in these situations is something more than shared heredity or exposure to local environmental carcinogens. The common element in such cancer clusterings may relate the presence of geopathic stress. This does not necessarily mean that geopathic stress, by creating this reverse polarity in the blood, is the cause of cancer. It is likely that the geopathic stress influence is one of many factors operating in the development of cancer. *The geopathic field probably acts in concert with a variety of other predisposing factors including diet, genetics, environmental carcinogens, viruses, abnormal electromagnetic radiation exposure, as well as the subtle-energy factors which affect general vitality and immune competence.*

There are a variety of methods available which can directly deal with neutralizing the influence of geopathic stress. The easiest way to remove such stress is to move the afflicted individuals and their belongings to different locations. Since this is not always economically feasible, individuals with experience in dowsing can examine the suspected deleterious home or work environment and make specific recommendations. The insertion of iron and steel rods at specific points in the earth, as well as the placement of crystals at specific field locations, can interrupt the abnormal energy patterns and neutralize the geopathic stress. In addition, there are electroacupuncture and radionic systems, such as the Mora device, which can be used to directly reverse the blood polarity in individuals and make sick persons with this condition more amenable to vibrational therapies.

Stresses Originating
Within the Human Multidimensional Energy Field

On yet a more ethereal level are the toxic dangers of working in an environment of negative thought energies. This last stress is perhaps one of the hardest to define, but it is worth mentioning as a potential source of unseen stress. Because thoughts are energy, and our thoughts create energy patterns in our auric fields, those individuals that come in contact with these energy fields may be subtly, yet unconsciously, affected. There appear to be certain individuals who, because of blockages or leaks in their own chakra system and auric field, are actually energy leeches. These people, either consciously or unconsciously, drain the energy and life-force from others that are around them. Many people know someone who makes them feel totally drained after spending only a short period of time with them. Oftentimes this draining person is an unconscious energy leech. Thus, our negative thought patterns and emotional disturbances may create health and energy problems not only in ourselves but in others around us.

Another spiritual malady, which is more of an inner than an outer stress, is something known as "divine discontent." It is a form of inner friction that will be seen with increasing frequency over the next ten or twenty years. This type of stress is due to an inner pushing from higher spiritual levels which seeks to subtly remind us (at conscious or unconscious levels) of the need to give greater expression to the divine qualities of the Higher Self. This form of subtle discontent is often a reflection of a person's movement toward higher consciousness, and is frequently seen in people who have spent years in daily spiritual practices such as meditation.

Divine discontent frequently comes after a gradual shift in thinking that moves people to listen to their intuitive inner directions and higher spiritual guidance. This inner guidance may provide avenues for alleviating inner conflict and discontent by suggesting a need for some type of personal change, whether it be in mental outlook, pattern of behavior, lifestyle, or even career direction. When one sees large differences between one's current lifestyle and the patterns of change suggested by one's higher guidance, further feelings of dissonance may be created, hence the term divine discontent. Sometimes people may simply feel that they are in a rut and are unsure of how they can get themselves out. They only know that there is something within which tells them that they are not following the inner direction of their soul. The only way to resolve the conflict is by slowly moving in a direction that is in greater accordance with their inner spiritual guidance.

It is important to understand that there are many invisible stresses that surround us throughout our daily lives. Psychological stress is only one type of stress that has been studied and its superficial physiological effects defined. My discussion of undefined (by traditional medicine) and unrecognized forms of stress which affect the human organism is an attempt to point out the many unseen influences upon human health. Vibrational medicine, with its attention to subtle-energy systems and higher dimensional anatomy, can provide, not only the physiological reasons behind these stressors' influence, but also the therapeutic methods for neutralizing their effects. By understanding at which levels humans are affected by stressful and disease-producing factors, future doctors will be able to treat patients at both the physical and subtle levels. Thus, physician/healers will be able to provide specific treatments that will correct the energy imbalances behind illness and naturally assist the healing process.

As we have seen, the current models of medical practice have promoted a level of patient-physician interaction which tends to deal mainly with superficial levels of diagnosis, therapy, and health maintenance. Traditional physicians are currently occupied with finding gross physical causes for illness, and with prescribing the right drug for the right disease in the shortest time course possible. Holistic medicine and its growing army of practitioners represents a gradual shift in medical approach. The holistic physician attends to the traditional physical ailments but also looks for less well-defined illness-producing factors, including emotional stress, food allergies, and nutritional deficiencies. Holistic practitioners address the issues of spiritual health as well as the emotional and physical determinants of health and illness, albeit frequently along the lines of traditional religious thinking.

Holistic medicine is a step in the right direction. But the somewhat conservative approaches of many holistic physicians must eventually be expanded upon with information and insights from the rapidly accumulating database of vibrational medicine. There are indications that this is already occurring, as many holistic practitioners are beginning to experiment with Bach Flower Remedies, homeopathic medicines, and electroacupuncture diagnostic systems. Vibrational medicine provides a scientific perspective of subtle physiology which will allow physicians to understand and treat the varied effects of stress on the human bioenergetic system. Utilizing new subtle-energy diagnostic technologies, we will begin to re-define exactly what stress is, and what the necessary elements are for health, growth, and wellness on a multiplicity of levels.

New Age technologies are beginning to grow in their abilities to image subtle disease states and to measure vibrational imbalances associated with illness on many energy levels. As these diagnostic systems become more widespread, physician/healers will become more proficient in their ability to detect potentially stressful and harmful factors in the life of each patient, whether it be food allergies, miasmatic tendencies, or reactions to subtle environmental pollutants. More importantly, having better defined those subtle stresses which may be having acute or chronic negative effects upon the patient's health, future physicians will be able to match the ap-propriate vibrational remedy to the patient's energetic needs. By correcting the patients' physical, emotional, mental, and spiritual imbalances through the use of vibrational treatments, meditative therapies, and personal growth techniques, the physician/healer of the future will be able to assist patients in moving beyond a state of neutrality to truly achieve a new level of health, personal growth, and wellness.

Key Points to Remember

1. We are on the verge of a major paradigm shift that extends across the sciences, from physics to medicine and biology. This shift involves a transition from the mechanistic Newtonian model to the acceptance of the Einsteinian paradigm of a complex, yet interconnected, energetic-field-like universe.

2. Consciousness is a form of energy. Consciousness evolves as it moves through and interacts with the physical vehicles of expression, as illustrated by reincarnational philosophy. It is the higher spiritual im-petus which drives the biological evolutionary process itself.

3. Human beings are mind/body/spirit complexes which exist in continuous dynamic equilibrium with higher energy dimensions of reality. These higher energies endow the physical vehicle with the pro-perties of life and creative expression.

4. The interface which regulates the flow of these higher energies into the physical framework is made up of the chakra-nadi system and the acupuncture meridian system, working in conjunction with the body's biocrystalline and bioelectronic networks.

5. Various approaches exist for treating heart disease. The orthodox medical model utilizes drugs, surgery, and various non-surgical tech niques of angioplasty to improve heart function. The holistic practitioners offer chelation therapy as an alternative medical therapy, in addition to visualization and stress reduction approaches. Vibrational practitioners would further deal with the subtle energetic predisposing factors (i.e. impaired heart chakra function) which contribute toward heart disease. This would include the use of various vibrational modalities such as flower essences and gem elixirs/crystal therapies, homeopathic remedies, and meridian-balancing treatments, in addition to inner spiritual-directed counseling. Ideally, each therapeutic option offered by the different schools of thought might be used to complement and augment the effectiveness of the others, as opposed to relying on any single technique. This integrated model is one which may eventually be extended toward treating all forms of disease in a multidisciplinary fashion.

6. The current medical model teaches a "problem-oriented approach" to doctors for dealing with illness. This means that a health problem can be identified and treated only if it is labelled as such by the health-care practitioner. As such, the ability to identify a health problem is a function of both the sensitivity of the medical systems used for diagnosis as well as the mind-set and clinical sensitivity of the individual practitioner.

7. As modern medicine continues to branch out into health maintenance organizations where medical care becomes more time-limited, practitioners will seek to focus on the treatment of more acute patient complaints and superficial problems. HMO doctors will tend to spend less time looking into minor complaints which are deemed not as important in their immediacy or significance. Such a focus is less conducive to examining health problems which are more subtle, yet may be of deeper long-term significance.

8. Part of the difference in approach between health-care practitioners has to do with the differences in defining health. Whereas the orthodox physician tends to focus on bringing the patient to the neutral

point or "OK" state as the endpoint of therapy, the vibrational and holistic health practitioner sees "wellness" as the goal of treatment. It also tends to take more individualized therapy and counseling time to get a person to a state of wellness than it does to get them "OK," but the long term consequences of assisting a person to that wellness point are greater health and the prevention of future illness.

9. There is an optimal amount of stress that human beings require for the maintenance of health and continued growth, sometimes referred to as "eustress." Dysfunction begins to occur in the system when the stress load is perceived by the mind/body as excessive, thus resulting in "distress." Oftentimes, pychological stress is only a function of the mindset of the individual perceiving the home or work situation as threatening to well-being.

10. Nutritional supplementation and proper diet, meditation, and stress-reduction techniques offer an easy way to deal with the common emotional and biological stresses of life.

11. There are many different types of unseen stress that pose health threats to the individual. These include psychological stress, nutritional stress, chronobiological stress (shifting sleep cycles), environmental stress from chemicals (drugs, pollutants, sensitivity reactions to foods and subtle toxins) and bacteria and viruses, EM radiation, geopathic stress (abnormal earth energies), and even negative psychic fields.

12. Vibrational diagnostic systems offer the only methods which can identify the influence of, and determine therapy for, many of these subtle, yet omnipresent stresses that impact upon human health.

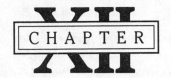

Personal & Planetary Evolution:

VIBRATIONAL HEALING
& ITS IMPLICATIONS FOR AN
EVOLVING HUMANITY

Humanity is in a state of perpetual evolution because human consciousness is constantly evolving and growing. At the present time, people are slowly changing their lifestyles and mindstyles in ways that reflect a greater awareness of the interrelationships between mind and body in both health and illness. However, human beings do not live in a vacuum. The way that we live and the environment we create for ourselves has psychological, biological, and subtle-energy effects upon ourselves and others in our environment. The issue of personal responsibility extends beyond the realm of the self to the very boundaries of our planet. Our personal decisions and patterns of spiritual expression are beginning to have increasing impact upon the global community in which we live.

When individuals change, the whole planetary consciousness also evolves. As above, so below. The evolving patterns of individual human awareness can eventually produce larger changes in the global macrocosm. As increasing numbers of human beings begin to grow spiritually through the inner understanding of their illnesses and energy blockages, and as they begin to realize their true divine nature, they will also start to recognize that all people are subtly connected to each other and to the world around them. As the enlightened consciousness of this small segment of humanity grows, it will have a ripple effect upon the minds of the greater planetary whole. The rising tide of increased spiritual awareness will begin to affect larger numbers of people through a kind of cosmic resonance effect. When enough minds have changed to reach the critical threshold necessary to move the entire global consciousness to a new level of healing and awareness, we will have arrived at the New Age.

The concept that human beings are dynamic energy systems which reflect evolutionary patterns of soul growth is the main tenet underlying vibrational medicine. The ideas that vibrational medicine aims to teach us are actually quite old. They only seem new because it has taken people this long to validate what the ancient priesthoods had already understood for milennia. It might be said that the physician/healers are evolving into a new type of priesthood. At the end of this evolutionary process, the eventual physician/healer/priests will combine the highest knowledge of both the ancient mystery religions and modern science to promote healing at all possible levels.

We have examined how the unique insights of vibrational medicine and the greater understanding of our extended subtle-energy anatomy may affect the evolution of future physicians. What we must now do is make sense of how these revelations about our connection to our Higher Selves and our spiritual bodies will affect the rest of humankind. How will the patients of the healer/physician come to change in the future? More appropriately, we must ask how individuals will need to change in order to achieve true healing at the physical as well as the emotional, mental, and higher spiritual dimensions of human existence.

Personal Responsibility & Spiritual Growth: Our Innate Potential for Self-Healing

In the last chapter we discussed how medicine has become extremely time limited, and has focused on solving specific problems for patients in the most succinct and efficient manner. The consciousness of physicians has often come to conceptualize health care as a system for finding the right drug for the sick patient to alleviate ills. Conversely, patients have come to expect an easy and quick solution to any problem that they bring into the doctor's office. They want to be "fixed-up" with the least amount of discomfort, expense, and time spent away from their busy lives. Taking a pill to solve one's ills has become an ingrained belief and expectation among many people. It is much easier to take a drug for a quick-fix solution than it is to change potentially unhealthy lifestyle habits which may be contributing to the health problem. In other words, given the chance, most people will always elect to take the easier way out.

The desire for an easier, quicker solution is a reflection of the deficiency of self-responsibility that has crept into many an individual's thinking patterns. Sure, life is stressful, and it is hard to eat a proper diet and exercise regularly. The easier way is always to eat whatever and whenever you can, to have a few drinks or smokes with the guys from the office over lunch, and to sit around and space out with the television at night in order to relax from the aggravations of the day.

Seen from the perspective of the concerned traditional physician who is legitimately trying to help his or her patients to a healthier life, it has always been a struggle to get people to change their lifestyles. Frequently, people do not take up healthier life habits until something catastrophic occurs, such as a heart attack or the diagnosis of some other serious illness which forces them to reevaluate their lifestyle. Most people tend to take an attitude with their physicians that says, "Here's my body, fix it up and get it back to me by six o'clock." They do not want to take responsibility for getting their own lives back into shape. They see it as the doctor's responsibility to make them healthy, regardless of their personal habits. This attitude is slowly beginning to shift due to greater patient education and to increased public awareness about the concept of wellness.

The issue of self-responsibility in life is an important one in relation to personal health. It is a subject which has been tackled in various degrees by even the most conservative traditional physicians, often with great frustration. On the subject of prescribing drugs, a physician can give a prescription to a patient for a particular medication, as with the administering of an antibiotic for an infection, but it is the responsibility of the patient to get the prescription filled and to take it according to directions. If the patient does not take the responsibility to follow the doctor's advice, and subsequently does not become well, it is not the fault of the physician, although many patients have assumed otherwise. Thus, personal responsibility plays an important role in even the most mundane of patient-physician interactions. The physician is in many ways an adviser and an educator as well as a healer. It is up to the patient to take the advice of the physician if he or she is to achieve the state of health that is sought.

Many early Western medical models of disease saw threats to health and well-being as originating from outside the self. Illness was due to trauma, poisoning, or infection from some external toxic source. As we have examined throughout the last chapter and much of this book, disease is a multifactorial condition. The state of illness is a culmination of the effects of negative external as well as internal factors. We have discussed those internal factors predisposing individuals to illness under the general category of "host resistance." It is apparent that our capacity for homeostasis and immunologic competence is affected not only by physical factors, such as nutritional status and general physical condition, but also by our level of emotional and mental well-being.

This last category, the effects of emotions upon our level of health, is one that has been underestimated by traditional medicine until very recently. Emotional stress is being increasingly recognized by both holistic and orthodox physicians as a significant contributor to illness. In the last chapter we examined how emotional conflicts, feelings of powerlessness, and lack of self-love can have detrimental effects upon the functioning of the major chakras. Because the chakras supply subtle-energy sustenance to the organs of the body, emotional blockages and conflicts can result in abnormal energy flow to various physiologic systems. Over time, this abnormal energy flow may result in minor or possibly serious illness in any organ system of the body.

Of the chakra blockages that are known to occur, dysfunction in the heart chakra can be the most devastating. *The heart chakra is the central energy center in the chakra/nadi system.* It is an integral link between the three higher and the three lower chakras. In another sense, it is also the center of human existence, because it is the major chakra from which we are able to express love. *The expression of love is perhaps one of the most important lessons that humans have incarnated upon the physical plane to learn. Without love, existence can be dry and meaningless. It is necessary that we learn to love not only those around us but also ourselves.*

We must learn to be more giving to others in various forms of service not only to make money for keeping a roof over our heads and acquiring the material niceties of life, but also to reflect our dedication to the betterment of our fellow human beings. As has been pointed out, it is critical that we learn to love ourselves first before we can truly learn to love others. When we do not love ourselves and our self-image is poor, blockages can occur in the heart chakra which may secondarily affect the functioning of the thymus gland and thus our immune defenses. A weak immune system opens us up to illnesses from any number of internal or external invaders including common viruses, bacteria, and deadly cancer cells. Lack of subtle-energy flow from the heart chakra to the physical heart may actually weaken the heart, making us more susceptible to coronary artery disease, heart attacks, and strokes. The heart chakra also supplies nutritive energy to the lungs, therefore blockages within this critical center may also contribute to many pulmonary diseases.

It might be said that many of the diseases we bring to the physician are not strictly an indication of exposure to negative external factors. *Our illnesses are often a symbolic reflection of our own internal states of emotional unrest, spiritual blockage, and dis-ease.* From both the vibrational and reincarnational perspectives, we know that this viewpoint is indeed accurate. This suggests that the prescription of quick-fix drugs, which may only temporarily relieve the acute condition or discomfort, are not the ideal solutions to alleviating illness. Perhaps one of the most important things that future spiritual physicians will be able to do in moving people toward a state of greater wellness is to teach their patients to recognize those subtle emotional and energetic factors which may predispose them to particular disease states. The evolving spiritual physician will be more adept at detecting dysfunction in the meridians and chakras, and in the emotional, astral, and mental bodies. Future physician/healers will also be able to detect negative thought forms in their patient's auric field which may reflect deeper levels of psychospiritual imbalance.

What will be important in the coming New Age is that people will begin to recognize that their states of emotion and degree of spiritual attunement to their Higher Selves can play an important part in their health and well-being. As people become more aware that their emotions and level of inner attunement can create either health or illness, they will learn to become more responsible for the ways they relate to themselves and others. As people start to work with vibrationally oriented physicians, they will learn methods for changing dysfunctional patterns of behavior, thinking, and feeling, in order to create an inner environment that is more conducive to wellness. Today's proliferation of stress-reduction classes and the attention being focused upon the negative health effects of stress is a step in the right direction. But relaxation is only the tip of the iceberg in really learning to change the deeper psychospiritual elements that open us up to illness in the first place.

The orthodox medical community is having a hard time dealing with the idea that our thoughts and emotions might contribute to the causation of illness. Many have reacted by stating that "physicians who propound these philosophies of the emotions creating disease do a disservice to patients because they make them feel guilty at having fallen ill." Many physicians fear having to address the issue of emotional contributions to illnesses like cancer. Scientists' attitudes have been so negative to the mind/body issue in cancer that funding for health agencies who are trying to study the connections between emotions and health has all but dried up. The painstakingly slow acceptance of research in the newly evolving field of psychoneuroimmunology is a direct demonstration of this reluctant attitude on the part of many within traditional medicine.

Orthodox physicians would rather disregard the notion of emotional contributors to illness because these factors are more difficult for them to get a handle on and to treat. In addition, the psychosocial and spiritual precursors to disease are even harder to diagnose, especially within the limited time interval that physicians usually spend with patients. Many of the orthodox medical surveys of cancer patients, which examined the influence of emotional factors upon their illness, have been based on questionnaires or superficial interviews with patients. One of the difficulties in establishing the link between emotional blockages and the production of illnesses is that patients may not always be truthful or cognizant enough of their own psychological shortcomings to give adequate insight via superficial surveys. Also, people may sometimes not admit to problems that occur within the context of their family unit. To them, such questions may be trivial or have little relevance to the illness that the physician is supposed to be treating. This is true of patients in general, not just those with cancer.

There is, however, data accumulating in the orthodox medical literature, as seen in Dr. Caroline Thomas' landmark study on personality traits and emotional attitudes, which suggests that family relationships and psychological factors do have a predictive value in foretelling the occurrence of diseases such as cancer and heart disease.[1] Thomas followed a sample of 1300 Johns Hopkins Medical School students who graduated between 1948 and 1964, and continued to update their medical histories over the years. She gathered elaborate information about each person's family history and administered a battery of physical and psychological tests to all participating students during the period that they were still attending Johns Hopkins. Years later, as the now older physicians began to succumb to various illnesses, she looked back at her data on the medical students to see whether there were common psychological factors among students with particular types of diseases.

There were, indeed, common psychological factors among those students who had succumbed to cancer. Interestingly, the traits of the group that later developed cancer were similar to those who eventually committed suicide. They typically described themselves as emotionally detached from their parents. Members of the cancer group also felt that their parents had often been emotionally disagreeable toward one another. In fact, more students who eventually developed cancer had described negative early family relations than any other group in her study. Other work by psychologist Lawrence LeShan[2] has also suggested that many cancer patients habitually bottle up their emotions, especially negative ones. In many, this sense of alienation from family contributes to periods of overpowering depression in later life.

All of these negative emotional patterns revolve around the individual's inner capacity to express love toward self and others. Many individuals had been conditioned by early negative relations with their parents, which eventually created a diminished sense of self. The distorted self-image later affected their ability to relate to others freely, and created patterns of unexpressed anger and hostility that were never released. Thus we see powerful confirmation of how various types of emotional blockage, especially those which impair the capacity to love self and others, create abnormal energy patterns within the heart chakra. These dysfunctional energy patterns diminish the vitality of the immune system and other organ systems, and may eventually manifest as a serious illness within the physical body.

Therapists like Dr. Carl Simonton, who have worked with cancer patients to change negative attitudes and self-images, have found that aggressive attitudes toward survival, and a strong will to live, have a positive effect on survival from advanced maligancies.[3] Their treatment programs sought to not only mobilize patients' immune systems but to change dysfunctional emotional patterns and attitudes which contributed to their illnesses via meditation, imagery, and a variety of other techniques. Some physicians have attempted to study whether attitude alone can have an effect on survival from advanced malignancy, as Simonton's results have suggested. Unfortunately, it is not really possible to compare survival statistics between cancer patients who are hopeful and those who are positive but also actively stimulate their immune systems through visualization. It is difficult to generalize the results of Simonton's work strictly by examining the effect of positive attitudes on survival. Nor is it possible to dismiss Simonton's work solely on the basis of the effects of positive or negative attitudes.

A study which was reported in the June 13, 1985 issue of *The New England Journal of Medicine* claimed to have found no relationship between emotional attitudes and survival in patients with advanced high-risk cancers. The authors of the study *did not claim* that positive emotional attitudes had no effect upon quality of life nor upon survival in patients with less advanced cancer. However, many superficially minded lay people and physicians who read this article *interpreted* it as meaning that there were no significant psychological factors operating in the survival of any cancer patients. One of the primary authors of the study, Dr. Barrie Cassileth, has since been quick to point out these misconceptions. Dr. Cassileth believes that emotions do affect health and illness, and that the will to live is an important factor in some diseases. She was disturbed that the results of her study were being used to refute the claims of people like Norman Cousins who believe that positive emotions, faith, laughter, and the will to live have a direct influence on healing outcome. Unfortunately, the media's coverage of this article and their incorrect interpretations about the real influence of emotions on health and illness has created further false confirmation of the beliefs of many traditional physicians, who were already dubious of suggested links between emotions and serious illnesses such as cancer.

The evidence is mounting, even in the traditional medical literature, that our emotions affect our health.[4] If this is so, then people must begin to take responsibility for their thoughts and emotions if they are to positively influence their health. It is only by working cooperatively with enlightened physicians, sensitive to these subtle contributors to illness, that people may achieve high levels of wellness and an integration and balance of the interlocking elements of body, mind, and spirit. All people have within their inner natural resources a powerful ally, their Higher Self, which sometimes tries to teach them things about themselves by manifesting particular types of illness or dysfunction. The adversities that illnesses impose upon us interfere with the enjoyment of our normal lifestyles. Diseases may be viewed as obstacles in our paths which have been positioned by our Higher Selves so as to make us slow down and reexamine where we are going with our lives. Illness is a subtle warning sign which tells us that something is wrong and must be corrected before more serious consequences occur. If we could only learn to listen to the inner wisdom that exists within each of us, we could surmount these self-imposed obstacles and grow to become happier, healthier, more spiritually aware beings.

When disease occurs, it is a signal that we are constricting the natural flow of life energy through our multidimensional bodies. Health and wellness are a reflection of the normal unimpeded flow of higher vibrational energies through the body/mind/spirit. Each person may be viewed as a channel or conduit of many different kinds of energy. We each take in food, water, air, light, sound, and various types of sensory stimulation, as well as other less-well-recognized inputs including prana, chi, and psychospiritual energies of a more subtle nature. Within the many levels of our multidimensional anatomy, we transform these energy inputs, using them to maintain, rebuild, and heal our bodies. In turn, we release or express a variety of outputs. These outputs include the more obvious biological or physical wastes in the form of carbon dioxide, sweat, urine, and feces— the by-products of energy metabolism. In addition, we express a number of other outputs such as physical work and communication in the forms of speech, touch, emotion, and various intellectual and artistic forms of creative expression. On a higher level, we are also expressing psychospiritual energies and communication through our subtle bodies and chakras.

For good health to be enjoyed, one must have constant and unimpeded energy flow through each of the many simultaneous levels of internal processing. If we are blocked in some way and thus impair the flow of energy at any level of the system, disease results. Abnormalities can occur at a single or even at multiple levels of energy input simultaneously. Also, blocking the energy outflow can be just as detrimental to the system. The resultant buildup of pressure must be eventually released. Often, the built-up stresses are vented through overactivity of various bodily systems, which can create abnormal physiologic reactions and eventually disease. In the past, traditional physicians have tended to pay more attention to problems stemming from blockage of basic inputs at the physical level. Diseases caused by contaminated air and water and poor nutritional intake are given prime attention by traditional doctors. Orthodox medicine's recognition of the emotion/illness link is a reflection of the newly evolving awareness among health-care professionals that psychological energies can also affect physical health. Thus, proper energy output at the level of our emotional energy structure is also essential for the attainment and maintenance of high-level wellness.

Seen from the perspective of a plumbing analogy, one must have adequate water input, lack of sewage or blockage in the pipes, and also an opened release valve for water to optimally flow through the system. Blockages at any of these levels will result in a shutdown of water flow. The same is true of human beings. In addition to our requirements for a proper energy intake via the various physical and subtle nutrients, we must have clean pipes in the form of disease-free arteries and veins, symmetrically balanced acupuncture meridians, unblocked chakras and nadis, and healthy organ structures for the life energy to flow and be properly utilized. Lastly, human beings must be able to express their stored-up energy properly, or dangerously high levels of stress will build up in the system.

This implies that we must not only release our biological wastes, but as human beings we need to dump our emotional garbage as well. If we do not allow ourselves to forgive others for their mistakes and if we continue to hold onto old hostilities, unresolved anger, guilt, and the psychic wounds of previous hurts, then negativity will build up and eat away at us like seeping toxic wastes. Ill health will occur if we continuously allow emotional negativity to block the inflow of our higher spiritual energies. When we surround ourselves with negative emotions and do not allow love to penetrate, we are only hurting ourselves. We must learn to express our emotions properly so that we do not build up unreleased angers, tensions, and resentments. If these emotions are unexpressed, and are left to boil silently and build unconscious pressures, they may finally vent their way through our systems via disruption of the weakest link in our complex chain of interactive energy levels. It is most important that we learn to express love in our relationships to others, including our parents, our families, our significant others such as spouses and children, and also especially toward ourselves. This is perhaps the greatest lesson that human beings need to learn. There would be far less suffering and illness if we could all learn to love each other and to love and forgive ourselves for our mistakes.

In addition to expressing emotional outputs, humans are by nature creative and intelligent beings who must allow themselves to channel their natural talents for writing, painting, invention, and artistic endeavor into various forms of expression. We must not block the flow of creative energies through our systems. If the flow of creative kundalini energies is impeded, undue pressure may build in the chakras, creating blockages, physiological dysfunction, and eventually illness. In order that each level of energy input and output be maintained in proper working order, people must take self-responsibility by periodically reexamining personal habits and lifestyles.

When illness occurs, it is an important message that blockage is occurring at some level of the multidimensional self. In addition to being conduits of physical and conventional forms of energy, we are also channels of information and guidance that originates from the higher levels of our spiritual awareness. Some of the messages sent from our Higher Selves are symbolically manifested in the form of disease, and are not intended to make us feel guilty that we are sick. The illness may be an indication from our higher levels of consciousness that changes need to occur in our lives if we are to find and maintain our health and happiness. Sometimes the only change that is needed is rest and rebalancing. Other times the necessary change will be that of nutritional alteration, emotional reassessment, or the avoidance of some toxic environmental influence. Sometimes the lesson is that we must seek greater spiritual awareness and attunement. As we approach the New Age, the divine discontent that many are beginning to feel is a reflection of the greater human need for spiritual awakening and fulfillment. The crucial thing to be learned is that we must begin to look more closely at our bodies. We need to listen to each pattern of physical distress as a kind of message that the Higher Self is trying to communicate to us through the right-brain language of body symbolism.

When we are sick and in pain, we seek help from authorities who are more experienced in understanding the causes of illness. Oftentimes it is important to seek professional assistance to obtain help in getting back to states of greater balance and ease. It is one thing to ask for help. It is another to expect the physician to cure all of our ills without any need for our own active participation. We cannot relinquish all control and responsibility to our authority figures. People must begin to work with physicians as a cooperative team. The more enlightened vibrational physicians, with their various subtle energetic methods of detection, will be able to diagnose both the superficial and deeper reasons for the problems that patients bring to their doctors. Future physicians will begin to teach patients that if optimal health is to be achieved, then the deeper causes of illness must also be adequately addressed. Patients will begin to learn that quick-fix solutions, even when strongly desired, may only further mask the deeper problems of chronic energetic imbalance.

Enlightened physicians will be able to work with patients to try and alter dysfunctional patterns of emotion via counseling, vitamins, stress-reduction techniques, and meditation. Patients will modify the higher elements of their consciousness using flower essences, gem elixirs, homeopathic remedies, and various other subtle-energy modalities. However, it will still be important that people use these therapies adjunctively while they are implementing other changes in their modes of thinking, feeling, nutritional habits and general lifestyle, if a more lasting healing and inner balance is to occur. *Once we have learned the real reasons for feeling ill, we must begin to make lasting changes that will result in a healing on many simultaneous levels. We must learn to accept responsibility for our own lives.*

Throughout life, we make choices and take actions in particular directions. It is necessary that people begin to take responsibility and become more aware of the consequences of their actions. Certainly we have only recently become cognizant of how simple things like our thoughts and our emotions can adversely affect our health. Having been armed with this new knowledge by their physicians, patients must begin to realize that their emotional relationships, thinking patterns, and their capacity for expressing love towards themselves and others do have significant effects upon their health. How one goes about changing these things is another story. We have described a number of psychological techniques and psycho-energetic methods for doing so throughout this book.

The important lesson is that people must be taught and educated about the crucial interrelationships between their bodies, minds, emotions, and spiritual energies. Once we begin to understand that we are primarily spiritual beings working through the limitations of physical bodies, our consciousness begins to change. As people reach the level of enlightenment where they begin to comprehend the real reasons for their illnesses, they must slowly change toward a more positive direction. To ignore the true source of our suffering after knowing its effect upon us would only serve to exacerbate our distress. The physician cannot do it all by him or herself. He or she needs the cooperation and energetic assistance of the patient if health is to be the long-term result. Doctors cannot absolve people of their responsibility simply by giving them a prescription or having them undergo an operation.

The physician/healer will be better able to counsel people on the ways that their actions, emotions, or environment may be affecting them in a negative way. After knowing those negative influences, the individual must go about making changes that will remove the source of constricted energy flow through his or her multilevel system, or further distress and disease will eventually occur.

Some of the major emotional issues that people are trying to work through at this time involve the basic lessons of the chakras that were discussed in Chapter 10. Each of these issues is an obstacle along the transformational path to spiritual enlightenment that each human being must eventually resolve. The most basic issues, affecting the lower three chakras, involve the aspects of grounding, sexuality, and personal power. In a way, grounding is the most primal of these because it involves our relationship to the planet that we live upon. Our connectedness to the Earth and its beauty affects our ability to work together cooperatively as humans to promote greater environmental safety, preservation of our natural resources, and attunement to the higher forces of nature.

Sexuality has become of increasing importance over the last few decades. Sexual expression and comfortability with one's sexuality is not a new issue. It has been with us since the dawn of time. However, the physical problems that are now arising due to conflicts involving our sexual appetites can result in a constricted or accentuated energy flow through the second chakra. The affliction of many with sexually transmitted illnesses can be seen as a reflection of an improper focus upon sexuality at a time when there is renewed spiritual awakening occurring over the face of the planet. There is too much time being spent on the older focus of lower-chakra-based sexuality and not enough attention being paid to sixth and seventh-chakra-associated issues of spiritual seeking.

The issue of personal power has been of importance in the past. But it is perhaps more accentuated at this time because at no other point in human history have personal freedoms and the ability to work one's way up in the world become so easily obtainable in Western society. The ability to gain power over one's life, regardless of sex or race, has never been so great as it is in today's modern world. Conflicts arise when people who have less than what they want out of life look enviously at those who have achieved the status, position, and material wealth that they have dreamed of but never obtained. This sense of powerlessness is especially evident in those people who work in boring or thankless jobs, and who perceive that they have little chance for advancement. Other difficulties associated with personal power, such as self-aggrandizement or overinflated egos, can also arise in managerial types of people or in authority figures who delegate tasks to others. Personal power and the ability to work together cooperatively in the home and workplace are basic developmental tasks of societal integration. These three basic issues of grounding, sexuality, and personal power need to be addressed and resolved before one can truly concentrate on working through the psychospiritual goals of the higher chakras.

The abilities to express and receive love are fundamental qualities of the heart chakra. We have discussed throughout the latter two chapters of this book how important the lesson of the heart chakra is. If imbalances in this center constrict the life energy flow through the body, there can be serious consequences. The heart, lungs, bronchial tubes, and thymus gland are all energized and strengthened by the heart chakra. When this important subtle energy center is closed and emotionally blocked, then we may develop heart diseases, breathing problems, and a general susceptibility to environmental, infectious, and cancerous diseases. Also, if there are any blockages in the heart chakra from early childhood traumas or issues from past lives, the heart is often stressed as this chakra opens. The lesson of love is one of the most important things that we must try to learn during our brief incarnations upon the physical plane. Higher levels of personal sacrifice and selfless service to our fellow human beings are as much a part of the lesson of love as are loving family and personal relationships, and the inner love of self-acceptance. Once we have opened up our heart chakras, and the energies of love and joy can truly flow, the higher chakras and their special lessons come within easier reach. *Personal and spiritual transformation are dependent upon the opening of the heart chakra.* As our heart centers open wider and we begin to feel greater compassion and empathy for all living things, we move closer to expressing the divine unconditional love of the Christ Consciousness, which is the supreme facet of spiritual awakening towards which we are all gradually evolving.

Learning self-discipline and the controlled expression of the will is another important issue of the higher chakras, specifically the throat center. At a time when self-indulgence has become commonplace, the development of discipline in one's life is an important steppingstone toward any type of personal or spiritual transformation. Modification of dietary habits, forcing oneself to exercise, and the daily practice of meditation are all crucial facets of self-discipline that one must acquire in order to truly achieve health and wellness of the total mind/body/spirit.

Communication is another important issue of the throat chakra. It is an ability which we all demonstrate but which we do not always express with the clarity and honesty that may be required. Communication is more than just exchanging words. We also communicate through our vocal tones, our body language, our facial expressions, our touch, and through many other unspoken subtle energetic routes. We each need to learn how to better communicate our thoughts and feelings to the people around us, especially to those significant others in our relationships. When we do not communicate adequately with those around us by leaving important things unspoken, we constrict our vital energy flow. We build up tensions and stresses that eventually work their way outward through the body and manifest in various forms of physical illness and distress. The clarity and depth of our personal relationships, marriages, family relations, and work roles are dependent upon concise, effective, and honest communication in all its many forms of expression.

The final issues of the higher psychic centers, the brow and crown chakras, relate to the search for spiritual fulfillment and personal transformation through the attainment of higher consciousness. The development of inner vision, intuition, and spiritual awareness are issues that are slowly growing in importance throughout the Western world as more and more people begin to search for the path toward enlightenment. This can be seen in many different outward manifestations as people seek for spiritual fulfillment through the more conventional Western religions of Christianity and Judaism, and the Eastern faiths of Buddhism, Taoism, Sufism, and Hinduism. The tremendous surge of interest in meditation and prayer over the last twenty years is a growing sign of people's quest for greater spiritual direction.

We are moving toward a period in human history when we will begin to see the spiritual transformation of thousands of people upon the Earth. It is a time when a more enlightened higher consciousness is desperately needed to work through and solve our many social, economic, ecological, and diverse planetary problems. There is a powerful driving force at work from the higher dimensional planes which is accelerating the process of spiritual transformation and enlightenment for many. As more people begin to meditate and explore the inner guidance of their Higher Selves, they will kindle a tremendous energy for self-healing and wellness. Through meditation, the latent kundalini forces of many people will begin to awaken and unleash the stress-releasing capacities of the nervous system. In addition, these powerful psychic forces will begin to open and cleanse the chakras and the human brain itself to activate the hidden psychic potentials of higher consciousness.

As the New Age vibrations begin to affect more and more people, the spiritual awakening of thousands of sleeping minds will begin to kindle the energies of love and healing that may eventually be able to transform the planet Earth into a place of greater peace and balance. When we begin to heal ourselves and learn that fear and misunderstanding is the root cause of much illness, distress, and suffering, we will begin to replace hate, prejudice, and distrust with love and cooperation. When we are functioning in the lower mind of conscious awareness, we tend to project our own dissatisfactions and inabilities onto the world. Seeing our own problems and inabilities reflected in the faces of those around us, we exaggerate our fears and prejudices in a viciously expanding cycle. We are often afraid of owning up to our own fears, anxieties, and shortcomings. To cope with this frightening inner environment, *we begin to project our fear and insanity onto the world,* making it seem that the problem is coming from out there when, in fact, it originates from within our own egos. *The only way to break this vicious cycle of confused thinking and illness is through love and forgiveness and a greater awareness of the healing potential of love.* When we start to forgive ourselves for our perceived faults, and honestly admit that we still have a ways to grow, we begin to heal ourselves from the highest level of spirit on down to the physical. Only then can we truly love and accept ourselves. Once we love ourselves, it becomes easier to love those around us.

That is not to say that there is not chaos and unrest occurring in many places throughout the world, and that there is not much discord in these times of crisis. There will likely be a worsening of the world situation before it becomes better. In order to cope with a world that has seemingly gone mad at times, we must find an inner center of peace within ourselves so that we may begin to expand our own energy of peace and harmony to encompass the troubled needy world around us. As we begin to find that center of peace and spiritual understanding, healing naturally follows. We become better citizens and servants of world order and fellowship. We must heal ourselves before we can go out and heal the planet on which we live. The first step of this long journey begins at home.

The Cosmic Cycle of Regeneration & Rebirth: Ancient Philosophies for a New Age

We have seen that vibrational medicine holds the potential to truly revolutionize the field of healing and spiritual development. Subtle-energy medicine has the ability to not only heal illness at the physical level but also to change the consciousness of the individual that helped to create the disease in the first place. By changing the psychoenergetic elements of the personality which interact with toxic environmental agents to produce illness, we create a cure that is more permanent than that which is achieved through the mere palliation of symptoms at the physical level. Vibrational medicine is critically important to furthering our knowledge of the healing process, especially because it is predicated upon a fuller understanding of the multidimensional nature of the self.

Vibrational healing modalities are effective because of their ability to impact upon the subtle unseen hierarchical levels of human physiology, which include the physical and etheric bodies, the acupuncture meridians, the chakras and nadis, and the astral, mental, causal, and higher spiritual bodies. Having described the function and integration of these many levels of energetic and spiritual physiology, we must now ask how all of this information fits in with our divine purpose upon the planet Earth. An understanding of the higher levels of subtle anatomy and their influence upon our daily lives and health will help us to comprehend how we are all intimately linked with the continually evolving divine energies of the soul.

Our physical and higher bodies are specialized vehicles which allow the expression of the soul's consciousness upon the dense Earth plane. The consciousness of each soul is actually a particularization of that greater spiritual consciousness which we refer to as God. Various spiritual philosophies look to the time of our universe's creation as the period when God created all souls simultaneously. Mixing cosmic evolution with theology, one might view the Big Bang as more than just the creation of primordial interstellar hydrogen and light. It was also the time at which the Creator gave birth to the billions of human souls that would inhabit the new universe through an explosive particularization of the divine conscious energies. It is said that God created human beings in the divine image. As each soul was created in that first moment, God separated into smaller beings of light which were energetic representations of the original vast beingness. Through the conscious evolution of these lesser gods and the holographic connectivity of the universe, God could enrich and develop the tremendous potential for diversity and self-knowledge inherent in supreme consciousness. These primal beings of light, or souls, developed ways of manifesting the ethereal energies of their consciousness through denser forms of expression. The denser forms, called physical bodies, would allow them to experience through their senses the wonders and beauties of the evolving planets. Also, it would allow them to experiment with the expression of their emotional nature through interactions and relationships between themselves, their environment, and the other sentient life forms manifesting upon the planets on which they chose to incarnate.

Because no entity could develop itself in all possible ways through the course of a single life span of these dense vehicles of expression, a continuous cycle of regeneration and rebirth, known as reincarnation, was created. During each lifetime, the incarnating soul is able to partake of many diverse experiences which allow it to explore the wonders, joys, and sorrows of human existence. Through hit or miss, and reward or punishment, the consciousness of the soul, projected through earthly bodies, can learn and experience planetary life through every conceivable variation of the human form. Via the reincarnational cycle, each soul comes to know the splendor and achievements, as well as the difficulties and sadnesses, of each of the existing races and colors of peoples. All souls come to experience life as the pinnacle of high society as well as the simplicity and daily toil of the farms and fields. All conscious entities find out how life differs between being male and female in the different societies. Through each of these varied experiences, the soul comes to know itself and to better understand its own emotional, physical, and spiritual nature, as well as the many different expressions that physical human life allows. Perhaps most importantly in its earthly sojourns, the soul comes to appreciate and experience the nature of love in its many different forms, and develops a greater compassion and caring for all of God's creations.

All souls are spiritual beings of light which remain energetically connected to the Creator and the Creator's universe through a holographic connectivity relationship. All souls have evolved as unique but diverse manifestations of the single divine principle (also known as the Law of One). As the souls become enriched through their experiences, so too does the Creator come to grow and evolve in a greater knowing of self in infinite expression. In spite of this unity with God and the universe, the souls temporarily lose the memory of their spiritual origins after incarnating into dense physical bodies. In reality, the higher spiritual bodies of the souls maintain a cosmic awareness and connection to the God-force. Only the projected fragment of the soul's total consciousness which inhabits the dense physical form loses the memory of its origins.

The earthly personalities forget that they are manifestations of the one supreme intelligence, as the perceptual mechanisms of their brains and bodies create a physical sense of separation from each other as well as from their Creator. Partly because of this sense of separation from God, human beings have created religion and its rituals in an attempt to reunite themselves with the creative forces of nature and the physical universe which seemed outside of themselves. Human beings forget that the kingdom of God is already within each of us. Jesus incarnated to teach and remind us of this simple forgotten truth.

Because of this built-in forget mechanism which activates shortly after incarnating into the physical form, all memories of previous existences are removed from the conscious awareness of the ego. This allows each entity to develop according to new rules and environments without the contaminating influence of knowledge or habits acquired in previous lives. Each of the individual personalities projected into physical incarnation are actually fragments of one single greater soul. The total soul, or higher spiritual self, acquires the complete knowledge of all the incarnations of its soul fragments in a way that might be compared to the unified collective awareness of a single bee hive. Through the gestalt consciousness of its community of many workers, drones, and the queen, the hive functions as a single great entity or as a larger brain composed of many smaller mobile information gatherers. Seen in another light, the soul is like a cosmic tree. Each incarnating personality or soul fragment sent out from the original cosmic soul is like one of many individual flowers that blossom on the branches of a large tree. Every ego flower on each branch of the soul tree remains in constant communication with the total plant as it is fed by the sap lifelines of a common trunk and root system.

The total soul is therefore a collective consciousness of many individual incarnations or personalities whose knowledge and experiences are woven together like a colorful tapestry through a networking of many subtle threads of psychic communication. From experiences in the many differing expressions of humanity, each soul is able to grow in understanding of its emotional capacity, intellectual creativity, and physical limitations, and to eventually develop a greater awareness for its own higher spiritual nature.

The reincarnational cycle has special built-in safeguards that prevent the perpetuation of wrong thinking and negative actions toward fellow journeyers upon the soul quest of self-discovery and enlightenment. This system of energy credits and debits, based on positive and negative deeds and actions, has been referred to as the Law of Karma. The subtle nature of higher dimensional anatomy and its controlling influence upon the creation and physiological maintenance of the physical body, allows the negative energies of past-life misdeeds to be carried over to future lifetimes by causing subtle abnormalities in the human physical and emotional structure.

By working through physical handicaps and illnesses, individuals are able to "burn away the karma" of their negative deeds and redeem their souls for the evils, torments, and suffering that they may have caused others in previous lives. Often the ways that people torment others come back to haunt them in future lives in a fashion that is symbolically reminiscent of the original negative act. For instance, torturers of the Spanish inquisition who blinded their heretical victims with red hot iron swords might themselves develop incurable blindness in a later life. Various clairvoyant studies[5,6] and hypnotic past-life regressions[7,8] have suggested the validity of this form of karmic expression in understanding the reasons behind certain types of illnesses and phobias. The nature of this type of karmic expression is that it allows the tormenters to eventually understand the true nature of the suffering that they have inflicted by experiencing a form of it themselves. Additionally, by overcoming the obstacles of self-inflicted handicaps, the individuals may grow stronger in the face of adversity and develop in ways that they might not have had a chance to had they not had to fight so hard to overcome the stumbling blocks in their paths. This is not to say that all handicaps are past-life carryovers. Many are, but some are chosen by the soul as an experience which can have positive growth effects if correctly utilized. Simonton's work with cancer patients has demonstrated that life-threatening illnesses can produce transformational outcomes.

Although this is not a subject that we have dealt with extensively throughout this book, karmic illness is worth mentioning because it is an area of disease upon which vibrational medicine is able to have certain impacts, at least in creating an awareness of the reasons behind some diseases and handicaps. Again, this returns us to the concept of self-responsibility in accepting the consequences of our actions, whether they originate from this life or a past one. Few would dream that the negative emotions and malicious deeds of their previous lives would come back to haunt them in their present lives as some form of illness. But it is possible, nonetheless.

In spite of the fact that the incarnating personality loses the memory of its past lives at the time of birth, the personality remains tied to the spiritual energies of its Higher Self through the connection of its higher vibrational bodies. Through various methods, the soul tries to bring greater self-awareness to the incarnating personality via symbolic dreams, the manifestation of certain illnesses or bodily dysfunctions, and occasionally through direct inner communication during the meditative state. The Higher Self is always able to perceive what the conscious personality cannot. The consciousness of the causal body is able to observe the directions of the personality and ego from the higher level of causes, and not just the effects perceived upon the physical plane. Each person's Higher Self knows how emotional dysfunctions create abnormal energy physiology in their physical body. The Higher Self tries to relay warnings to the ego before serious illness results. The Higher Self always knows what is really going on in our lives, as well as how our suffering and distress could be transformed into peace, joy, and satisfaction. If we could tap into that inner resource of the Higher Self, we would find a limitless storehouse of power, knowledge, love, and wisdom.

The Higher Self or causal body contains all of the memories and knowledge of the soul through its sojourns in many past-life incarnations. Within that body of knowledge exists the transformational wisdom which could elevate the consciousness of the individual to an understanding of its true spiritual origins, the transitory nature of life, death, and rebirth, and the cosmic signficance of its existence and its connection to the Creator. As our consciousness elevates to a higher vantage point, we are better able to perceive the reasons for our suffering and self-imposed obstacles. When we become more spiritually aware and in tune with the inner guidance of our Higher Selves, the mechanisms by which we can change our emotions, our minds, our bodies, and our lives, become more apparent. For instance, flower essences contain the very energies of pure consciousness that allow the connections between the lower and higher selves to be reestablished. These types of vibrational healing modalities can help the higher qualities of the soul manifest more easily at the physical level, thus allowing for healing and increased awareness.

Humanity has evolved through many civilizations that once accepted as truth the spiritual knowledge spoken by the healers, priests, and physicians of their time. Many thousands of years ago, when humans existed on the continent known as the motherland of Lemuria, or Mu, people were more directly linked with their higher spiritual selves. Lemuria existed at an early time in human history when the reincarnational cycle of dense physical forms had only recently begun. In early Lemuria, people lived simple lives. Spirituality and the recognition of the God-force in all things was a part of daily life. Because of an attunement with nature and themselves, Lemurians were healthy and almost disease-free. They were also extremely psychic, and could see auras and the spiritual light around all living things quite easily. Information flowed from their Higher Selves into waking consciousness with great ease. Telepathic communication was commonplace. The Lemurians were aware of the various subtle structures of consciousness linking the physical form and its basic lower awareness with the sensibility of the middle or conscious waking personality and with the cosmic consciousness of the higher spiritual self. Flower essences were utilized primarily for psychic and spiritual development because there was little illness that required healing. The Hawaiians, and especially the Kahuna priests with their knowledge of the lower, middle, and higher selves, appear to be descendents of this lost race of peoples. The Hawaiian Islands are the peaks of the submerged mountains and lands of Lemuria which sank beneath the ocean waters many centuries ago. Prior to the loss of Lemuria, many migrated to the land mass known as Atlantis, where one of the greatest civilizations of all time was evolving.

Atlantis actually began as an agrarian culture many centuries before it developed into the pinnacle of technology and advancement that the legends record. Eventually, the simple Lemurians blended into the high-tech cities of Atlantis. This assimilation of people was probably similar to rural Americans being absorbed into huge urban complexes. *Because of the need to adapt to the faster paced life of Atlantean society, many Lemurians suffered from what one would consider the very first stress-related disorders.* In Atlantis there were three different schools of thought on the treatment of illness. There were those healers who treated illness through more spiritual methods, using flower essences, crystals, and color therapies. Those in the priesthood used homeopathy as an integration of spiritual and scientific methods. The allopathic healers of the day utilized herbs, drugs, and surgical treatments as most doctors would tend to use today.

The more natural healers who used flower essences, color, crystals, and homeopathy were considered the majority thinkers of the Atlantean medical establishment. The allopaths were a minority faction. The allopaths were considered to be quite radical by the natural healers of the time, to the extent that certain allopathic physicians were actually persecuted for their thinking. From a reincarnational or karmic perspective this is quite interesting, considering that today there is a reversal of the old Atlantean focus on natural and spiritual healing systems toward a greater emphasis on allopathic treatment methods. It is likely that many in the Atlantean natural healing movement who persecuted allopathic physicians are today holistic healers who have come under fire for their radical treatment methods. One might say that, from a karmic viewpoint, the shoe is on the other foot now. The torments of the Atlantean persecutors may have come back to haunt them.

The Atlantean culture grew to become a pinnacle of civilization. Atlantean scientists were extremely skilled in the art of healing and the manipulation of the life-force itself. Like the Lemurians before them, the Atlanteans were also quite adept at psychic communication and perception. They even developed their psychoenergetic technologies to the point where they were able to experimentally manipulate the genetic expression of lifeforms, somewhat like science is beginning to rediscover today. Today's experiments in the area of recombinant DNA in bacteria would be considered primitive in comparison.

As the Atlanteans' power over nature grew, there occurred a gradual shift in their society. People began to lose sight of their original harmony with nature and the spiritual dimensions of life. Many became self-indulgent by utilizing their new-found capabilities to cater to every whim of the senses, without respect for the natural order of living things.

In the latter days of Atlantis, prior to its final destruction, evil and perversity grew to new levels among certain sectors of the population. The Atlantean society had slowly separated into two, large, opposing factions. The original spiritual group, who still followed what was known as the Law of One, i.e. the teachings of the one God and the oneness of all life, remained true to their higher orientations and fought to maintain balance and equality amongst all peoples. The other group, known as the Sons of Belial, were the power mongers and debaucherers of that society. The Sons of Belial utilized the technologies of the crystals to torture and gain power. In the end, the power-mad leaders of the Sons of Belial wreaked environmental havoc upon the people and the continent of Atlantis itself. Eventually, Atlantis was totally destroyed and sank beneath the waves.

Those of the more spiritual accord could see the end of Atlantis coming, and prepared to carry away from the continent the best of its achievements in healing, philosophy, technology, and the following of the Law of One. They planned, even before the final submergence of their land, to carry away the important records on the greatest developments of Atlantean civilization to places of safety, where the information and technology could be preserved for future civilizations when people could again learn to use such spiritual powers over nature wisely. Of those who escaped the destruction, there were three major groups who carried the records and teachings to distant lands. They brought with them the most basic of their spiritual practices and ways of life, in the hopes that they would be able to carry on the highest traditions of Atlantean life and spiritual teaching, including the ideas of unity in consciousness between all living things and their loving Creator.

The first of these groups went to the land of Egypt, with splinter groups going still further in to Europe, Asia, and places like Tibet. Another group travelled to the coast of Peru in what we now know as Central and South America. Still a third group migrated to North America. Evidence of the ancient influence of Atlantean culture can be seen in the commonly used symbols among stone carvings of early South American Indians, the hieroglyphics of ancient Egyptians, and the works of Native American Indians. In addition, the propagation of the pyramidal form of architecture as a structure of worship and initiation can be seen in the ancient ceremonial buildings of the Aztec culture, the Egyptian pyramids, and the pyramid-like structures built by a group of Native American Indians known as the mound builders. The ancient legends of the South American Indians, the North American Indians, and the old Egyptians still tell about the terrible deluge that occurred when Atlantis was submerged beneath the ocean's waves. The ocean into which the continent disappeared, the Atlantic, still bears its name.

In the case of those who migrated to Egypt, the influx of ancient vibrational systems of healing knowledge into the Egyptian culture resulted in a high point of civilization that had not previously been seen in those lands. The intermingling with the old Atlanteans and their specialized knowledge of the healing arts and spiritual practices changed certain aspects of Egyptian society. Many of the old Egyptian legends of the elder gods, including the story of Thoth, who brought the knowledge of science and healing to Egypt, are based upon translations of the original stories of the migrating Atlanteans, who came to that land in the year 10,000 B.C. For a period of more than several hundred years, there was a new level of culture and civilization in ancient Egypt which was based upon alignment with humanity's higher dimensional nature and the activation of the innate potential for psychic and spiritual awareness.

That was a time when science and religion were actually united under one roof in Egypt. Initiates within the priesthood were dedicated to the healing arts, and carried on many of the Atlantean traditions in healing with flower essences, color, and various other subtle-energy modalities. Healers were divided into three main types. There were those who were known as the healers with the herbs. They applied various herbal and medicinal preparations to assist in the healing process. There were also those who were called the healers of the knife, the surgeons of ancient Egypt. Some of the ancient papyruses which have survived from these times suggest that their surgical skills were great. For instance, their surgical technique of craniotomy, which was used to remove traumatically induced blood clots which were pressing against the brain, is very similar to modern-day approaches. But instead of sutures they used melted wax to seal the skin surrounding the incision. In addition, the surgical site was then wrapped in cotton dressing that was charged by priests with "the life of Ptah." This was a form of psychic healing similar to that which is used today by nurse practitioners of Therapeutic Touch. The healer-charged cotton was applied in order to promote rapid wound closure without infection.

The last of the three groups was perhaps the most interesting. This was the group of healers who worked with psychic and clairvoyant skills of diagnosis and healing. Some of these were the high priests of Anubis. They had the ability to see with the eyes of spirit, and could look into the body as well as the external auric field to diagnose physical abnormalities, injuries, psychological problems, and past-life or karmic influences. Some priests, as we have already mentioned, had the ability to heal directly with their hands or with their minds at great distances. Others had the ability to psychically lift the individual out of the physical body and into the astral form if surgery needed to be performed. This was a unique form of drugless anesthesia. The priests were carefully trained to use their abilities wisely and to assist the people of the land of Egypt in growing towards greater health and balance within their minds, bodies, and spirits. Thus, the scientists and the priests were of a single group. The doctrines of religion and science were based upon the integral knowledge and psychic perception of human multidimensional anatomy and its relationship to the reincarnational process. The ancient wisdom was carefully safeguarded by the priesthood because they knew that the inherent power of psychic abilities and psychoenergetic technologies could again be misused by those of a less-than-spiritual consciousness, as had been the case with the Sons of Belial in the latter years of old Atlantis.

This time of greater spiritual integration covered more than several thousand years of Egyptian history. Unfortunately, corruption eventually settled into the priesthood and societal structures. There resulted an eventual loss of much knowledge and spiritual wisdom. The elder priests anticipated that a corrupt priesthood would eventually misuse the powerful old Atlantean knowledge. Thus, the old records were safeguarded in special places such as the Pyramid of Records. This ancient chamber is described in the Edgar Cayce readings. As yet it has not been discovered by archaeologists. These records were to be secreted away until a future time when people of the correct spiritual orientation could responsibly deal with the powerful ancient knowledge of Atlantean technology. Stories of the miraculous deeds of the old Atlantean elders and their gifts of knowledge and science to Egyptian culture have gradually come down through the ages via Egypt's legends and mythology, which survive to this day in the hieroglyphics covering the walls of Egyptian temples. Because of the multiple symbolic meanings in certain sets of hieroglyphics, some of the original esoteric translations of ancient Egyptian writings have remained undisclosed even to modern-day Egyptologists. The Pyramid of Records has yet to be discovered. It is possibly a hidden crystal chamber within the great pyramid of Cheops. But the time is gradually approaching when these secret caches of Atlantean knowledge will be unearthed and revealed after many centuries of silence. The opening of the chamber is dependent upon a raising of the spiritual consciousness of enough people upon the planet to allow the powerful knowledge stored within the entombed records to be understood and utilized responsibly. When these hidden records are made public, perhaps much of ancient history will have to be rewritten. The records should confirm much of what many individuals already know within their hearts and minds.

After the fall of the spiritual dynasties of Egypt, some of the ancient wisdom did survive and was translated into what later became known as the ancient mystery schools of Greece. Again, the knowledge of people's spiritual origins and their vibrational subtle anatomy continued to be taught, albeit in secret, for many years. The teachings of the ancient wisdom instructed many esoteric initiates in the powerful ways that emotions could affect the subtle bodies. Those that taught within the mystery schools demanded that aspirants be of the purest motivation in their hearts as well as in their spiritual orientations. Many of the teachings were actually very simple things, such as the golden rule of "do unto others as you would have them do unto you." They were shown the so-called Law of Correspondences, sometimes known as the principle of "as above, so below," which states that events upon the physical plane are mirrored by actions taking place within higher vibrational spheres of influence.

Over the succeeding centuries there incarnated in different areas of

the world special teachers, who came to rekindle for humankind the ancient spiritual wisdom in a form that the simple peoples of the time could
understand. To the Far East there came Lao-Tze, Confucius, as well as Buddha,
Zoroaster, Mohammed and others to teach the wisdom of following the
spiritual way. Following the incarnations of these mighty souls, new schools
of philosophy and entirely new religions sprang into being to carry forth
the greatest of their teachings to a world that was hungry for spiritual knowledge. To the Middle East there came one of the world's greatest teachers,
who literally changed the course of history. Of course, that teacher was
Jesus, otherwise known as Yeshua ben Joseph, a simple Hebrew rabbi who
came to show the way and remind us of the beauty of our spiritual heritage.

Although the Bible and history books do not record it (as some of
these sources have been altered by people throughout the centuries), Jesus
actually spent a period of his life travelling to Egypt, Greece, and other
places to learn of the mystery religions and spiritual philosophies of other
cultures.[9] Jesus became an adept, proficient in demonstrating various
spiritual powers. He did healing through the laying-on-of-hands, as has
been documented in the Bible. Because of the primitive desert peoples
with whom he was dealing, Jesus translated his lessons on spirituality into
symbolic parables. These stories were not meant for literal translation, as
many have come to interpret them, but for their symbolic significance.

Unbeknownst to many modern-day Christians, Jesus also taught
about reincarnation. But portions of the original Bible that alluded to reincarnation were deleted in 555 A.D. by a powerful Catholic pope who felt
that such information on past and future lives would interfere with the
religious power of the church.[10] Jesus' resurrection was a demonstration of
the reincarnational principle of consciousness continuing beyond the
death of the physical body. He tried to teach people not to fear death, but
to understand it as a natural process of the cycle of life, death, and rebirth
of the soul's consciousness through its many incarnations. Jesus came to
demonstrate to the world of lost and forgotten souls that the most crucial
lesson they must learn was *love*. He told people that they must learn to
forgive others and try to send love and light to all individuals. Of his many
miracles, Jesus said, "These things I do, so too can you do."

People through the centuries have accepted Jesus as the one true son
of God. This is, in fact, a misinterpretation. What Jesus came to teach us
is that *we are all* the children of God. In the beginning, when God particularized the divine beingness into many smaller units of consciousness

which eventually became the souls of humankind, this was done through the creative power of thought. These souls might be called the products of God's act of tremendous creative thought. A colloquial term for a thought or idea which becomes manifest in physical reality is a brainchild. In point of fact, we who are the evolving souls or fragments of God's consciousness are divine brainchildren. *We are the sons and daughters of God.* This is what Jesus was trying to say. But his truths have been lost and confused through the literalization of what was meant to be only an allegory.

The most important things that Jesus taught—learning to love ourselves and others, to forgive, and to pray and give thanks to the Creator—are just as important today as they were 2000 years ago. We have seen how distortions of our emotional nature, and blockage of our ability to love and forgive, can cause disturbance and imbalance of our chakras and subtle-energy anatomy. When one combines weakness of the body's energetic physiology from emotional, mental, and subtle imbalances, with infectious or toxic environmental factors, illness is often the result. Through the sophisticated New Age technologies which spiritual scientists are using to document the existence of our subtle anatomic framework, we are finally beginning to understand the true spiritual significance of what Jesus and many others have taught throughout the centuries since the time of Lemuria and Atlantis. *The discoveries that we are making today are, in fact, reincarnational expressions of older spiritual knowledge which originated in these ancient yet advanced civilizations.*

The basic principles of holistic and natural healing, as well as vibrational medicine, are actually thousands of centuries old, dating back to the times of Atlantis and Lemuria. Through the continuous cycle of regeneration and rebirth, these ideas have surfaced once again to produce methods of spiritual healing that may help to alleviate much of the dis-ease that humanity seems to have inflicted upon itself. Homeopathy, flower essences, the use of sunlight, color, and crystals in healing are actually a very ancient art. It is only because of a gradual shift in consciousness within the new guard of the medical and scientific community that the intellectual and spiritual environment has ripened to the point that these powerful healing modalities may again surface to see the light of day.

Vibrational Medicine
As the Spiritual Science of the Future:
The Next Evolutionary Step in Personal and Planetary
Transformation

Vibrational or energy medicine has finally found modern-day scientific validation in our Einsteinian understanding of matter as energy, especially as it is applied to the examination of biological systems from the perspective of interactive energy fields. More simply stated, the Einsteinian viewpoint sees human beings from the higher dimensional perspective of fields within fields within fields. Matter itself, from the infinitessimal subatomic particle to the level of the physical and higher vibrational bodies, is now seen as dynamic energy contained within the constraints of fluctuating energy fields. We have observed that experimentation in the fields of high-energy particle physics, Kirlian photography, holography, and the study of the effects of psychic healing on biological systems, have converged to teach us new ways of understanding the energetic field nature of all life processes. As we begin to think about human beings as multidimensional spiritual beings of light, we can start to comprehend the powerful effects of vibrational healing modalities which deliver specified quanta of subtle energy to promote healing through reintegration and realignment of our mind/body/spirit complexes. Vibrational healing methods work by rebalancing disturbances of structure and energy flow within the context of our multilevel interactive energetic fields.

Many of the energies that make up the etheric and higher dimensional worlds of human subtle anatomy vibrate at speeds faster than ordinary light. The physics of so-called magnetoelectric energy, predicted by Einstein's equations, holds the keys to deciphering the scientific principles which underlie the behavior of higher vibrational phenomena. Our thoughts and our emotions are indeed manifestations of this special energy. For medicine and psychology to truly advance over the next several decades, we must begin to think about our emotional problems as energetic imbalances that affect the functioning of our subtle and physical anatomy. If we can accept that these emotional disturbances are partly due to problems within the subtle fields of human physiology, then we can begin to utilize other natural forms of subtle energy that can remove or correct the problematic imbalances. Because homeopathic remedies, flower essences, gem elixirs, crystals, and color energies affect the subtle-energy fields of the human body, such vibrational therapies can have powerful impacts on stress and illness. Over the next twenty years, we will see the creation of a whole new science of energy as it applies to human consciousness and subtle physiology. Spiritual scientists will begin to extend the limits of known science to incorporate higher energetic phenomena.

Humankind is at a unique turning point in history. The development of new technologies in pharmacology, surgery, and electronic imaging systems for diagnosis has allowed traditional medicine to evolve in this century toward tremendous breakthroughs in the treatment of serious illness. We have come far in treating many common infectious diseases, in providing relief from various types of cancer and heart disease, as well as in knowing better ways of controlling hypertension and kidney ailments. Orthodox medicine is truly a marvelous field of continual discovery. We cannot deny that modern medicine has uplifted the human condition significantly, for many people would have died prematurely had it not been for some of the miracles of its scientific discoveries and applications. The problem lies in the fact that orthodox medical approaches still fall short of treating the *true causes* of illness. Traditional physicians can treat the *effects* of disease; but can they really approach the emotional, mental, bioenergetic, and spiritual precursors of disease?

At the present time, we simply cannot do without conventional drugs or surgery. Our expertise in the field of vibrational healing is still at an early stage. The current structure of health care in America is such that one may have difficulty obtaining insurance coverage for any type of medical treatment other than that provided by orthodox practitioners of medicine. Seen from an economic standpoint, third-party payer organizations who reimburse physicians for medical treatment are still locked into the Newtonian medical model as the only mode of therapy. As such, those who have their health care provided by health insurance providers and the growing organizations of PPO's and HMO's can only have their health-care dollars spent on traditional approaches. Holistic medical practitioners are slowly becoming more prevalent, but the system is slow to change.

Of course, one can always pay out-of-pocket for vitamins, flower essences, and homeopathic remedies, but not everyone can afford the expense. Generally speaking, however, many subtle energy and natural healing remedies tend to be much less expensive than conventional drug treatments. Holistic and vibrational medicine is not something that should be strictly for the upper middle class. It is a type of healing system which should apply to everyone, should they be open and interested enough to try it. Unfortunately, the increasing cost of health care in this country has made it necessary for many to obtain health insurance to provide for the medical needs of their families. Because of the third-party payer's attitudes toward reimbursement for services, the tendency is still to encourage orthodox medical approaches. An optimistic note can be derived from the observation that a number of third-party payers, including Blue Cross, are opting toward the promotion of wellness programs of prevention. These third-party payers have learned that it is significantly more economical to prevent than to treat illness. Hopefully, this is a positive sign of things to come.

As practitioners of vibrational medicine begin to acquire greater amounts of clinical data on the efficacy of their treatment approaches, and as more holistically directed physicians become inclined to use such subtle energetic methods, we may eventually see the proliferation of New Age health insurance companies which will not only cover orthodox medical and surgical treatments, but also flower essences, homeopathy, Voll and other electroacupuncture diagnostic workups, and many similar procedures. Unfortunately, the insurance company of the future is still a long way off, mainly because of the political power and dogmatic opinions of antagonistic organizations like the American Medical Association. Much of vibrational medicine is still considered quackery by the Newtonian minds of the AMA. That is why it is so crucial that vibrational medicine and the subtle anatomical connections between health and illness become scientifically established through medical research utilizing new etheric scanners and imaging systems, which can prove the validity of this system of diagnostic theory and practice.

Orthodox medicine has been an important and necessary stepping stone in the evolution of our modern healing sciences. Newtonian physics was also an important stepping stone toward the eventual recognition of Einsteinian models of relativity and energetic field theory. Modern medicine, as we discussed in the first three chapters, is largely based upon Newtonian models of mechanistic behavior. It is a system of understanding that must now expand and grow by incorporating the newer discoveries in science. Just as Einstein was initially thought to be crazy when he first expounded upon his radical theories, many of today's proponents of energetic and vibrational physiology are also considered to be too far out. This is often the case with far-sighted thinking that is a little too ahead of its time. It took more than 60 years for scientists to begin to validate what Einstein had told them. Now he is heralded as a genius. Such examples of common roadblocks to progress suggest some of the difficulties in acceptance encountered by pioneers like vibrationally minded healers who are also just a little too ahead of their time. Unfortunately, growth is often painful not only for individuals but for human cultures and civilizations as well. As we evolve toward new paradigms in science, and embrace the Einsteinian understanding of matter as energy and physiological systems as interactive energy fields, doctors will begin to slowly replace older drug and surgical techniques with more subtle and less invasive methods of treatment. The newer systems of subtle-energy medicine will not only relieve the symptoms of illness, as does traditional medicine, but they will also address the emotional, mental, bioenergetic, subtle environmental, and spiritual causes of disease.

The future vibrational physicians will be more than doctors who dispense pills and potions. They will be healers and sensitives. They will diagnose the emotional imbalances and bioenergetic disturbances which may eventually manifest as illness within their patients. They will be able to identify those biopsychoenergetic factors which can predispose to sickness, and assist their patients in preventing illness by teaching them to modify these elements of imbalance. Physician/healers will instruct their patients in ways that can promote greater wellness through improved nutritional and exercise habits, healthier patterns of emotional response, stress reduction techniques that promote relaxation, and self-awareness meditations which help an individual discover the real causes of their dis-ease and distress.

Spiritual health-care practitioners will also be able to diagnose imbalances in the body at the levels of the chakras and the meridians through a variety of intuitive and instrumentational techniques. In addition to prescribing the vibrational tinctures already mentioned, they will also direct sound and laser energy into acupuncture points, and move healing energies into the body through the laying-on-of-hands. However, in order for vibrational physicians to be successful at healing illness, people must begin to accept responsibility for their lives and for their recovery. They must work as a team with physicians in moving their lives into patterns of greater balance and an integration of the interactive elements of mind, body, and spirit.

As difficult as it will be for some to accept, we must begin to acknowledge the validity of reincarnation as a system by which the soul evolves to gain experience. For it is through the reincarnational process that illness is often created as a teaching experience for the soul. It is only when disease is understood in this context, and when we grasp the true spiritual nature of the consciousness that seeks to manifest through the transitory physical body, that we can correct our patterns of emotional imbalance and work through the obstacles and lessons that our soul has chosen for us. We have seen that orthodox medicine does not hold all the answers to dealing with illness in our high-tech industrial nations. Subtle-energy medicine does contain solutions to many of the problems that orthodox treatment methods cannot hope to correct. Vibrational medicine is revolutionary in both its theory and its methods of application. It is a healing system whose time has finally come.

The discord and unrest occurring upon the planet at this time is a higher reflection of the emotional and spiritual imbalances that exist in many people throughout the world. We must begin to heal dis-ease and distress at the level of causes and not just at the superficial world of physical effects. In order to accept and work with vibrational healing methods, one must begin to make the transition toward personal transformation that is necessary before true physical and spiritual healing can occur. Already we are seeing how certain segments of humanity have begun to manifest the transformational consciousness necessary to assist the Earth and the people upon it in making the critical leap from planetary distress to peace and global healing that is critical if this small blue sphere is to survive.

Vibrational medicine appears to hold some of the answers for a world that seems quite ill, but it will only work if we can work with it. If utilized correctly, subtle-energy methods of healing promise to create a new wave of healing, balance, and peace upon the planet as has not been seen for thousands of years. That which we are beginning to use in the form of vibrational treatments have had their origins in ancient systems of healing which have been held in secret for many centuries. Perhaps humanity has finally begun to accept enough responsibility for its actions that the knowledge and grace of our ancient spiritual teachers may again be visited upon many needy people in this, the dawning of a New Age.

Key Points to Remember

1. Human beings are dynamic energy systems which reflect evolutionary patterns of soul growth. Human consciousness is constantly learning, growing, and evolving. As spiritual awareness of this dynamic process of change becomes more prevalent, there will be a ripple effect that will shift the energetic dynamics of the human race as a whole.

2. In general, most people go to physicians to be treated for their ills without thinking about the need for themselves to somehow change their lifestyles or mindstyles. The physician-patient interaction is only healing to the extent that there is mutual cooperation and increased awareness on the parts of both parties. People must take responsibility for their own lives, in part by following the advice of their physicians.

3. Our illnesses may often be a symbolic reflection of our own internal states of emotional unrest, spiritual blockage, and dis-ease. Although there may be external factors operating which have negative effects, these effects are only able to create disease where there is an underlying susceptiblity. Our subtle energetic components, i.e. the chakras and the meridian system, translate our emotional and spiritual difficulties into physiological weaknesses which may eventually result in a localized system breakdown in the physical body, i.e. disease.

4. When disease occurs, it is a sign that we are constricting the natural flow of creative consciousness and subtle life-energies through our multidimensional body/mind/spirit complexes. It is a symbolic warning message that something has gone wrong in the system. The area of constriction needs to be rebalanced if lasting health is to be achieved.

5. Many of the basic emotional/spiritual issues that human beings are trying to work through are reflections of the key lessons of the chakras. These chakric issues relate to grounding, sexuality, personal power, love, will, creative expression, inner vision, and spiritual seeking.

6. When the individual has a blockage in working through one of these key life issues, it may result in a blocked flow of energy in the corresponding major chakra, thus constricting the flow of life-energy to the associated bodily organ system(s). Such blockages may eventually express themselves as illnesses if the problem becomes chronic and is an important learning experience for the incarnating personality.

7. Of the chakric issues, none is more important than the lesson of the heart chakra, for it involves being able to freely express love toward oneself, as well as to others, both strangers as well as meaningful others. Personal and spiritual transformation are ultimately dependent upon the opening and blossoming of the flower-like heart chakra.

8. Fear and misunderstanding are the root causes of much illness, distress, and suffering in the world. Often, when we are functioning in the lower aspects of our awareness, we are blind to our own fears and we project them onto the world, when in fact the problem lies within. The key toward dissolving and healing these fears is to release the blockages of the heart chakra and to operate from a position of love and forgiveness. As we open our heart center and the higher spiritual energies can more easily flow through us, it is a catalyst to healing not only ourselves, but also those around us.

9. Reincarnation is a system by which souls, the particularizations of God's own energy, can evolve, learn, and spiritually mature, thus adding to the total knowledge and experience banks of both God and the individuated consciousnesses that are the souls. Because of the holographic connectivity between God and all aspects of creation, the vast consciousness which is God is always aware of everything that happens in the universe.

10. The system of reincarnation allows souls to learn by trial and experience through many lifetimes in physical bodies. Both positive and negative life experiences are stored in the causal body, and through karma, may affect the outcome of future lives.

11. The misdeeds and tormenting behavior of one lifetime may be translated into an appropriate handicap in future lifetimes, thus teaching the lesson of seeing both sides of the issue. Similarly, the incarnating personality may achieve wealth, position, and social advancement partly as a consequence of the grace of their positive deeds in previous lives. The philosophy of reincarnation allows one to see the various physical and socioeconomic handicaps as learning experiences chosen by the soul for the growth and spiritual maturation of the physical personality. How each person chooses to act in a particular setting, as to whether or not they will use that circumstance as an opportunity for soul growth, will vary according to the free will of the individual.

12. There have been many past civilizations which knew the truth

about reincarnation and human multidimensional anatomy. These included Atlantis, Lemuria, and the various mystery schools of Egypt and
Greece. In spite of human perversion, wars, and corruption, there have
always been secret outposts teaching the divine nature of humanity and
the full range of extended human potential.

13. Over the centuries, there have incarnated great teachers who
came to rekindle the ancient spiritual wisdom. These included Lao-Tze,
Confucius, Buddha, Zoroaster, Mohammed, and Jesus of Nazareth. In
their wake have sprung up many world religions, each teaching the
same basic principles in a slightly different tongue and version, but all
speaking the same truth. What has been lost over the years is the symbolic nature of the lessons they came to teach. Their metaphorical
words have been literalized, often to the extent that the basic spiritual
meanings have been altered or lost.

14. Vibrational medicine is a healing approach which is based
upon the Einsteinian concept of matter as energy, and of human beings
as a series of complex energy fields in dynamic equilibrium. The
physical matter field is in equilibrium with these negative space/time,
higher dimensional fields. These fields of etheric, astral, mental, causal
and even higher frequency matter operate to provide energetic information, structure, and higher knowledge to the incarnating personality
from its spiritual source. The purpose of the entire structural arrangement is to provide a vehicle of expression for the soul to grow through
experiences in the worlds of matter.

15. Vibrational medicine seeks to reunite the personality with the
Higher Self in a more meaningful, connected way. Vibrational
modalities help to strengthen the energetic connections between the
personality and the soul itself, by rebalancing the body/mind/spirit
complex as a whole. Not all vibrational healing tools work at the higher
energetic levels, but it is the intent and goal of the vibrational
healer/physician to seek and assist this alignment within his or her
patients.

16. As the New Age technologies evolve, and imaging systems are
developed which can substantiate this author's picture of extended
multidimensional human anatomy, vibrational medicine will become
more widely accepted by those within the more orthodox medical
establishment.

APPENDIX

The Tiller-Einstein Model of Positive-Negative Space/Time

The reason I call this model the Tiller-Einstein Model is because its insights are basic to the Einsteinian equation relating energy to the matter from which it is derived. The form most familiarly expressed for this equation is $E=mc^2$, however this is not the entire expression. The true equation is modified by a proportionality constant known as the Einstein-Lorentz Transformation that describes how different parameters of measurement, from time distortion to alteration of length, width, and mass, will vary according to the velocity of the system being described. The true Einsteinian equation is:

Diagram 13.
EINSTEIN-LORENTZ TRANSFORMATION

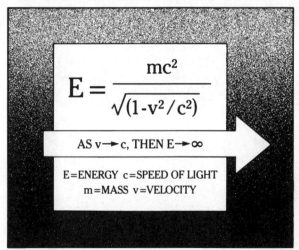

$$E = \frac{mc^2}{\sqrt{(1 - v^2/c^2)}}$$

AS $v \rightarrow c$, THEN $E \rightarrow \infty$

E=ENERGY c=SPEED OF LIGHT
m=MASS v=VELOCITY

In describing the kinetic energy of a system, one may utilize the equation: kinetic energy = ½ mv². As a particle moves faster, its kinetic energy increases according to the given equation. The relativistic factor given by the Einstein-Lorentz Transformation demonstrates mathematically that as a particle moves at velocities approximating the speed of light, the mass of that particle increases exponentially. The proportionality constant which

503

describes this increase in mass is shown in the denominator of the above diagramatic equation. The only thing which is affected by the proportionality constant is mass. The rest of the variables, such as "c," which is a constant, are unaffected. A graphic representation of this relationship betwee. the energy of a particle and its velocity is shown in Diagram 14. A demonstration of how this proportionality constant mathematically increases mass, and the total energy of a system as given by Einstein's equation $E=mc^2$, is as follows.

In the above equation, labelled the Einstein-Lorentz Transformation, we see that energy is related to matter according to a proportionality constant containing the ratio v^2/c^2. As velocity (v) of a particle approaches the speed of light (c), then this ratio approaches the number 1. If one substitutes into (v) a velocity equalling 99.995 percent of the speed of light, then the ratio v^2/c^2 is close to 1 (actually 0.9999). The figure within the square root sign shows that we must subtract our previous solution from 1: 1-0.9999= 0.0001. The square root of 0.0001 is equal to 0.01. This solution must now be inverted because it exists in the equation as the denominator of the frac-

Diagram 14.
RELATIONSHIP OF ENERGY TO VELOCITY

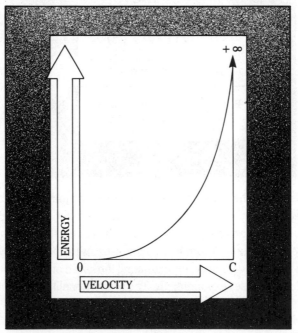

tional expression, therefore $1/0.01 = 100$. This means that at a velocity of 99.995 percent of the speed of light, the associated energy calculated from the expression mc^2 must be multiplied by a factor of 100. If one were dealing with only the mass of the particle, then the Einstein-Lorentz Transformation would cause the mass to be greater by a factor of 100. As velocity goes even higher, and even closer to light velocity, the amplification factor becomes exponentially greater. The visual expression of this relationship is displayed in Diagram 14.

This diagram illustrates the exponential relationship between matter and energy at velocities approaching the speed of light. To those interpreting this relationship, it would seem that it is physically impossible to accelerate particles beyond the speed of light. For instance, high-energy particle physicists are aware that as one tries to accelerate a subatomic particle faster and faster, close to the speed of light, large amounts of energy are needed. This is because as the particle accelerates faster and faster, its mass increases proportionately, until the energy needed for further acceleration to light velocity becomes tremendous.

This is, of course, the energy necessary to accelerate a "physical" particle. Let us examine the equation again but this time substituting a velocity greater than light, where v is greater than c. Because the ratio v^2/c^2 is now greater than 1, 1 minus a number greater than 1 is equal to a negative number. One ends up with an equation that has a denominator containing the square root of a negative number. This may be factored out to a positive number times the square root of -1. This number has been called "i" by mathematicians. It is a factor which can be substituted for the square root of -1 (for ease in dealing with difficult equations). The square root of -1 is considered an imaginary number by most individuals dealing with numbers.

As mentioned in Chapter 4, certain pioneering mathematicians, such as Charles Muses, consider square the root of -1 to be one of a category of numbers he describes as "hypernumbers." These hypernumbers, he believes, are necessary in developing equations which mathematically describe the behavior of higher dimensional phenomena (such as the subtle energetic interactions of living systems that we have been describing throughout this book). Although at first glance imaginary numbers like the square root of -1 might seem to be impossible to fathom, Muses points out that they are necessary for finding solutions to the equations of electromagnetic and quantum theory.

What happens to the behavior of matter and energy, as described by the Einstein–Lorentz Transformation, when we are dealing with systems whose velocities exceed the speed of light?

Diagram 15.
POSITIVE-NEGATIVE SPACE/TIME MODEL

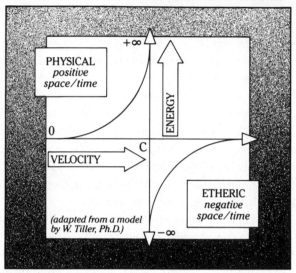

To the left of c (light velocity), we observe the familiar exponential curve we have just demonstrated. However, when we substitute velocities greater than light in the equation, a second inverted curve appears with a mirror-like symmetry to the first. Whereas the first curve begins at the zero axis and climbs toward positive infinity ($+\infty$), the second curve begins at negative infinity ($-\infty$) and returns back toward the zero axis. Tiller refers to matter described by the curve to the left of c, (at velocities less than the speed of light) as the world of *positive space/time* (+S/T). This is the familiar world of physical matter. In Tiller's model, the curve to the right of c (at velocities greater than that of light), is the world of *negative space/time* (−S/T), where energy is magnetoelectric and negatively entropic, and substance is of a subtle magnetic character.

Negative space/time is the dimension of the etheric world of energies, which includes the human etheric body. The substance which makes up our etheric bodies vibrates at speeds faster than light, making it difficult to directly measure with conventional electromagnetic sensing equipment. In addition, it is my opinion that the astral world also exists within the negative space/time dimension, at vibrational speeds exceeding those of the etheric. The exact dividing line between the two cannot yet be measured, as the graph coordinates of the Tiller-Einstein model are still theoretical. The fact that both etheric and astral energies move faster than light explains their common subtle magnetic nature as well as their resistance to measurement with our usual systems of sensing. The developed clairvoyant is able to perceive these subtle energies because he or she does so through energy taken in via the etheric and astral chakras, which act as organs of perceptions on the appropriate levels of reality.

NOTES

CHAPTER 1

1. H. S. Burr, *The Fields of Life* (New York: Ballantine Books, 1972).
2. S. Kirlian and V. Kirlian, "Photography and Visual Observations by Means of High Frequency Currents," *Journal of Scientific and Applied Photography*, vol. 6 (1961), pp. 145-148.
3. W. Tiller, "Present Scientific Understanding of the Kirlian Discharge Process," *Psychoenergetic Systems*, vol. 3, nos. 1-4 (1979).
4. S. Mallikarjun, "Kirlian Photography in Cancer Diagnosis," *Osteopathic Physician*, vol. 45, no. 5 (1978), pp. 24-27.
5. "Kirlian Photography Fighting for Toehold in U. S. Medicine," *Medical News*, March 6, 1978, p. 24.
6. T. Moss, "Puzzles and Promises," *Osteopathic Physician*, February, 1976, pp. 30-37.
7. "The Ghost Effect," *IKRA Communications* (Brooklyn, N.Y.: International Kirlian Research Association, June,1978).
8. T. Moss, *The Body Electric* (Los Angeles: J.P. Tarcher, Inc., 1979) p. 219.
9. "Life Energy Patterns Visible Via New Technique," *Brain/Mind Bulletin*, vol. 7, no. 14 (August 23, 1982).
10. J. Briggs and F. Peat, "David Bohm's Looking-Glass Map," in *Looking Glass Universe: The Emerging Science of Wholeness*, (New York: Simon and Schuster, Inc., 1984).
11. R. Targ and H. Puthoff, *Mind Reach: Scientists Look at Psychic Ability* (New York: Dell Publishing Co., Inc., 1977).
12. P. Levine et al, "EEG Coherence During the Transcendental Meditation Technique," in *Scientific Research on the Transcendental Meditation Program: Vol. I*, ed. Orme-Johnson and Farrow (Livingston Manor, NY: Maharishi European Research University Press, 1977), pp. 187-207.
13. J. Whitton, "Ramp Functions in EEG Power Spectra During Actual or Attempted Paranormal Events," *New Horizons*, vol. 1 (1974), pp. 174-183.
14. M. Cade and N. Coxhead, *The Awakened Mind* (New York: Delacorte Press, 1979), pp. 242-246.
15. T. Kuhn, *The Structure of Scientific Revolutions* (Chicago: University of Chicago Press, 1970).

16. C. Tart, "State-Specific Sciences," in *States of Consciousness* (New York: E. P. Dutton & Co., 1975), pp. 206-228.

CHAPTER 2

1. B. Griggs, Green Pharmacy: *A History of Herbal Medicine* (New York: Viking Press, 1981).

2. S. Hahnemann, *Organon of Medicine* (1810; reprint, Los Angeles: J. P. Tarcher, Inc., 1982).

3. B. Grad, "Some Biological Effects of Laying on of Hands and Their Implications," in *Dimensions in Wholistic Healing: New Frontiers in the Treatment of the Whole Person*, ed. Otto and Knight (Chicago: Nelson-Hall, 1979), pp. 199-212.

4. "New Technologies Detect Effects of Healing Hands," *Brain/Mind Bulletin*, vol. 10, no. 16 (September 30, 1985).

5. R. Miller, "Methods of Detecting and Measuring Healing Energies," in *Future Science*, ed. White and Krippner (New York: Doubleday & Co., Inc., 1977), pp. 431-444.

6. D. Dean and E. Brame, "Physical Changes in Water by Laying-on of Hands," in *Proceedings of the Second International Congress of Psychotronics*, (Monte Carlo, 1975).

7. S. Schwartz et al., "Infrared Spectra Alteration in Water Proximate to the Palms of Therapeutic Practitioners," (unpublished technical report, 1987).

8. D. Shepherd, *The Magic of the Minimum Dose: Experiences and Cases* (1938; reprint, Wellingborough, Northamptonshire: Health Science Press, 1973).

9. L. Bendit and P. Bendit, *The Etheric Body of Man* (Wheaton, IL: Theosophical Publishing House, 1977).

10. S. Karagulla, *Breakthrough to Creativity* (Santa Monica, CA: DeVorss & Co., 1967).

11. R. Grossinger, *Planet Medicine* (Garden City, NY: Anchor Press, Doubleday, 1980), pp. 165-175.

12. Gurudas, *Flower Essences and Vibrational Healing*, channeled by Kevin Ryerson, (Albuquerque, NM: Brotherhood of Life, 1983), p. 35.

CHAPTER 3

1. N. Shealy, "Wholistic Healing and the Relief of Pain," in *Dimensions of Wholistic Healing: New Frontiers in the Treatment of the Whole Person*, ed. Otto and Knight (Chicago: Nelson-Hall, 1979), pp. 391-399.

2. R. Melzack and P. Wall, "Pain Mechanisms: A New Theory," *Science*, vol. 150 (1965), pp. 971-979.

3. B. Sjolund and M. Eriksson, "Electro-Acupuncture and Endogenous Morphines," *Lancet*, Nov. 2 1976, p. 1085.

4. R. Becker, "An Application of Direct Current Neural Systems to Psychic Phenomena," *Psychoenergetic Systems*, vol. 2 (1977), pp. 189-196.

5. R. Becker et al., "The Direct Current System: A Link Between the Environment and the Organism," *New York State Journal of Medicine*, vol. 62 (1962), pp. 1169-1176.

6. "Healing Intransigent Fractures," *Medical World News*, April 17, 1978, p. 32.

7. J. Hurtak, *The Book of Knowledge: The Keys of Enoch* (Los Gatos, CA: The Academy for Future Science, 1977), pp. 382.

8. L. Weymouth, "The Electrical Connection," *New York Magazine* November 24, 1980, p. 24.

9. G. Taubes, "An Electrifying Possibility," *Discover*, April 1986, pp. 23-37.

10. S. Stavish and N. Horwitz, "Pioneering Cancer Electrotherapy," *Medical Tribune*, March 11, 1987, p. 1.

11. R. Rose, "Magnetic Pulses in RA: Less Pain and Mobility Gain," *Medical Tribune*, June 3, 1987, p. 1.

12. R. Leichtman, *Nikola Tesla Returns* (Columbus, OH: Ariel Press, 1980), pp. 41-43.

CHAPTER 4

1. S. Rose-Neil, "The Work of Professor Kim Bong Han," *The Acupuncturist*, vol. 1 (1967), p. 15.

2. W. Tiller, "Some Energy Field Observations of Man and Nature," in *The Kirlian Aura* (Garden City, NY: Anchor Press/Doubleday, 1974), pp. 129-135.

3. P. De Vernejoul et al, "Etude Des Meridiens D'Acupuncture Par Les Traceurs Radioactifs," *Bull. Acad. Natle. Med.*, vol. 169 (Oct. 22,1985), pp. 1071-1075.

4. E. Russell, *Design For Destiny* (New York: Ballantine Books, 1971).

5. S. Karagulla, "Energy Fields and Medical Diagnosis," in *The Human Aura*, ed. N. Regush (New York: Berkeley Publishing, 1974).

6. Gurudas, *Flower Essences and Vibrational Healing,* channeled by Kevin Ryerson (Albuquerque, NM: Brotherhood of Life, Inc., 1983), p. 29.

7. W. Tiller, "Energy Field Observations," pp. 125-128.

8. I. Dumitrescu and J. Kenyon, *Electrographic Imaging in Medicine and Biology* (Suffolk, Great Britain: Neville Spearman Ltd., 1983).

9. C. W. Leadbeater, *The Chakras* (1927; reprint, Wheaton, IL: Theosophical Publishing House, 1977).

10. Gurudas, *Flower Essences*, p. 83.

11. R. Stanford, *The Spirit Unto the Churches* (Austin, TX: Association for the Understanding of Man, Inc., 1977).

12. Gurudas, *Flower Essences*, p. 85.

13. H. Motoyama and R. Brown, *Science and the Evolution of Consciousness: Chakras, Ki, and Psi* (Brookline, MA: Autumn Press, Inc., 1978), pp. 93-98.

14. I. Bentov, personal communication, November, 1977.

15. "Electronic Evidence of Auras, Chakras in UCLA Study," *Brain/Mind Bulletin*, vol. 3, no. 9 (March 20, 1978).

16. R. Miller, "Bridging the Gap: An Interview with Valerie Hunt, Ed.D.," *Science of Mind*, October 1983.

17. A. Bailey, *Esoteric Healing* (New York: Lucis Publishing Co., 1953), pp. 195-196.

18. A. Bailey, *Esoteric Healing*, p. 625.

19. J. Gray, *The Psychology of Fear and Stress* (New York: McGraw-Hill, 1971).

20. P. Maclean, "Psychosomatic Disease and the 'Visceral Brain': Recent Developments Bearing on the Papez Theory of Emotion," *Psychosomatic Medicine*, vol. 11, pp. 338-353.

21. Near Death Experience in Children: A First Report," *Brain/Mind Bulletin*, vol. 9, no.2 (December 12, 1983).

22. R. Moody, *Life After Life* (New York: Bantam Books, 1975).

23. K. Ring, *Heading Toward Omega: In Search of the Near Death Experience* (New York: William Morrow & Co., 1984).

24. R. Monroe, *Far Journeys* (Garden City, NY: Doubleday & Co., Inc., 1985).

25. I. Swann, *To Kiss Earth Good-Bye* (New York: Dell Publishing Co., Inc., 1975).

26. R. Morris, "PRF Research on Out-Of-Body Experiences, 1973," *Theta*, Summer 1974.

27. H. Puthoff and R. Targ, "Psychic Research and Modern Physics," in *Psychic Exploration: A Challenge For Science*, ed. J. White (New York: G. P. Putnam's Sons, 1974), pp. 536-53.

28. C. Muses, "Working with the Hypernumber Idea," in *Consciousness and Reality*, ed. C. Muses and A. Young (New York: Avon Books, 1972), pp. 448-469.

29. L. Feldman, "Short Bibliography On Faster-Than-Light Particles (Tachyons)," *American Journal Of Physics*, vol. 42 (March 1974).

30. R. Miller, "Methods of Detecting and Measuring Healing Energies," in *Future Science*, ed. S. Krippner and J. White (New York: Doubleday & Co., 1977), pp. 431-444.

31. Smith J., "The Influence on Enzyme Growth by "Laying-on-of-Hands," *The Dimensions of Healing: A Symposium* (Los Altos, CA: Academy of Parapsychology and Medicine), 1972.

32. "New Technologies Detect Effects of Healing Hands," *Brain/Mind Bulletin*, vol. 10, no. 16 (September 30, 1985).

33. A. Besant and C. W. Leadbeater, *Thought-Forms* (1925; reprint, Wheaton, IL: Theosophical Publishing House, 1969).

34. Leichtman, R., *Einstein Returns* (Columbus, OH: Ariel Press, 1982), pp. 48-49.

35. J. Leo, "I Was Beheaded in the 1700s," *Time*, September 10, 1984, p. 68.

36. W. Tiller, "Theoretical Modeling on the Function of Man," in *Healers and the Healing Process*, ed. G. Meek (Wheaton, IL: Theosophical Publishing House, 1977), p. 192.

37. Hodson, G., *The Miracle of Birth: A Clairvoyant Study of a Human Embryo* (1929; reprint, Wheaton, IL: Theosophical Publishing House, 1981), pp. 85-86.

38. O. C. Simonton et al, *Getting Well Again* (Los Angeles: J.P. Tarcher, Inc., 1978).

CHAPTER 5

1. I. Veith, *The Yellow Emperor's Classic of Internal Medicine* (Berkeley & Los Angeles: University Of California Press, 1966).

2. R. Melzack and P. Wall, "Pain Mechanisms: A New Theory," *Science*, vol. 150 (1965), pp. 971-979.

3. "Frequency a Factor in Electroacupuncture," *Brain/Mind Bulletin*, vol. 5, no.10 (April 7, 1980).

4. W. Tiller, "Some Physical Network Characteristics of Acupuncture Points and Meridians," in *Transcript of the Acupuncture Symposium* (Los Altos, CA: Academy of Parapsychology and Medicine, 1972).

5. G. Luce, *Biological Rhythms in Human and Animal Physiology* (New York: Dover Publications, Inc., 1971).

6. H. Motoyama and R. Brown, *Science and the Evolution of Consciousness* (Brookline, MA: Autumn Press, 1978), pp. 99-119.

7. The initial electrical measurements from the acupoints are referred to as "BP" or "before polarization." This BP value reflects the body's basic constitutional state or metabolic level. Following the initial measurement of the meridian termination points, the AMI device delivers a three-volt DC electrical stimulus sequentially to each of the acupoints connected to the monitoring circuit. Following the electrical stimulus, the AMI device registers a second set of readings for each of the meridian acupoints known as "AP" or "after polarization." The AP values reflect the temporary or acute condition of the meridians. The difference between the two recorded values (BP-AP) is known as "P" or "polarization." The P value indicates the amount of resistance to the external environment which the body is able to manifest. Motoyama has discovered that devices such as GSR meters

(which measure Galvanic Skin Resistance) measure only AP values which are subject to alteration under the influence of temperature, as well as the acute mental and physical status of the individual. The BP and P values have been found to be relatively constant, revealing more reliable information about the chronic status of the organism. The AMI Machine measures all three of these values (BP, P, and AP) which the computer prints out on paper within minutes of assimilating electrical information about the individual.

8. J. Pizzo et al., "Fingertips to Faces," *Osteopathic Physician*, vol. 43, no. 2 (February 1976), pp. 41-47.

9. I. Dumitrescu and J. Kenyon, *Electrographic Imaging in Medicine and Biology* (Suffolk, Great Britain: Neville Spearman, Ltd., 1983), p. 158.

10. J. Hurtak, *The Book of Knowledge: The Keys of Enoch* (Los Gatos, CA: The Academy for Future Science, 1977), pp. 526, 380.

11. B. Pomeranz, "Do Endorphins Mediate Acupuncture Analgesia?" in *Advances in Biochemical Psychopharmacology*, vol. 18, ed. Costa and Trabucchi (New York: Raven Press, 1978), pp. 351-359.

12. L. Barchas et al., "Behavioral Neurochemistry: Neuroregulators and Behavioral States," *Science*, vol. 200 (May 26, 1978), pp. 964-973.

13. T. Hokfelt et al., "Peptidergic Neurones," *Nature*, vol. 284 (April 10, 1980).

14. R. Becker, "An Application of Direct Current Neural Systems to Psychic Phenomena," *Psychoenergetic Systems*, vol. 2 (1977), pp. 189-196.

15. W. Tiller, "The Positive and Negative Space/Time Frames as Conjugate Systems," in *Future Science*, ed. White and Krippner (Garden City, NY: Doubleday & Co., Inc., 1977), pp. 257-279.

16. I. Oyle and J. Wexler, "Acupuncture with High Frequency Sound: A Preliminary Report," *Osteopathic Physician*, September 1973.

17. H. Gris and W. Dick, *The New Soviet Psychic Discoveries* (New York: Warner Books, 1978), p. 397.

18. G. Playfair and S. Hill, *The Cycles of Heaven* (New York: Avon Books, 1978), p. 281.

CHAPTER 6

1. H. Motoyama and R. Brown, *Science and the Evolution of Consciousness* (Brookline, MA: Autumn Press, 1978), pp. 99-119.

2. H. Burr, *The Fields of Life* (New York: Ballantine Books, 1972).

3. W. Tiller, "The Positive and Negative Space/Time Frames as Conjugate Systems," in *Future Science*, ed. White and Krippner, (Garden City, NY: Doubleday & Co., Inc., 1977), pp. 257-279.

4. "German Device Is Used to Detect Changes at Acupuncture Points," *Brain/Mind Bulletin*, vol. 7, no.14 (August 23, 1982).

5. I. Bell, *Clinical Ecology: A New Medical Approach to Environmental Illness* (Bolinas, CA: Common Knowledge Press, 1982).

6. A. Ber, "Neutralization of Phenolic (Aromatic) Food Compounds in a Holistic General Practice," *Journal Of Orthomolecular Psychiatry*, vol.12, no.4 (1984).

7. J. McGovern et al., "The Role of Naturally Occurring Haptens in Allergy," *Annals of Allergy*, vol.47, no.123 (1981).

8. J. McGovern, "Apparent Immunotoxic Response To Phenolic Compounds," *Food and Chemical Toxicology*, vol. 20, no. 4 (1982), p.491.

9. J. McGovern et al., "Natural Foodborne Aromatics Induce Behavioral Disturbances in Children with Hyperkinesis," *International Journal of Biosocial Diseases*, vol. 3 (December 1982).

10. Abrams, A., *New Concepts in Diagnosis and Treatment* (San Francisco, CA: The Philopolis Press, 1916).

11. L. Day and G. de la Warr, *New Worlds Beyond the Atom* (London: Vincent Stuart, Ltd., 1956).

12. L. Day and G. de la Warr, *Matter In The Making* (London: Vincent Stuart, Ltd., 1966).

13. D. Tansley, M. Rae, and A. Westlake, *Dimensions of Radionics: New Techniques of Instrumented Distant-Healing* (Essex, England: C.W. Daniel Co. Ltd., 1977).

14. R. Targ and H. Puthoff, *Mind-Reach: Scientists Look at Psychic Ability* (New York: Dell Publishing Co., 1977).

15. E. Baerlein and A. Dower, *Healing with Radionics: The Science of Healing Energy* (Wellingborough, Northamptonshire: Thorsons Publishers Ltd., 1980), pp. 48-49.

16. D. Dean, "Plethysmograph Recordings as ESP Responses," *International Journal of Neuropsychiatry*, September/October 1966.

17. W. Tiller, "Radionics, Radiesthesia, and Physics," in *The Varieties of Healing Experience: Exploring Psychic Phenomena in Healing* (Los Altos, CA: The Academy of Parapsychology and Medicine, 1971), pp. 55-78.

18. A. Mermet, *Principles and Practice of Radiesthesia* (London: Vincent Stuart Co., 1959).

19. D. Tansley, *Radionics and the Subtle Anatomy of Man* (Essex, England: Health Science Press, 1972).

CHAPTER 7

1. E. Bach, "Heal Thyself," in *The Bach Flower Remedies* (1931; reprint, New Canaan, CT: Keats Publishing Co., 1977).

2. R. Armstrong, "Radiesthesia: A Tool of Intuitive Perspective," *The Flower Essence Journal*, no. 2 (July 1980), pp. 7-9.

3. Gurudas, *Flower Essences and Vibrational Healing*, channeled by Kevin Ryerson (Albuquerque, NM: Brotherhood Of Life, Inc., 1983).

4. Ibid., pp. 29-30.

5. I. Bentov, "Micromotion of the Body as a Factor in the Development of the Nervous System," in *Kundalini: Psychosis Or Transcendence?* by L. Sannella (San Francisco, CA: H.S. Dakin Co., 1976), pp. 71-95.

6. Gurudas, *Flower Essences and Vibrational Healing*, pp. 30-31.

7. Ibid., p. 35.

8. D. Dean, "Plethysmograph Recordings as ESP Responses," *International Journal Of Neuropsychiatry*, September/October 1966.

9. Gurudas, *Flower Essences and Vibrational Healing*, p. 31.

10. Ibid., p. 41.

11. Ibid., pp. 42-43.

12. Ibid., p. 44.

13. Ibid., p. 139.

14. Ibid., p. 125.

15. Ibid., p. 164.

16. Ibid., pp. 144-145.

17. Ibid., p. 140.

18. Ibid., pp. 133-134.

19. Ibid., p. 36.

20. E. Babbitt, *Principles of Light and Color* (1878; reprint, Secaucus, NJ: Citadel Press, 1967).

21. D. Ghadiali, *Spectro-Chrome Metry Encyclopedia*, 2nd ed. (Malaga, NJ: Spectro-Chrome Institute, 1939).

22. R. Hunt, *The Seven Keys to Color Healing* (New York: Harper & Row Publishers, 1971), p. 103.

23. Gurudas, *Flower Essences and Vibrational Healing, p. 201.*

CHAPTER 8

1. B. Grad, "Healing by the Laying On Of Hands: A Review of Experiments," in *Ways of Health: Holistic Approaches to Ancient and Contemporary Medicine*, ed. D. Sobel (New York: Harcourt Brace Jovanovich, 1979), p. 267.

2. A. Westlake, "Vis Medicatrix Naturae," *Proceedings of the Scientific and Technical Congress of Radionics and Radiesthesia* (London: May 1950).

3. A. Debus, *The English Paracelsians* (New York: Franklin Watts, 1965), p. 114.

4. M. Goldsmith, *Franz Anton Mesmer* (Garden City, NY: Doubleday, 1934).

5. B. Grad, "The Biological Effects of the 'Laying On Of Hands' on Animals and Plants: Implications for Biology," in *Parapsychology: Its Relation to Physics, Biology, Psychiatry, and Psychiatry*, ed. G. Schmeidler (Metuchen, NJ: Scarecrow Press, 1967).

6. B. Grad et al., "An Unorthodox Method of Treatment on Wound Healing in Mice," *International Journal of Parapsychology*, vol. 3 (Spring 1961), pp. 5-24.

7. R. Miller, "Methods of Detecting and Measuring Healing Energies," in *Future Science*, ed. White and Krippner, (Garden City, NY: Doubleday & Co., Inc., 1977), pp. 431-444.

8. J. Smith, "The Influence on Enzyme Growth by the "Laying On Of Hands," in *The Dimensions of Healing: A Symposium* (Los Altos, CA: The Academy of Parapsychology and Medicine, 1972).

9. C. Panati, *Supersenses: Our Potential for Parasensory Experience* (Garden City, NY: Anchor Press/Doubleday, 1976), p. 121.

10. W. Tiller, "The Positive and Negative Space/Time Frames as Conjugate Systems," in *Future Science*, ed. White and Krippner (Garden City, NY: Doubleday & Co., Inc., 1977), pp. 257-279.

11. "New Technologies Detect Effects of Healing Hands," *Brain/Mind Bulletin*, vol. 10, no. 16, September 30, 1985.

12. "Healer Speeds Up Self-Organizing Properties," *Brain/Mind Bulletin*, vol. 7, no. 3 (January 4, 1982).

13. I. Prigogine and I. Stengers, *Order Out Of Chaos: Man's New Dialogue With Nature* (New York: Bantam Books, 1984).

14. B. Grad, "A Telekinetic Effect on Plant Growth, Part 2; Experiments Involving Treatment of Saline in Stoppered Bottles," *International Journal Of Parapsychology*, vol. 6 (1964), pp. 473-498.

15. D. Krieger, "The Response of In-Vivo Human Hemoglobin to an Active Healing Therapy by Direct Laying-on of Hands," *Human Dimensions*, vol. 1 (Autumn 1972), pp. 12-15.

16. D. Krieger, "Healing by the Laying-On Of Hands as a Facilitator of Bioenergetic Change: The Response of In-Vivo Hemoglobin," *International Journal of Psychoenergetic Systems*, vol. 1 (1976), p. 121.

17. S. Karagulla, *Breakthrough To Creativity* (Los Angeles, CA: DeVorss Publishers, 1967), pp. 123-146.

18. D. Krieger, "Therapeutic Touch: The Imprimatur of Nursing," *American Journal Of Nursing*, vol. 75 (1975), pp. 784-787.

19. L. LeShan, *Alternate Realities: The Search for the Full Human Being* (New York: Ballantine Books, 1976).

20. R. Miller, "The Positive Effect of Prayer on Plants," *Psychic*, April 1972.

21. J. Rindge, "The Reality of Healing Energies," in *Healers and the Healing Process*, ed. G. Meek (Wheaton, IL: Theosophical Publishing

House, 1977), pp. 136-137.

22. C. M. Cade and N. Coxhead, *The Awakened Mind: Biofeedback and the Development of Higher States of Awareness* (New York: Dell Publishing Co., 1979).

23. R. Leichtman, *Einstein Returns* (Columbus, OH: Ariel Press, 1982), pp. 50-51.

CHAPTER 9

1. R. Boling, "Superman's Hologram," *Omni*, vol. 7, no. 1 (October 1984), p. 52.

2. R. Steiner, *Cosmic Memory: Atlantis and Lemuria* (Blauvelt, NY: Rudolph Steiner Publications, 1971), p. 45.

3. Gurudas, *Flower Essences and Vibrational Healing*, channeled by Kevin Ryerson (Albuquerque, NM: Brotherhood of Life, 1983), p. 8.

4. *The Revelation of Ramala* (Suffolk, Great Britain: Neville Spearman, Ltd., 1978), p. 245.

5. Ibid., p. 246.

6. Ibid., p. 246.

7. "Biblical Floods," *Nature/Science Annual: 1977 Edition* (New York: Time-Life Books, 1976), p. 180.

8. R. Baer and V. Baer, *Windows of Light: Quartz Crystals and Self-Transformation* (San Francisco, CA: Harper & Rowe Publishers, 1984), p. 54.

9. R. Miller, "The Healing Magic of Crystals: An Interview with Marcel Vogel," *Science Of Mind*, August, 1984.

10. Ibid., p. 74.

11. M. Harner, *The Way of the Shaman* (New York: Bantam Books, 1982), p. 139.

12. N. Gardner and E. Gardner, "Oh Shinnah Speaks," in *Five Great Healers Speak Here* (Wheaton, IL: Theosophical Publishing House, 1982), p. 123.

13. Gurudas, *Flower Essences and Vibrational Healing*, pp. 30-31.

14. R. Baer and V. Baer, *Windows of Light*, p. 82.

15. F. Alper, *Exploring Atlantis: Volume 2* (Phoenix, AZ: Arizona Metaphysical Society, 1983), pp. 25-33.

16. W. Richardson and L. Huett, *The Spiritual Value of Gem Stones* (Marina del Ray, CA: DeVorss & Co., 1980), p. 15.

17. Ibid., pp. 19-24.

18. Ibid., p. 40.

19. Ibid., p. 107.

20. Ibid., p. 50-51.

21. A. Bhattacharya, *Teletherapy and Allied Science* (Calcutta: Firma KLM Private Limited, 1977).

22. V. Neal and S. Karagulla, *Through the Curtain* (Marina Del Ray, CA: DeVorss & Company, 1983), pp. 171-2, 177, 180,191-2.

CHAPTER 10

1. R. Trubo, "Stress and Disease: Cellular Evidence Hints at Therapy," *Medical World News*, January 26, 1987.

2. Gurudas, *Flower Essences and Vibrational Healing*, channeled by Kevin Ryerson, (Albuquerque, NM: Brotherhood of Life, Inc., 1983), p. 83.

3. L. LeShan, *You Can Fight for Your Life: Emotional Factors in the Causation of Cancer* (New York: Jove Publications, Inc., 1977).

4. R. Leichtman and C. Japikse, *Active Meditation: The Western Tradition* (Columbus, OH: Ariel Press, 1982).

5. J. Schwarz, *The Path of Action* (New York: E. P. Dutton, 1977).

6. *The Rainbow Bridge: First and Second Phases Link with the Soul Purification* (Escondido, CA: The Triune Foundation, 1981).

7. J. Schwarz, *Voluntary Controls: Exercises for Creative Meditation and for Activating the Potential of the Chakras* (New York: E. P. Dutton, 1978).

8. D. Walker, *The Crystal Book* (Sunol, CA: The Crystal Company, 1983), p. 57.

9. Hilarion, *Body Signs* (Toronto, Ontario: Marcus Books, 1982), p. 31.

10. L. Hay, *You Can Heal Your Life* (Farmingdale, NY: Coleman Publishing, 1984), pp. 147-182.

11. P. Levine et al, "EEG Coherence During the Transcendental Meditation Technique," in *Scientific Research on the Transcendental Meditation Program: Vol. I*, ed. Orme-Johnson and Farrow (Livingston Manor, NY: Maharishi European Research University Press, 1977), pp. 187-207.

12. I. Bentov, "Micromotion of the Body as a Factor in the Development of the Nervous System," in *Kundalini: Psychosis or Transcendence?*, by L. Sanella (San Francisco, CA: H. S. Dakin Co., 1976), pp. 71-92.

13. "Pain May Cause Lasting Change in Neuromachinery," *Brain/Mind Bulletin*, vol. 2, no. 4, January 3, 1977.

14. "Kindling, Once Epilepsy Model, May Relate to Kundalini," *Brain/Mind Bulletin*, vol. 2, no. 7, February 21, 1977.

15. M. Chia, *Awaken Healing Energy Through the Tao* (New York: Aurora Press, 1983).

CHAPTER 11

1. "Theory Relates to Brain Processes, Altered Awareness," *Brain/Mind Bulletin*, vol. 4, no. 13, May 21, 1971.

2. K. Pribram, "The Holographic Hypothesis of Brain Function: A Meeting of Minds," in *Ancient Wisdom and Modern Science*, ed. S. Grof (Albany, NY: State University of New York Press, 1984), pp. 167-179.

3. F. Capra, "The New Vision of Reality: Toward a Synthesis of Eastern Wisdom and Western Science, in *Ancient Wisdom and Modern Science*, ed. S. Grof (Albany, NY: State University of New York Press, 1984), pp. 135-148.

4. M. Talbot, *Mysticism and the New Physics* (New York: Bantam Books, Inc., 1980).

5. D. Baker, "The Occult Anatomy and Physiology of the Heart," in *Esoteric Healing* (High Road, Essendon, Herts., England: Dr. Douglas Baker).

6. N. Rosenberg, "Laser Bursts Appear to Help Revascularize Myocardium," *Medical Tribune*, vol. 27, no. 8, March 19, 1986.

7. E. Cranton and A. Brecher, *Bypassing Bypass: The New Technique of Chelation Therapy* (New York: Stein & Day Publishers, 1984).

8. M. Lesser, *Nutrition and Vitamin Therapy* (New York: Bantam Books, Inc., 1980).

9. R. Johnson, "Vitamins Reverse Smokers Lesions," *Medical Tribune*, vol. 28, no. 2, January 14, 1987, pp. 4-5.

10. R. Johnson, "Vitamins for Cervical Cells," *Medical Tribune*, vol. 28, no. 2, January 14, 1987, p. 5.

11. A. Gaby, *The Doctor's Guide to Vitamin B6* (Emmaus, PA: Rodale Press, 1984), pp. 125-129.

12. S. Ziff, *Silver Dental Fillings: The Toxic Time Bomb* (New York: Aurora Press, 1984).

13. K. Mason, *Radionics and Progressive Energies* Essex (England: C. W. Daniel Co. Ltd., 1984), p. 42.

14. Gurudas, *Flower Essences and Vibrational Healing*, channeled by Kevin Ryerson (Albuquerque, NM: Brotherhood of Life, 1983), p. 45.

15. D. Edwards, "ELF Under Suspicion in New Report," *Science News*, vol. 132, July 18, 1987, p. 39.

16. T. Graves, *Needles of Stone* (Great Britain: Turnstone Press, Ltd., 1978), pp. 71-81.

17. J. Kenyon, *Modern Techniques of Acupuncture: Vol. 3* (Wellingborough, Northamptonshire: Thorson's Publishers Limited, 1985), pp. 61, 89.

CHAPTER 12

1. C. Thomas and D. Duszynski, "Closeness to Parents and the Family Constellation in a Prospective Study of Five Disease States: Suicide, Mental Illness, Malignant Tumor, Hypertension, and Coronary Heart Disease," *The Johns Hopkins Medical Journal*, vol. 134 (1973),

pp. 251-270.

2. L. LeShan, "Psychological States as Factors in the Development of Malignant Disease: A Critical Review," *Journal of The National Cancer Institute*, vol. 22 (1959), pp. 1-18.

3. O. Simonton and S. Simonton "Belief Systems and Management of the Emotional Aspects of Malignancy," *Journal of Transpersonal Psychology*, vol. 7, no. 1 (1975), pp. 29-47.

4. R. Trubo, "Stress and Disease: Cellular Evidence Hints at Therapy," *Medical World News*, January 26, 1987, pp. 26-41.

5. G. Hodson, *The Science Of Seership* (London: Rider & Company), pp. 61-63.

6. M. Woodward, *Scars of the Soul: Holistic Healing in the Edgar Cayce Readings* (Columbus, OH: Brindabella Books, 1985).

7. F. McClain, *A Practical Guide to Past Life Regression* (St. Paul, MN: Llewellyn Publications, 1986).

8. B. Clow, *Eye of the Centaur: A Visionary Guide into Past Lives* (St. Paul, MN: Llewellyn Publications, 1986).

9. Levi, *The Aquarian Gospel of Jesus The Christ* (1907; reprint, Marina Del Rey, CA: DeVorss & Co., 1979).

10. Guru R.H.H., *Talk Does Not Cook the Rice: A Commentary on the Teaching of Agni Yoga*, Vol. 1 (York Beach, ME: Samuel Weiser, Inc., 1982), p. 133.

RECOMMENDED READING

CHAPTER 1

Holography, Consciousness & Reality

Briggs, J., and F. Peat. *Looking Glass Universe: The Emerging Science of Wholeness*. New York: Simon and Schuster Inc., 1984.

Loye, D. *The Sphinx and the Rainbow: Brain, Mind, and Future Vision*. Boulder & London: Shambhala/New Science Library, 1983.

Pelletier, K. *Toward a Science of Consciousness*. New York: Dell Publishing Co., 1978.

Electrophotography & the Kirlian Effect

Dumitrescu, I., and J. Kenyon. *Electrographic Imaging in Medicine and Biology*. Suffolk, Great Britain: Neville Spearman Ltd., 1983.

Moss, T. *The Body Electric*. Los Angeles: J. P. Tarcher, Inc., 1979.

Remote Viewing & Psi Abilities

Targ, R., and H. Puthoff. *Mind-Reach: Scientists Look at Psychic Ability*. New York: Dell Publishing Co., Inc., 1977.

Targ, R., and K. Harary. *The Mind Race: Understanding and Using Psychic Abilities*. New York: Villard Books, 1984.

Consciousness & the New Physics

Capra, F. *The Tao of Physics*. New York: Bantam Books, 1977.

Postle, D. *Fabric of the Universe*. New York: Crown Publishers, Inc., 1976.

Talbot, M. *Mysticism and the New Physics*. New York: Bantam Books, 1980.

Toben, B. *Space-Time and Beyond*. New York: E. P. Dutton and Co., 1975.

Zukav, G. *The Dancing Wu Li Masters: An Overview of the New Physics*. New York: William Morrow and Co., Inc., 1979.

CHAPTER 2

Blackie, M. *The Patient, Not the Cure: The Challenge of Homeopathy*. Santa Barbara, CA: Woodbridge Press Publishing Co., 1978.

Coulter, H. *Divided Legacy: The Conflict Between Homeopathy and the American Medical Association*. Richmond, CA: North Atlantic Books, 1973.

Coulter, H. *Homoeopathic Science and Modern Medicine: The Physics of Healing with Microdoses*. Richmond, CA: North Atlantic Books, 1980.

Hahnemann, S. *Organon of Medicine*. 1810. A New Translation by Kunzli, Naude, and Pendleton. Los Angeles, CA: J. P. Tarcher, Inc., 1982.

Tiller, W. "Towards A Scientific Rationale of Homeopathy." *Journal of Holistic Medicine*, 6, no. 2 (Fall 1984).

Vithoulkas, G. *Homeopathy: Medicine of the New Man*. New York: Arco Publishing Co., Inc., 1979.

Vithoulkas, G. *The Science of Homeopathy*. New York: Grove Press, Inc., 1980.

Whitmont, E. *Psyche and Substance: Essays on Homeopathy in the Light of Jungian Psychology*. Richmond, CA: North Atlantic Books, 1980.

CHAPTER 3

Becker, R., and G. Selden. *The Body Electric: Electromagnetism and the Foundation of Life*. New York: William Morrow and Company, Inc., 1985.

Playfair, G., and S. Hill. *The Cycles of Heaven*. New York: Avon Books, 1978.

Weymouth, L. "The Electrical Connection (Part 1)." *New York Magazine*, November 24, 1980, pp. 26-47.

Weymouth, L. "The Electrical Connection (Part 2)." *New York Magazine*, December 1, 1980, pp. 44-58.

CHAPTER 4

The Physical-Etheric Interface

Bendit, J., and P. Bendit. *The Etheric Body of Man: The Bridge of Consciousness*. Wheaton, IL: Theosophical Publishing House, 1977.

Powell, A. E. *The Etheric Double: The Health Aura of Man*. Wheaton, IL: Theosophical Publishing House, 1969.

Tiller, W. "Some Energy Field Observations of Man and Nature." *The Kirlian Aura*. Edited by Krippner and Rubin. Garden City, NY: Anchor Press/Doubleday, 1974.

The Chakra-Nadi System

Leadbeater, C. W. *The Chakras*. 1927. Reprint. Wheaton, IL: Theosophical Publishing House, 1977.

Motoyama, H. *Theories of the Chakras: Bridge to Higher Consciousness* Wheaton, IL: Theosophical Publishing House, 1981.

Rendel, P. *Introduction to the Chakras*. Wellingborough, Northamptonshire: The Aquarian Press, 1979.

Stanford, R. *The Spirit unto the Churches: An Understanding of Man's Existence in the Body Through Knowledge of the Seven Glandular Centers*. Austin, TX: Association for the Understanding of Man, 1977.

The Astral Body & Astral Projection

Greenhouse, H. *The Astral Journey*. New York: Avon Books, 1974.

Monroe, R. *Far Journeys*. Garden City, NY: Doubleday & Co., Inc.,1985.

Monroe, R. *Journeys Out of the Body*. Garden City, NY: Anchor Press/ Doubleday, 1977.

Powell, A. E. *The Astral Body*. Wheaton, IL: Theosophical Publishing House, 1965.

Rogo, D. *Mind Beyond the Body: The Mystery of ESP Projection*. New York: Penguin Books, 1978.

Swann, I. *To Kiss Earth Good-Bye*. New York: Dell Publishing Co., Inc., 1975.

Our Higher Subtle Bodies & the Evolution of Consciousness

Bentov, I. *Stalking the Wild Pendulum: On The Mechanics of Consciousness*. New York: E.P. Dutton, 1977.

Powell, A.E. *The Causal Body and the Ego*. 1928. Reprint. Wheaton, IL: Theosophical Publishing House, 1978.

Powell, A.E. *The Mental Body*. Wheaton, IL: Theosophical Publishing House, 1967.

Death as a Transition & Beyond

Holmes, J. *As We See It From Here*. Franklin, NC: Metascience Corporation, 1980.

Meek, G. *After We Die, What Then? Answers to Questions about Life after Death*. Franklin, NC: Metascience Corporation, 1980.

Taylor, R. *Witness From Beyond*. South Portland, ME: Foreword Books, 1975.

White, S. *The Unobstructed Universe*. New York: E. P. Dutton & Co., 1940.

The Positive-Negative Space/Time Frame & the Theories of Dr. William Tiller Ph.D.

Tiller, W. "Consciousness, Radiation, and the Developing Sensory System" *The Dimensions of Healing: A Symposium*. Los Gatos, CA: Academy of Parapsychology and Medicine, 1973.

Tiller, W. "Creating a New Functional Model of Body Healing Energies." *Journal of Holistic Health* 4 (1979): 102-114.

Tiller, W. "Energy Fields and the Human Body." *Frontiers of Consciousness*, Edited by J. White. New York: Avon Books, 1974.

Tiller, W. "Homeopathy: A Laboratory for Etheric Science?" *Journal of Holistic Medicine* 5, no. 1 (Spring/Summer 1983).

Tiller, W. "A Lattice Model of Space and Its Relationship to Multidimensional Physics." *A Holistic Approach to Etiology and Therapy in the Disease Process* (Proceedings of the 10th Annual Medical Symposium). Phoenix, AZ: A.R.E. Clinic, Inc., January 19-23, 1977.

Tiller, W. "The Positive and Negative Space/Time Frames as Conjugate Systems." *Future Science*. Edited by White and Krippner. Garden City, NY: Doubleday & Co., 1977.

Tiller, W. "The Simulator and the Being." *Phoenix*. Stanford, CA: Phoenix Associates, Fall/Winter 1978.

Viewpoints on Reincarnation

Cerminara, G. *Many Mansions: The Edgar Cayce Story on Reincarnation*. New York: New American Library, Inc., 1950.

Goldberg, B. *Past Lives Future Lives: Accounts of Regressions and Progressions Through Hypnosis*. North Hollywood, CA: Newcastle Publishing Co., Inc., 1982.

Head, J., and S. L. Cranston. *Reincarnation: The Phoenix Fire Mystery*. New York: Warner Books, 1977.

Lenz, F. *Lifetimes: True Accounts of Reincarnation*. New York: Fawcett Crest Books, 1979.

Perkins, J. *Experiencing Reincarnation*. Wheaton, IL: Theosophical Publishing House, 1977.

CHAPTER 5

The Chinese Philosophy of Healing

Haas, E. *Staying Healthy with the Seasons*. Millbrae, CA: Celestial Arts, 1981.

Kaptchuk, T. *The Web That Has No Weaver: Understanding Chinese Medicine*. New York: Congdon & Weed, 1983.

Acupuncture Therapy

Chang, S. *The Complete Book of Acupuncture*. Millbrae, CA: Celestial Arts, 1976.

Langone, J. "Acupuncture: New Respect for an Ancient Remedy." *Discover*, August 1984, pp. 70-73.

McGarey, W. *Acupuncture and Body Energies*. Phoenix, AZ: Gabriel Press, 1974.

Omura, Y. *Acupuncture Medicine: Its Historical and Clinical Background*. Tokyo: Japan Publications, Inc., 1982.

Seem, M. *Acupuncture Energetics: A Workbook for Diagnostics and Treatment*. Rochester, VT: Thorsons Publishers Inc., 1987.

Wensel, L. *Acupuncture for Americans*. Reston, VA: Reston Publishing Co., Inc., 1980.

Woolerton, H., and C. McLean. *Acupuncture Energy in Health and Disease: A Practical Guide for Advanced Students*. Wellingborough, Northamptonshire, Great Britain: Thorsons Publishers Ltd., 1979.

CHAPTER 6

Electroacupuncture Diagnostic Methods

Ber, A. "Neutralization of Phenolic (Aromatic) Food Compounds in a Holistic General Practice." *Journal of Orthomolecular Psychiatry* 12, no. 4 (1984).

Kenyon, J. *Modern Techniques of Acupuncture/Volume 1: A Practical Scientific Guide to Electro-Acupuncture*. New York: Thorsons Publishers, Inc., 1983.

Kenyon, J. *Modern Techniques of Acupuncture/Volume 3: A Scientific Guide to Bio-Electronic Regulatory Techniques and Complex Homeopathy*. New York: Thorsons Publishers, Inc., 1985.

Tiller, W. "Homeopathy: A Laboratory for Etheric Science?" *Journal of Holistic Medicine* 5, no. 1 (Spring/Summer 1983).

Tiller, W. "What Do Electrodermal Diagnostic Acupuncture Instruments Really Measure?" *American Journal of Acupuncture* 5, no. 1 (January/March 1987).

Voll, R. "Twenty Years of Electroacupuncture Diagnosis in Germany: A Progress Report." *American Journal of Acupuncture* (March 1975).

Voll, R. "Twenty Years of Electroacupuncture Therapy Using Low-Frequency Current Pulses." *American Journal of Acupuncture* (December 1975).

Radionics & Radiesthesia

Reyner, J. et al. *Psionic Medicine: The Study and Treatment of the Causative Factors in Illness*. London: Routledge & Keegan Paul, 1974.

Russell, E. *Report on Radionics: Science of the Future*. Suffolk, Great Britain: Neville Spearman Ltd., 1973.

Tansley, D. et al. *Dimensions of Radionics: New Techniques of Instrumented Distant Healing*. Essex, England: C. W. Daniel Co. Ltd., 1977.

Tansley, D. *Radionics: Interface with the Ether-Fields*. Bradford, England Health Science Press, 1975.

Tansley, D. *Radionics: Science or Magic—An Holistic Paradigm of Radionic Theory and Practice*. Essex, England: C.W. Daniel Co. Ltd., 1982.

Tiller, W. "Radionics, Radiesthesia, and Physics." *The Varieties of Healing Experience: Exploring Psychic Phenomena in Healing*. Los Altos, CA: The Academy of Parapsychology and Medicine, 1971.

CHAPTER 7

Healing with Flower Essences & Gem Elixirs

Bach, E. "Heal Thyself." *The Bach Flower Remedies*. 1931. Reprint. New Canaan, CT: Keats Publishing, Inc., 1977.

Barnard, J. *Patterns of Life Force*. Great Britain: Bach Educational Programme, 1987.

Chancellor, P. *Handbook of the Bach Flower Remedies*. New Canaan, CT: Keats Publishing, Inc., 1971.

Gurudas. *Flower Essences and Vibrational Healing*, channeled by Kevin Ryerson. Albuquerque, NM: Brotherhood of Life, Inc., 1983.

Gurudas. *Gem Elixirs and Vibrational Healing: Volume I*, channeled by Kevin Ryerson. Boulder, CO: Cassandra Press, 1985.

Gurudas. *Gem Elixirs and Vibrational Healing: Volume II*, channeled by Kevin Ryerson and Jon Fox. Boulder, CO: Cassandra Press, 1986.

Hilarion. *Wildflowers: Their Occult Gifts*. Toronto, Canada: Marcus Books, 1982.

Scheffer, M. *Bach Flower Therapy: Theory and Practice*. Wellingborough, Northamptonshire, UK: Thorsons Publishers Ltd., 1986.

Vlamis, G. *Flowers to the Rescue: The Healing Vision of Dr. Edward Bach*. Wellingborough, Northamptonshire, UK: Thorsons Publishers Ltd., 1986.

Weeks, N. *The Medical Discoveries of Edward Bach, Physician*. New Canaan, CT: Keats Publishing, Inc., 1973.

Healing with Color

Babbitt, E. *The Principles of Light and Color: The Healing Power of Color*. 1878. Reprint. Secaucus, NJ: The Citadel Press, 1976.

Babey-Brooke, A., and R. Amber. *Color Therapy: Healing with Color*. New York: Santa Barbara Press, Inc., 1979.

Clark, L. *The Ancient Art of Color Therapy*. New York: Pocket Books, 1975.

David, W. *The Harmonics of Sound, Color, and Vibration: A System for Self-Awareness and Soul Evolution*. Marina Del Ray, CA: DeVorss & Co., 1980.

Gimbel, T. *Healing Through Color*. Essex, England: The C.W. Daniel Co., Ltd., 1980.

Hunt. R. *The Eighth Key to Color: Self Analysis and Clarification Through Color*. Chadwell Heath, Essex: L. N. Fowler & Co., Ltd., 1965.

Hunt, R. *The Seven Keys to Color Healing: Diagnosis and Treatment Using Color*. New York: Harper & Row, 1971.

MacIvor, V., and S. LaForest. *Vibrations: Healing Through Color, Homeopathy, and Radionics*. New York: Samuel Weiser, Inc., 1979.

Ousley, S. *The Power of The Rays: The Science of Colour-Healing*. Chadwell Heath, Essex: L. N. Fowler & Co., Ltd., 1951.

CHAPTER 8

Burke, G. *Magnetic Therapy: Healing in Your Hands*. Oklahoma City, OK: Saint George Press, 1980.

The Dimensions of Healing: A Symposium. Los Altos, CA: The Academy of Parapsychology and Medicine, 1972.

Hammond, S. *We Are All Healers*. New York: Ballantine Books, 1973.

Joy, W. B. *Joy's Way: A Map for the Transformational Journey, An Introduction to the Potentials for Healing with Body Energies*. Los Angeles, CA: J.P. Tarcher, Inc., 1979.

Krieger, D. *The Therapeutic Touch: How to Use Your Hands to Help or to Heal*. Englewood Cliffs, NJ: Prentice-Hall, Inc., 1979.

Krippner, S., and A. Villoldo. *The Realms of Healing*. Millbrae, CA: Celestial Arts, 1976.

Lansdowne, Z. *The Chakras and Esoteric Healing*. York Beach, ME: Samuel Weiser, Inc., 1986.

Meek, G. *Healers and the Healing Process*. Wheaton, IL: Theosophical Publishing House, 1977.

Pavek, R., *The Health Professional's Handbook of SHEN: Physioemotional Release Therapy*. Sausalito, CA: The SHEN Institute, 1987.

Regush, N. *Frontiers of Healing: New Dimensions in Parapsychology*. New York: Avon Books, 1977.

Wallace, A., and B. Henkin. *The Psychic Healing Book*. New York: Dell Publishing Co., 1978.

CHAPTER 9

Alper, F. *Exploring Atlantis: Volumes I and II*. Phoenix, AZ: Arizona Metaphysical Society, 1981, 1983.

Baer, R., and V. Baer. *Windows of Light: Quartz Crystals and Self Transformation*. San Francisco: Harper & Rowe, 1984.

Baer, R., and V. Baer. *The Crystal Connection: A Guidebook for Personal and Planetary Transformation*. San Francisco: Harper & Rowe, 1986.

Bhattacharya, A. *Gem Therapy*. Calcutta: Firma KLM Private Ltd, 1976.

Bonewitz, R. *Cosmic Crystals: Crystal Consciousness and the New Age*. Wellingborough, Northamptonshire: Turnstone Press Limited, 1983.

Bonewitz, R. *The Cosmic Crystal Spiral: Crystals and the Evolution of Human Consciousness*. Longmead, Shaftesbury, Dorset: Element Books Ltd., 1986.

Burka, C. F. *Clearing Crystal Consciousness*. Albuquerque, NM: Brotherhood of Life, Inc., 1985.

Calverly, R. *The Language of Crystals*. Toronto, Ontario: Radionics Research Association, 1986.

Chocron, D. S. *Healing with Crystals and Gemstones*. York Beach, ME: Samuel Weiser, Inc., 1986.

Gems, Stones, and Metals for Healing and Attunement: A Survey of Psychic Readings. Virginia Beach, VA: Heritage Publications, 1977.

Gold, G. *Crystal Energy*. Chicago, IL: Contemporary Books, Inc., 1987.

Gurudas. *Gem Elixirs and Vibrational Healing: Vol. II*, channeled by Kevin Ryerson and Jon Fox. Boulder, CO: Cassandra Press, 1986.

Harold, H. *Focus on Crystals*. New York: Ballantine Books, 1986.

Isaacs, T. *Gemstones, Crystals, and Healing*. Black Mountain, NC: Lorien House, 1982.

Lorusso, J., and J. Glick. *Healing Stoned: The Therapeutic Use of Gems and Minerals*. Albuquerque, NM: Brotherhood of Life, 1979.

Lorusso, J., and J. Glick. *Stratagems: A Mineral Perspective*. Albuquerque, NM: Brotherhood of Life, Inc., 1984.

Mella, D. *Stone Power: The Legendary and Practical Use of Gems and Stones*. Albuquerque, NM: Domel, Inc., 1976.

Peterson, S. *Crystal Visioning: A Crystal Workbook*. Nashville, TN: Interdimensional Publishing, 1984.

Richardson, W., and L. Huett. *The Spiritual Value of Gem Stones*. Marina del Ray, CA: DeVorss & Co., 1980.

Stewart, C. *Gem-Stones of the Seven Rays*. 1939. Reprint. Mokelumne Hill, CA: Health Research, 1975.

Raphaell, K. *Crystal Enlightenment: The Transforming Properties of Crystals and Healing Stones*. New York: Aurora Press, 1985.

Raphaell, K. *Crystal Healing: The Therapeutic Application of Crystals and Stones / Volume II*. New York: Aurora Press, 1987.

Rea, J. *Patterns of the Whole, Vol. I: Healing and Quartz Crystals*. Boulder, CO: Two Trees Publishing, 1986.

Silbey, U. *The Complete Crystal Guidebook*. San Francisco, CA: U-Read Publications, 1986.

Smith, M. *Crystal Power*. St. Paul, MN: Llewellyn Publications, 1985.

Walker, D. *The Crystal Book*. Sunol, California: The Crystal Company, 1983.

CHAPTER 10

The Chakras in Health & Illness

Gurudas. *Gem Elixirs and Vibrational Healing, Vol. I*, channeled by Kevin Ryerson. Boulder, CO: Cassandra Press, 1985, pp. 56-71.

Schwarz, J. *Human Energy Systems*. New York: E. P. Dutton, 1980.

Schwarz, J. *Voluntary Controls: Exercises for Creative Meditation and for Activating the Potential of the Chakras*. New York: E. P. Dutton, 1978.

Stanford, R. *The Spirit Unto the Churches: An Understanding of Man's Existence in the Physical Body Through Knowledge of the Seven Glandular Centers*. Austin, TX: Association for the Understanding of Man,Inc., 1968.

Young, M. *Agartha: A Journey to the Stars*. Walpole, NH: Stillpoint Publishing, 1984, pp. 205-221.

Active Meditation

Adair, M. *Working Inside Out—Tools for Change: Applied Meditation for Creative Problem Solving*. Berkeley, CA: Wingbow Press, 1984.

Hay, L. *You Can Heal Your Life*. Farmingdale, NY: Coleman Publishing, 1984, pp. 147-182.

Leichtman, R., and C. Japikse. *Active Meditation: The Western Tradition*. Columbus, OH: Ariel Press, 1982.

Mesher, A. *Journey of Love: A Formula for Mastery and Miracles*. Austin,

TX: Quartus Foundation, 1982.

Kundalini

Krishna, G. *The Awakening of Kundalini.* New York: E. P. Dutton & Co., 1975.

Krishna, G. *Kundalini: The Evolutionary Energy in Man.* Berkelely, CA: Shambhala Publications, Inc., 1967.

Radha, S. *Kundalini Yoga for the West.* Boulder, CO: Shambhala Publications, Inc., 1978.

Sanella, L. *Kundalini: Psychosis or Transcendence?* San Francisco, CA: H. S. Dakin Co., 1976.

Scott, M. *Kundalini in the Physical World.* London: Routledge & Kegan Paul, 1983.

White, J. *Kundalini, Evolution, and Enlightenment.* Garden City, NY: Anchor Press/Doubleday, 1979.

CHAPTER 11

Holistic Medicine & Vibrational Healing

Bauman, E. et al. *The Holistic Health Lifebook: A Guide to Personal and Planetary Well-Being.* Berkeley, CA: And/Or Press, Inc., 1981.

Bauman, E. et al. *The New Holistic Health Handbook: Living Well in a New Age.* Edited by S. Bliss. Lexington, MA: The Stephen Greene Press, 1985.

Gurudas. *Flower Essences and Vibrational Healing,* channeled by Kevin Ryerson. Albuquerque, NM: Brotherhood of Life, 1983.

Gurudas. *Gem Elixirs and Vibrational Healing, Vol. 1.* channeled by Kevin Ryerson. Boulder, CO: Cassandra Press, 1985.

Hastings, A., J. Fadiman and J. Gordon. *Health for the Whole Person: The Complete Guide to Holistic Medicine.* Boulder, CO: Westview Press, Inc., 1980.

Hill, A. *A Visual Encyclopedia of Unconventional Medicine.* New York: Crown Publishers, Inc., 1979.

Kaslof, L. *Wholistic Dimensions in Healing: A Resource Guide.* Garden City, NY: Dolphin/Doubleday & Co., Inc., 1978.

Moore, M., and L. Moore. *The Complete Handbook of Holistic Health.* Englewood Cliffs, NJ: Prentice-Hall, Inc., 1983.

Otto, H., and J. Knight. *Dimensions in Wholistic Healing: New Frontiers in the Treatment of the Whole Person.* Chicago, IL: Nelson-Hall, 1979.

Pelletier, K. *Holistic Medicine: From Stress to Optimal Health.* New York: Delacorte Press/Seymour Lawrence, 1979.

Sobel, D. *Ways of Health: Holistic Approaches to Ancient and Contemporary Medicine.* New York and London: Harcourt Brace Jovanovich, 1979.

Stress, Illness, & Wellness

Ardell, D. *High Level Wellness: An Alternative to Doctors, Drugs, and*

Disease. Revised Edition. New York: Bantam Books, 1977, 1979.

Arehart-Treichel, J. *Biotypes: The Critical Link Between Your Personality and Your Health*. New York: Time Books, Quadrangle/The New York Times Book Co., Inc., 1980.

Hay, L. *You Can Heal Your Life*. Farmingdale, NY: Coleman Publishing, 1984.

Jaffe, D. *Healing From Within*. New York: Alfred A. Knopf, 1980.

Pelletier, K. *Mind as Healer, Mind as Slayer: A Holistic Approach to Preventing Stress Disorders*. New York: Delta/Dell Publishing Co., Inc., 1977.

Ryan, R. and J. Travis. *The Wellness Workbook*. Berkeley, CA: Ten Speed Press, 1981.

Selye, H. *The Stress of Life*. Revised Edition. New York: McGraw-Hill Book Co., 1976.

Totman, R. *Social Causes of Illness*. New York: Pantheon Books, 1979.

Vibrational Healing & the Future of Medicine

Achterberg, J. *Imagery and Healing: Shamanism and Modern Medicine*. Boston & London: New Science Library/Shambhala Publications, Inc., 1985.

Bailey, A. *Esoteric Healing*. New York: Lucis Publishing Co., 1953.

Capra. F. *The Turning Point: Science, Society, and the Rising Culture*. New York: Bantam Books, 1982.

Dossey, L. *Beyond Illness: Discovering the Experience of Health*. Boulder, CO: New Science Library/Shambhala Publications, Inc., 1984.

Dossey, L. *Space, Time, and Medicine*. Boulder & London: Shambhala, 1982.

Ferguson, M. *The Aquarian Conspiracy: Personal and Social Transformation in the 1980's*. Los Angeles: J. P. Tarcher, Inc., 1980.

Locke, S. and D. Colligan. *The Healer Within: The New Medicine of Mind and Body*. New York: E. P. Dutton, 1986.

Oyle, I. *Time, Space, and the Mind*. Millbrae, CA: Celestial Arts, 1976.

Reyner, J., G. Laurence, and C. Upton. *Psionic Medicine: The Study and Treatment of the Causative Factors in Illness*. London: Routledge & Kegan Paul, 1974, 1982.

Siegel, B. Love, *Medicine, and Miracles*. New York: Harper & Row, 1986.

Tansley, D. *Radionics: Science or Magic? An Holistic Paradigm of Radionic Theory and Practice*. Essex, England: C. W. Daniel Company Ltd., 1982.

CHAPTER 12

Ancient Wisdom & Philosophies of Life & Healing

Babbitt, E., and C. Hapgood. *The God Within: A Testament of Vishnu, A Handbook for the Spiritual Renaissance*. Turner Falls, MA: Fine Line Books, 1982.

A Course In Miracles. Tiburon, CA: Foundation For Inner Peace, 1975.

Elkins, D., C. Rueckert, and J. McCarty. *The Ra Material: An Ancient Astronaut Speaks.* Norfolk, VA: The Donning Co., 1984.

Eisen, W. *The Agashan Discourses.* Marina del Rey, CA: DeVorss & Co., 1978.

Eisen, W. *Agasha: Master of Wisdom.* Marina del Rey, CA: DeVorss & Co., 1977.

Grant, J. *Winged Pharaoh.* 1937. Reprint. New York: Berkely Publishing Corp., 1977.

Haich, E. *Initiation.* Palo Alto, CA: Seed Center, 1974.

Herwer, C. *Dwellers in the Temple of Mondama.* Los Angeles, CA: DeVorss & Co., 1949.

Steiner, R. *Cosmic Memory: Atlantis and Lemuria.* Blauvelt, NY: Rudolph Steiner Publications, 1971.

Personal & Planetary Transformation

Moss, R. *The I That Is We: Awakening to Higher Energies Through Unconditional Love.* Millbrae, CA: Celestial Arts, 1981.

The Revelation of Ramala. Sudbury, Suffolk, England: Neville Spearman, Ltd., 1978.

Russell, P. *The Global Brain: Speculations on the Evolutionary Leap to Planetary Consciousness.* Los Angeles: J. P. Tarcher, Inc., 1983.

Williams, S. *The Practice of Personal Transformation: A Jungian Approach.* Berkeley: California Journey Press, 1984, 1985.

Young, M. *Agartha: A Journey to the Stars.* Walpole, New Hampshire: Stillpoint Publishing, 1984.

GLOSSARY

ACUPOINT: Abbreviation for acupuncture point. An energetic pore in the skin through which subtle energy from the surrounding environment is carried throughout the body via the meridians, supplying nutritive ch'i energy to the deeper organs, blood vessels, and nervous system.

ALLOPATHIC: Refers to contemporary medical approaches which utilize multiple drugs simultaneously to provide multi-symptom relief and treatment of illness.

AMI DEVICE: Computerized electroacupuncture diagnostic system developed by Dr. Hiroshi Motoyama which simultaneously measures bioelectrical imbalances in the twelve major meridians of the body, thus revealing organ systems that are potentially affected by illness or energetic disturbances.

AMYGDALA: A deep brain structure which is part of the limbic system (a larger network of brain nuclei which is involved in emotional expression and is rich in endorphins); also one of the sites of the so-called pleasure centers of the brain.

ANALGESIA: Relief of pain.

ANGIOPLASTY: A technique whereby obstructions in blood vessels are repaired in order to establish improved blood flow. The most common techniques involve either balloon compression or laser destruction of cholesterol plaques.

ANTIBODY: A specialized protein, produced by the immune system, which binds to the outer coating of invaders that have been identified as "nonself." The antibody-binding process initiates various immune mechanisms for destroying or removing the offending substance.

ANTIGEN: A protein substance or material which is recognized as either "self" or "non-self" by the body's immune system. If the antigen is felt to be foreign, antibodies are produced against the antigen.

ARRHYTHMIA: An abnormal rhythm of the heart beat, usually caused by electrical instability within the heart's muscle and electrical conduction system.

ASTRAL: Refers to the energy/matter octave or frequency band just beyond the etheric. Because the astral body is strongly affected by emotionality, astral energy is often emotionally-linked.

AURA: The energy envelope that surrounds and interpenetrates the physical body. The aura is made up of all the different energy shells that compose the physical, etheric, astral, mental, causal, and higher spiritual aspects of the multidimensional human form.

AUTOIMMUNE: A type of immune reaction in which the body attacks itself by producing antibodies against so-called "self antigens." It is now felt that the body's T-suppressor cells, a special type of lymphocyte, normally inhibit this kind of reaction. Therefore, autoimmune diseases may be a reflection of altered T-suppressor cell activity.

AUTONOMIC NERVOUS SYSTEM: The body's automatic/unconscious regulatory nervous system, which is divided into the sympathetic and parasympathetic nervous systems.

AXIATONAL LINES: Energetic lines which connect biocellular activities to higher energetic inputs. The axiatonal lines connect higher energetic informational grids to the physical body through the acupuncture meridian system.

BASAL GANGLIA: Specialized nerve centers within the brain which assist in controlling certain aspects of muscle coordination.

B-CELLS: Also known as B-lymphocytes, these cells produce antibodies which contribute to the body's immune response.

BIOCRYSTALLINE: Refers to the network of cellular elements in the body which have liquid crystal or quartz-like properties. These areas include cell salts, lymphatics, fatty tissue, red and white blood cells, and the pineal gland.

BIOELECTRICAL/BIOELECTRONIC: An electrical network of information transmission and cellular repair mechanisms in the body. Also refers to electronic switching and control mechanisms within and between cells.

BIOENERGETIC: Any type of electrical, electromagnetic, or subtle energetic forces which are generated by living organisms.

BIOFIELD: The energy field which surrounds and interpenetrates the physical body. The biofield is made up of magnetic and electromagnetic energies generated by living cells, as well as subtle energetic fields.

BIOMAGNETIC: The energy generated by living cells, including both conventional magnetic fields as well as subtle magnetic fields, i.e. etheric.

BIONOSODE: A homeopathic remedy prepared from the tissue of a diseased organ. Only the vibrational qualities of the pathogen are extracted for the remedy so that no physical, illness-causing agents remain.

CAUSAL: The energy frequency band or octave just beyond the mental level.

CAUSAL BODY: The subtle body which is composed of causal substance. It is the level at which human consciousness stores all experiences gained during its many incarnations on the physical plane.

CEREBRAL HEMISPHERES: The right and left halves of the cerebral cortex, the highest center of function within the brain. The left hemisphere controls analytical and linear thought, while the right hemisphere controls intuitive, symbolic, and non-linear thought processes.

CHANNELING: The phenomenon whereby an individual allows a higher level of consciousness to flow through them, often verbally, as in trance channeling, but also through automatic writing.

CHELATION THERAPY: A treatment for arteriosclerosis (hardening of the arteries) involving multiple intravenous infusions of a chelating agent known as EDTA.

CHAKRA: An energy center in the body which is a step-down transformer for higher frequency subtle energies. The chakras process subtle energy and convert it into chemical, hormonal, and cellular changes in the body.

CH'I: The ancient Chinese term for a nutritive subtle energy which circulates through the acupuncture meridians.

CHRONOBIOLOGY: The science which studies how biological processes are affected by the cyclical rhythms of day and night.

CLAIRAUDIENCE: The psychic ability of hearing at higher vibrational levels. It is mediated by energy processing at the level of the throat chakra.

CLAIRVOYANCE: The psychic ability of seeing higher subtle-energy patterns (from the French, literally meaning "clear seeing"). An aspect of the brow or ajna chakra.

CLAIRVOYANT REALITY: A state of seeing and feeling that transcends the superficial senses. It is an experience of reality beyond the confines of time and space boundaries, which can often allow one to experience the interconnectedness of all things.

CLINICAL ECOLOGY: The scientific discipline which studies the adverse effects of various common environmental agents, both natural and synthetic, upon human health.

CLONING: The production of a living replica of a life-form. This is usually accomplished by inserting an organism's complete chromosome set into a newly fertizilized egg of the same species, substituting one set of genes for another.

CORONA DISCHARGE: The phenomenon of spark discharge around a grounded object with conductive properties. It is another name for the Kirlian aura produced by electrophotographic devices.

CORPUS CALLOSUM: The large nerve bundle which connects the two cerebral hemispheres.

CRYSTAL GRIDWORK PATTERNS: Crystals arranged in geometric arrays which have an amplified or synergistic effect greater than the sum of the individual crystals, often used for specific healing and meditative practices.

CT SCANNING: A specialized computer-assisted x-ray technique which can be used to study thin cross-sectional slices of the body.

DERMATRON: An electroacupuncture device used in diagnosis and treatment of illness. Another name for a particular model of the Voll Machine.

DIS-EASE: A frequently used term for illness. It implies that sickness is the result of the individual being at "ill ease" with some aspect of his or her higher consciousness.

DISTRESS: A level of stress that causes dysfunction and disease in the organism.

DNA: Deoxyribonucleic acid, the helical macromolecule which encodes the genetic information that participates in cellular growth and development at the molecular level.

DOWSING: Another term for radiesthesia. An intuitive skill used for finding hidden or lost objects and mineral resources, and for diagnosing illness.

EAV: Electroacupuncture According to Voll. One school of electroacupuncture diagnosis.

EGO: The incarnating personality as expressed through the physical body.

ELECTROACUPUNCTURE: The use of electrical currents to stimulate acupuncture points and their corresponding meridians. Also refers to electronic systems used to measure electrical characteristics of the acupoints for use in diagnosis of illness and meridian imbalance.

ELECTROGRAPHY: A general term for Kirlian photography or corona discharge photography.

ELECTROMAGNETIC: In the context of this book, a wide spectrum of energy which moves at the speed of light.

EMR SCANNER: A hypothetical etheric body scanner based upon the Kirlian principle of electrographically imaging the Phantom Leaf Effect using energetic resonance, combined with the CT-scanning computer technology.

ENDORPHINS: A variety of morphine-like proteins that are found in the brain and nervous system and in the organs of the body. One particular type of endorphin may mediate pain relief in certain settings.

ENERGY BLOCKAGE: A general term referring to the interruption of the natural flow of subtle energy through the human energetic system, often due to abnormal function in one or several chakras.

ENTROPY: A scientific term that describes the state of disorder within a system. The higher the entropy, the more disordered the system; the lower the entropy, the more organized and orderly the system. Crystals, because of their mathematical regularity, are considered to have the lowest entropy.

ENZYME: A specialized protein molecule which acts to catalyze or accelerate a chemical reaction in the body in a particular direction.

ETHEREAL FLUIDIUM: That part of the etheric body which surrounds the physical body and carries the life-force to the individual cells.

ETHERIC: The frequency band or octave just beyond the physical octave. Etheric energy or substance vibrates at speeds beyond light velocity and has a magnetic character.

EUSTRESS: A term coined by Hans Selye referring to the optimal amount of stress needed for proper functioning of the human organism.

FERROUS: Refers to iron and iron-like metals which have particular ferromagnetic properties, as opposed to subtle or biomagnetic interactions.

GEOMANCY: A form of divination or dowsing skill used to locate particular geographical regions which may harbor water sources, mineral deposits, and natural focalizations of earth energies.

GLIAL CELLS: A type of cell found throughout the nervous system, often surrounding nerve cells such as the Schwann and microglial cells. Originally thought only to nourish the nerve cells they surround and to contribute to nerve conduction, it has now been discovered that the glial cells may form an alternative (DC/analog) information transmission system (in contrast to digital-type nerve messages).

HAPTEN: A chemical which binds to naturally occurring substances in the body, making them appear foreign to the body's own immune system, and thereby initiating adverse immunologic reactions.

HEMOGLOBIN: A complex macromolecule in red blood cells responsible for carrying oxygen to all the cellular systems of the body.

HEPATIC: Refers to the liver.

HIGHER DIMENSIONAL: A term that describes subtle-energy systems which vibrate at speeds faster than light, i.e., non-physical energies.

HOLISTIC: A synergistic approach which deals with the combined physical, mental, emotional, and spiritual aspects of human health and illness.

HOLOGRAM: A three-dimensional image created by an interference pattern of two interacting laser beams.

HOLOGRAPHIC PRINCIPLE: Holograms are unique in that they represent an energy interference pattern in which every piece of the hologram contains the information of the whole.

HOMEOPATHIC: A method of using microdoses of natural substances to treat illnesses. The homeopathic principle assigns treatments to patients by matching the illness symptom complex with the known "drug picture" of a homeopathic remedy (the so-called Law of Similars).

HOST RESISTANCE: The factors within an organism which, together, allow it to resist illness. These elements include general vitality as well as the overall strength of the various divisions of the immune system.

HYPERNUMBER: A term coined by mathematician Charles Muses to characterize certain numbers, typified by the square root of -1, which may be useful in describing the mathematics of higher dimensional phenomena.

HYPERTHYROID: A condition of hyperactivity of the thyroid gland, sometimes resulting in hyperactivity, nervousness, and excessive sweating.

HYPOADRENAL: A medical condition caused by underactivity of the adrenal gland, often leading to general fatigue and weakness.

IMMUNOSUPPRESSION: Suppression of the body's natural immune defenses (i.e., impairment of host resistance) which may be caused by a variety of chemical, emotional, and energetic factors.

KARMA: The reincarnational principle, sometimes stated as "as ye sow, so shall ye reap." An energetic system of credits and debits, or checks and balances, which allows the soul to experience the full range of perspectives on life.

KINDLING: A phenomenon which takes place in the limbic system whereby repeated low-level stimuli along a particular neural pathway help to establish that route as a path of least resistance for nerve transmission.

KIRLIAN PHOTOGRAPHY: An electrographic process, pioneered in Russia by electrical engineer Semyon Kirlian, which uses the corona discharge phenomenon to capture the bioenergetic processes of living systems on film.

KUNDALINI: The creative energy of spiritual illumination which is stored as potential energy within the root or base chakra in the coccygeal region of the spine. It is a subtle energy which, if properly released, can cause activation and alignment of all of the major chakras of the body.

LASER: A device which produces coherent light, i.e., light with waves that are all in step or in phase.

LASERPUNCTURE: A form of therapy whereby low-level laser light is directed to stimulate particular acupoints for relief of illness.

LAYING-ON-OF-HANDS: A general term for a type of direct, hands-on type of healing, sometimes referred to as psychic healing or magnetic healing.

LEFT BRAIN: Refers to the left cerebral hemisphere, which operates in analytical, logical, and linear modes of thought.

LIGHT BODY: Another term for subtle body.

LIMBIC SYSTEM: A unique complex of centers within the brain which are involved in the processing of emotional expression and certain aspects of memory. It is a brain complex which is rich in endorphins.

LYMPHOCYTE: A type of white blood cell which participates in the immune response.

MANTRA: A word or sound which, when repeated to oneself during meditation or relaxation, helps one to achieve an undistracted meditative state of consciousness.

MAGNETOELECTRIC: A type of energy which vibrates at speeds faster than light velocity, has magnetic qualities, and negative entropic properties. It is predicted by the Tiller-Einstein Model of Positive-Negative Space/Time and is sometimes referred to as negative space/time (-S/T) energy or substance.

MAGNETIC HEALING: A type of hands-on healing which works primarily at the etheric level. In another context, refers to the use of therapeutic pulsed magnetic fields to treat illness.

MENTAL: Refers to the energy band or octave of subtle energy which exists between the astral and mental levels.

MERIDIAN: A microtubular channel which carries a subtle nutritive energy (ch'i) to the various organs, nerves, and blood vessels of the body.

MIASM: An energetic state which predisposes the organism to future illness, often due to the subtle effects of a particular toxic agent or noxious microorganism. Miasms may be acquired, inherited, or planetary in nature.

MOTOR CORTEX: The strip of cerebral cortex which controls voluntary muscle activity in the body, adjacent to the region which processes sensation. Both are sometimes referred to collectively as the sensorimotor cortex.

MRI: Magnetic Resonance Imaging. A technique which uses magnetic fields and radio waves to resonantly stimulate and visualize certain molecular components of the physical body, thereby producing high resolution, cross-sectional images for study.

MULTIDIMENSIONAL: Refers to the total spectrum of human energies, i.e., physical, etheric, astral, mental, causal, and higher spiritual levels.

MYELIN: An insulator-type fatty substance found in the Schwann cells which surround nerves, and felt to be important to nerve impulse transmission.

NADIS: The thread-like subtle paths of energy flow from the chakras to the various regions of the body. Meridians have physical components, whereas nadis are non-physical.

NDE: Near Death Experience. An experience in which an individual is resuscitated from a near-death state and reports events viewed from outside of the physical body. A traumatically-induced form of astral projection.

NEGATIVE ENTROPY: The characteristic of negative space/time or magnetoelectrical energy which influences living and non-living systems to become more ordered and less random. Negative entropy is also a characteristic of the life-force.

NEGATIVE SPACE/TIME: Refers to that domain where energy and substance vibrate at speeds exceeding light velocity, and likely includes the etheric and astral worlds of matter.

NEURON: A nerve cell.

NEUROREGULATOR: A type of chemical or protein molecule found in the nervous system which fine-tunes or modulates the nerve transmission of existing nerve pathways. Most neuroregulators are either inhibitory (brake) or excitatory (accelerator) types.

NEUROTRANSMITTER: A chemical or protein substance which is released at the synaptic membrane in order to continue the transmission of impulses from one nerve to the adjacent nerve.

NEUROTRANSMISSION: The general process of information transmission throughout the brain and nervous system.

NMR: Nuclear Magnetic Resonance. The phenomenon employed in magnetic resonance imagers to selectively excite certain atoms for visualization.

OCTAVE: Refers to a frequency band of energy, i.e. physical octave, etheric octave, etc., which are analogous to octaves of notes on a piano keyboard.

ONION EFFECT: Trauma to the human organism via vibrational therapies.

OOBE: Out-Of-Body-Experience. Another name for astral projection.

ORTHOMOLECULAR MEDICINE: A form of therapy which uses large doses of specific nutrients like amino acids in order to produce therapeutic effects in certain illnesses.

PARANORMAL: A term used to describe psychic phenomena, i.e. telepathy, clairvoyance, psychokinesis, etc.

PARAPHYSICAL: Refers to non-physical or subtle energetic phenomena.

PET SCANNER: Positron Emission Tomography. An imaging device which uses particles emitted by radioactive analogues of naturally-occuring biological chemicals to visualize ongoing brain processes.

PHANTOM LEAF EFFECT: The phenomenon in Kirlian photography by which a physically destroyed leaf fragment reappears in the image taken of the amputated leaf. The phantom image represents the etheric body of the missing leaf fragment.

PHARMACOKINETIC: Medical model which uses mathematical calculation of drug dosages, derived from patient's body mass, metabolism, and drug excretion rates, in order to achieve a desired therapeutic effect.

PHYSICAL-ETHERIC INTERFACE: The interface between the physical and etheric bodies, made up largely of the acupuncture meridian system. This interface serves to link physical with non-physical structural information fields and life-forces.

PHYSIO-KUNDALINI SYNDROME: An observed syndrome of left-sided body pains and dysfunction, likely caused by spontaneous or meditation-related stress release from the cerebral cortex.

PIEZOELECTRIC: A phenomenon observed in crystals whereby physical pressure is converted into electrical fields and vice versa. For instance, in a phonograph needle, a crystal translates vibrational pressures into electrical signals, which are then converted back into music and speech.

POSITIVE SPACE/TIME: The physical universe of energy and matter which vibrates at speeds less than (or equal to) light velocity.

POTENTIZATION: A process by which homeopathic remedies are made. A small amount of substance in a solvent (i.e., water) is forcefully shaken in a machine called a succussion device. Repeated dilutions are made using the same process to further potentize the remedy. The higher the dilution, the more potentized the remedy.

PRANA: An ancient Hindu or yogic term for a nutritive subtle-energy thought to be taken in during breathing.

PSI: General term for psychic phenomena.

PSYCHIC HEALING: Refers to various types of hands-on healing. Psychic healing can be subcategorized into various types of energetic interaction, i.e., magnetic healing, spiritual healing, psychic surgery, etc.

PSYCHONEUROIMMUNOLOGY: Medical term for the evolving discipline which studies the interaction between the mind, body, and the immune system in health and illness.

PSYCHOSPIRITUAL: Refers to the interdependent aspects of mind, emotion, and spirit.

PSYCHOTRONIC: A general term often used to describe devices which utilize various types of psychic or subtle energies to perform their function. In another definition, "psychotronics" is a term sometimes used to describe the science of studying subtle energies.

QI: The Japanese term for ch'i, sometimes spelled "qi" or "ki." The subtle nutritive energy which flows through the acupuncture meridians.

QUANTUM PHYSICS: The branch of physics which studies the energetic characteristics of matter at the subatomic level.

RADIESTHESIA: A psychic perceptual ability of being able to sense various types of subtle energetic radiation.

RADIONICS: Sometimes referred to as psionics, that branch of esoteric science which seeks to psychically diagnose energy imbalances in the human multidimensional system using instrumentation at a distance from the patient. A typical radionic device operates on the principle of resonance, using a "witness" as a vibrational focal point for the radionic operator to tune in to.

REINCARNATION: A philosophy of the soul having multiple lives (incarnations upon the physical plane) in order to achieve a higher level of integration and spiritual maturation.

RELAXATION RESPONSE: A term coined by Dr. Herbert Benson referring to a relaxed, meditative state to which the mind/body can attune when applying the appropriate relaxation techniques.

RELAXATION TECHNIQUE: A mental or physical practice which can allow the mind and body to enter into a more relaxed state. This includes various mental techniques such as mantra repetition, progressive relaxation affirmations, and muscle contraction/relaxation approaches.

REMOTE VIEWING: A more recent scientific term for clairvoyance. Refers to the ability to psychically perceive visual information about targets separated from the subject by either distance or appropriate shielding.

RESONANCE: The phenomenon of sympathetic vibration between two similarly tuned oscillators, e.g., the resonant vibration of the E strings of two Stradivarius violins. Resonance occurs at higher and lower harmonics as well (between similar notes in higher and lower octaves, i.e., middle C resonates with both high C as well as low C).

RIGHT BRAIN: The right cerebral hemisphere, associated with spatial, intuitive, artistic, symbolic, and non-linear thought.

RNA: Ribonucleic acid. A large molecule of so-called nucleic acid which carries information from the DNA and translates it into a protein structural assembly within the cell.

SCHWANN CELL: A type of glial cell which surrounds most peripheral nerves in the body. It may function both to nourish the adjacent nerve and to assist in normal nerve impulse transmission, as well as to carry information through a network of similar glial cells by varying the DC charge on its surface membrane.

SENSORY CORTEX: That area or strip of the cerebral cortex which processes the information of sensations coming from the body.

SLOW VIRUS INFECTION: A type of late viral manifestation caused by a delayed reaction to an earlier virus infection. Some slow viruses cause their primary illness manifestations fifteen to twenty years after the initial infection.

SONOPUNCTURE: An energetic form of acupuncture which uses high-frequency sound waves instead of needles to stimulate acupoints.

SPIRITUAL HEALING: A form of healing which operates on the lower physical and etheric levels, but also corrects energetic disturbances at the emotional or astral, mental, and higher spiritual levels.

STATE-SPECIFIC SCIENCES: A term coined by Dr. Charles Tart suggesting the development of sciences which would require that the scientist/observer enter into specially receptive states of consciousness.

SUBCONSCIOUS: That part of the personality which dwells below the surface of waking consciousness and controls automatic human functions. It subliminally records all information taken in by the senses and is conditioned/programmed by rewards, punishments, and messages that subtly build up our internal pictures of self-worthiness.

SUBTLE BODY: A term referring to any of the subtle-energy bodies which exist in the higher frequency octaves beyond the physical, i.e. the etheric, astral, mental and causal bodies.

SUBTLE ENERGY: A general term denoting energy that often exists outside the ordinary or positive space/time frame, i.e. magnetoelectric (ME) energy which moves faster than light.

SUPERCONSCIOUS: That part of the higher soul structure which is usually unconscious but accessible to the personality. The superconscious contains higher wisdom, whereas the subconscious relates with the personality of a six-year-old child.

SYNAPSE: A specialized meeting point between two nerve cells which allows the impulse/message from one cell to be carried on to the next nerve cell. The synaptic junction is an extremely close meeting place between two adjacent nerve cell membranes where an electrical message is changed into neurotransmitter release and then converted back into an electrical message.

T-CELL: A special type of white blood cell known as a T-lymphocyte which participates in certain aspects of the immune response. T-cells are further subdivided into T-helper cells (which process information), killer T-cells (which may kill cancer cells), and T-suppressor cells (which keep the body from attacking itself).

THERAPEUTIC TOUCH: A term coined by Dr. Dolores Krieger denoting a type of hands-on healing technique, sometimes used interchangeably with the term psychic healing.

THOUGHTFORM: A manifestation of a strong thought or emotion as an actual energetic structure within an individual's auric field.

THYMUS GLAND: An important gland, nourished by the heart chakra, which helps to regulate the immune response.

THYROID GLAND: A small butterfly-shaped gland in the neck region which produces thyroxine, a hormone that regulates the body's metabolic rate.

TILLER-EINSTEIN MODEL: A scientific model of positive and negative space/time domains which are predicted by the relativistic version of Einstein's mass/energy equation. According to Dr. William Tiller, the leading proponent of the model, positive space/time energy and substance vibrate at speeds less than or near the speed of light, and have electrical or electromagnetic qualities. Negative space/time energy and substance vibrate or move at speeds faster than light, are magnetic in quality, and are of an energetic nature referred to as magnetoelectric.

TNS: Transcutaneous Nerve Stimulator. An electrical device applied via a skin electrode which operates by shutting off the pain control gate in order to interrupt the flow of pain messages to the brain.

TRANSDUCTION: The interconversion, transformation, or translation of energy or information from one form into another. Signal transduction implies that an energetic or electrical signal may be converted into a chemical signal or vice versa, e.g. signal transduction at a nerve's synaptic site.

VENTRICLE: A hollow chamber of the heart or brain. In the heart, the muscular right and left ventricles pump blood to the lungs and body, respectively.

In the brain, the hollow third, fourth, and lateral ventricles produce and circulate cerebrospinal fluid.

VIBRATIONAL: Refers to subtle or electromagnetic energy in varying frequencies and amplitudes.

VIBRATIONAL MEDICINE: That healing philosophy which aims to treat the whole person, i.e. the mind/body/spirit complex, by delivering measured quanta of frequency-specific energy to the human multidimensional system. Vibrational medicine seeks to heal the physical body by integrating and balancing the higher energetic systems which create the physical/cellular patterns of manifestation.

VIRUS: A tiny infectious agent made up mostly of a specialized protein coat enclosing a strand of virus genetic material (either DNA or RNA).

VIRAL: Referring to aspects of a virus.

VOLL MACHINE: An electroacupuncture diagnostic device developed by Dr. Reinhold Voll which operates by taking electrical measurements of the various acupoints on the body.

WELLNESS: A term referring to health, happiness, vitality, and wholeness of the entire mind/body/spirit complex. A state of balanced health which is reflected in continued learning, growth, and ongoing creative expression.

WITNESS: A biological specimen or other energetic signature of a patient used as a focal point for attunement by a radionic practitioner. Oftentimes a blood spot is used, but a lock of hair, a photograph, or even a piece of paper with the patient's signature can sometimes be utilized. The witness is inserted into the witness well of the radionic device so that the subtle-energy signature of the patient is fed into the circuitry of the analytical radionic instrument.

INDEX

crystals used to recharge, 358-359
disease patterns and, 66, 82, 115,
    120-121, 177, 317, 341
  imaging systems for, 108, 111, 115-116
  vibrational medicines, effects on, 241
Etheric energy fields
  crystals and, 350, 365
  nature of, 302-303
Etheric matter. *See* Matter, etheric
Eustress, 440
Evolution, spirit as driving force of, 418

F

Feng-shui and earth energies, 460
Fertilization, 49
FES flower essences, 248
Five Element Theory, 178-182
Flower essences
  alignment of chakras and subtle bodies
    using, 269
  Atlantean origins of, 329-330
  Bach, 242-248
  biocrystalline network and, 251-252
  EAV testing and, 280
  healing properties of, 244-272
  Lemurian use of, 488
  mental illness and, 265
  meridians and life-energies of, 251-252
  miasms and their treatment by, 263-264
  personality stability via integration with
    Higher Self and, 259
  strokes, neurological diseases and,
    264-266, 269
Flower Essence Society, 247-248
Flowers, biomagnetic properties of, 250
Fludd, Robert, 287
Fluidum, 287-289
Fluoride, heavy metal miasm and, 263, 456
Fluorite, subtle energetic properties of, 353
Food allergies
  EAV diagnosis of, 216-222
  phenolics and, 217-218
  stress and, 448-449
Forgiveness: love, healing and, 476, 482
Fracture healing
  crystals and, 353
  electricity used in, 97
Franklin, Benjamin, 289, 304
Frequencies of energy, 364, 421. *See also*
  Matter, frequency characteristics of
Frequency domains, 156-159

G

Gallic acid sensitivity, food allergies
  and, 270
Gardner, Robert, 217
Garnet, subtle energetic properties of, 353
Gate Control Theory, 93, 174-175
Gem elixirs
  acupuncture meridians, effects on, 273
  meditation and, 345
  modification of consciousness, 273-274,
    345
  preparation of, 251, 271
  vibrational characteristics of, 271-274
Gems and stones, healing properties of,
  271-272. *See also* references to in-
  dividual gems
Genitourinary tract, chakras and, 388
Geomancy, 460
Geometrical energy patterns, crystals and,
  364
Geopathic stress, 459-462
Ghadiali, Dinshah, 275
Glial cells, 96-97, 189-190, 192, 195-197
God, creation of souls and their link with,
  483-484
Gold as trace element, 448
Gonadal chakra. *See* Sacral chakra
Gonads
  association with root chakra, 390
  association with sacral chakra, 387
Grad, Bernard, 77, 290-299, 301, 306
Green, Elmer, 320
Gurudas, 248-251, 253, 259, 264, 266,
  268, 270-271, 280

H

Hahnemann, Samuel, 74-76, 84-85, 210,
  262
Haptens, 217
Harary, Keith, 140-141
Healers
  laser effect of quartz crystals and, 338,
    366
  energies of, 315-320.
  See also Healing
Healing
  biorhythm entrainment effects of, 320
  crystallization effects and, 297

ABOUT THE AUTHOR

Richard Gerber, M.D., received his medical degree from Wayne State University School of Medicine, and currently practices internal medicine in a suburb of Detroit.

Medical school was a personal and professional revolution for Dr. Gerber. Although he had always considered himself to be an analytical and left-brained person, he commenced his education with strong metaphysical leanings. During the period of his medical training, he maintained and nurtured these views, and discovered how to harmoniously complement his keen intellect with a strong intuitive sense. For the last twelve years, he has been researching alternative methods for diagnosis and healing, including the use of Kirlian photography for cancer detection, while continuing to advance his career in orthodox medicine. The compilation of his progressive research forms the basis for this book—an amazing accomplishment for a man who is only 33 years old.

Vibrational Medicine is a revolutionary bridge between the metaphysical and medical communities, and creates a personal resolution to Dr. Gerber's long-standing sense of paradox between these two fields. His current vision is to found a multidisciplinary healing research center which will study, and objectively verify through new technologies, the model of health elaborated upon in *Vibrational Medicine*.

"If we are beings of energy, then it follows
that we can be affected by energy."

BOOKS OF RELATED INTEREST
BY BEAR & COMPANY

EARTH ASCENDING
An Illustrated Treatise on the Law Governing Whole Systems
by José Argüelles

ECSTASY IS A NEW FREQUENCY
Teachings of The Light Institute
by Chris Griscom

HILDEGARD OF BINGEN'S MEDICINE
by Dr. Wighard Strehlow and Gottfried Hertzka, M.D.

THE MAYAN FACTOR
Path Beyond Technology
by José Argüelles

MIDNIGHT SONG
Quest for the Vanished Ones
by Jamie Sams

THE UNIVERSE IS A GREEN DRAGON
A Cosmic Creation Story
by Brian Swimme

Contact your local bookseller or write:
BEAR & COMPANY
P.O. Drawer 2860
Santa Fe, NM 87504